Families and Mental Disorders

Families and Mental Disorders
From Burden to Empowerment

Edited by

Norman Sartorius
University of Geneva, Switzerland

Julian Leff
*Royal Free and University College Medical School,
London, UK*

Juan José López-Ibor
Complutense University of Madrid, Spain

Mario Maj
University of Naples, Italy

Ahmed Okasha
Ain Shams University, Cairo, Egypt

WILEY

Other Wiley Editorial Offices

John Wiley & Sons Inc., 111 River Street, Hoboken, NJ 07030, USA

Jossey-Bass, 989 Market Street, San Francisco, CA 94103-1741, USA

Wiley-VCH Verlag GmbH, Boschstr. 12, D-69469 Weinheim, Germany

John Wiley & Sons Australia Ltd, 33 Park Road, Milton, Queensland 4064, Australia

John Wiley & Sons (Asia) Pte Ltd, 2 Clementi Loop #02-01, Jin Xing Distripark, Singapore
129809

John Wiley & Sons Canada Ltd, 22 Worcester Road, Etobicoke, Ontario, Canada M9W 1L1

Wiley also publishes its books in a variety of electronic formats. Some content that appears in
print may not be available in electronic books.

British Library Cataloguing in Publication Data

A catalogue record for this book is available from the British Library

ISBN 0-470-02382-1

Typeset in 10/12pt Palatino by Dobbie Typesetting Limited, Devon.
Printed and bound in Great Britain by T.J. International Ltd, Padstow, Cornwall
This book is printed on acid-free paper responsibly manufactured from sustainable forestry
in which at least two trees are planted for each one used for paper production.

Contents

Contributors

Christine Barrowclough   Academic Division of Clinical Psychology, School of Psychological Sciences, University of Manchester, Education & Research Centre (2nd Floor), Wythenshawe Hospital, Manchester M23 9LT, UK

Paul E. Bebbington   Department of Mental Health Sciences, Royal Free and University College London Medical School, 48 Riding House Street, London W1N 8AA, UK

Francesca Brambilla   Department of Psychiatry, University of Naples SUN, Largo Madonna delle Gzazie, 80138 Naples, Italy

Henry Brodaty   Academic Department of Psychogeriatrics, University of New South Wales, Euroa Centre, Prince of Wales Hospital, Randwick, NSW 2031, Australia

Claudine Bryan   Section of Adolescent Psychiatry, Academic Unit, University of Liverpool, 79 Liverpool Road, Chester CH2 1AW, UK

Ian R.H. Falloon   Department of Psychiatry, University of Auckland, Park Road, Auckland, New Zealand

Angela Favaro   Department of Neuroscience, Psychiatric Clinic, Via Giustiniani 3, 35128 Padova, Italy

Jason Fogler   Boston University School of Social Work, 264 Bay State Road, Boston, MA 02215, USA

Susanna Galea   Department of Mental Health Sciences, St. George's Hospital Medical School, Cranmer Terrace, London SW1 0RE, UK

A. Hamid Ghodse   St George's Hospital Medical School, University of London, International Centre for Drug Policy, 6th Floor Hunter Wing, Cranmer Terrace, London SW17 0RE, UK

Simon G. Gowers   Section of Adolescent Psychiatry, Academic Unit, University of Liverpool, 79 Liverpool Road, Chester CH2 1AW, UK

Alison Heru   Department of Psychiatry and Human Behavior, Box G-BH, Brown University, Providence, RI 02912-G, USA

Gabor I. Keitner Department of Psychiatry, Rhode Island Hospital, 593 Eddy St, Potter Bldg, 3rd Floor, Providence, RI 02903, USA

Elizabeth Kuipers Department of Psychology, Box PO77, Institute of Psychiatry, King's College London, De Crespigny Park, Denmark Hill, London SE5 8AF, UK

Julian Leff Department of Mental Health Sciences, Royal Free and University College Medical School, London and TAPS Research Unit, 69 Fleet Street, London NW3 2QU, UK

Margaret Leggatt World Fellowship for Schizophrenia and Allied Disorders, 29 Mary Street, North Carlton, Victoria 3054, Australia

Palmiero Monteleone Department of Psychiatry, University of Naples SUN, Largo Madonna delle Grazie, 80138 Naples, Italy

Kiran Rao NIMHANS, Hosur Road, Bangalore 560029, India

Christine E. Ryan Department of Psychiatry and Human Behavior, Box G-RIH, Brown University, Providence, RI 02912-G, USA

Paolo Santonastaso Department of Neuroscience, Psychiatric Clinic, Via Giustiniani 3, 35128 Padova, Italy

Radha Shankar 16 First Cross Street, Indira Nagar, Chennai 600020, India

Gail Steketee Boston University School of Social Work, 264 Bay State Road, Boston, MA 02215, USA

Janet Treasure Department of Psychiatry, King's College London, 5th Floor, Thomas Guy House, Guy's Hospital, London SE1 9RT, UK

Preface

The presence in a family of a person with a severe mental disorder is often associated with a significant objective and subjective burden on the other family members, especially those who have a caregiving role. The entity of this burden depends on several factors, including the relative's age and gender, the quality of his/her premorbid relationship with the patient, the nature of the patient's problems, the coping strategies adopted by the relative as well as his/her appraisal of the situation and perception of the patient's illness, the emotional and practical support available to the family, and cultural and ethnic variables. An important component of the family burden are the consequences of the stigma attached to mental illness: stigma does not stop at those who are close to the patient; it extends across generations and reaches far away parts of families. The burden experienced by the family members may not only affect their own mental and physical well-being, but also have an impact on the course of the patient's disorder (well documented especially in the case of schizophrenia).

In the past, the family of a patient with a severe mental disorder was often blamed for the patient's disease and deliberately excluded from its management. Today, this happens more rarely, but the emotional and practical problems experienced by the relatives of people with severe mental disorders are not always a major focus of attention for mental health services. The family is not always provided with sufficient information on the patient's condition and how to deal with it. The involvement of families in structured intervention programmes is still rare, in spite of the research evidence that family-based interventions have a positive impact on the outcome of several mental disorders. Self-help groups based on mutual support, usually initiated by family organizations, are still not extensively available and are attended by a limited number of families, in spite of the emerging evidence of their usefulness. Legal provisions that could support the families are only rarely in place, and health and social services usually have no special provision for work with families of people with mental illness and for their support.

This volume portrays what is defined in one of its chapters "the journey of families from burden to empowerment", currently ongoing in several countries of the world. An overview is provided of the various dimensions of family burden, as well as of the possible positive consequences of caring for a person with a severe mental disorder, in terms of development of personal attitudes and skills, increase of self-confidence and strengthening of family bonds. The variables which modulate family burden (with a special focus on relatives' coping strategies, appraisal and illness perception) are described. Family-based interventions available for the various mental disorders are reviewed, including the evidence of their effectiveness, the barriers to their implementation and the methodological problems of the relevant research. The recent achievements of family organizations in developed as well as developing countries are outlined.

A distinctive feature of the volume is its focus on all the most prevalent mental disorders, including those—such as anxiety disorders, eating disorders and childhood mental disorders—which have been rarely considered in this specific context. Substance abuse, a remarkably neglected area as far as family problems are concerned, is also covered.

We hope that this book will contribute to sensitize not only psychiatrists, but all mental health professionals, to a dimension of mental health care which has been neglected for far too long, although it holds a major promise of improvement of quality of life of patients and all those involved in their care.

Norman Sartorius
Julian Leff
Juan José López-Ibor
Mario Maj
Ahmed Okasha

This volume includes several chapters developed from presentations delivered at the 12th World Congress of Psychiatry (Yokohama, Japan, 24–29 August, 2002).

Families of People with Schizophrenia

Christine Barrowclough

School of Psychological Sciences, University of Manchester, UK

INTRODUCTION

Families play an essential role in supporting people with long-term mental illness in the community and are focal in the social networks of people with schizophrenia [1]. Over 60% of those with a first episode of a major mental illness return to live with relatives [2], and this would seem to reduce only by 10–20% when those with subsequent admissions are included [3]. The carer role is often not without difficulties, and may be associated with considerable personal costs. In schizophrenia, many family members experience significant stress and subjective burden as a consequence of their caregiver role. Not only is such stress likely to affect the well-being of the relatives and compromise their long-term ability to support the patient, but it may also have an impact on the course of the illness itself and on outcomes for the client. This chapter describes research which has examined the impact of schizophrenia on families and the impact of family stress on patient outcomes. It then outlines the background to the development of family interventions in schizophrenia, summarizes the research findings including the evidence base for such interventions, and concludes by drawing attention to important areas for future development.

THE IMPACT OF SCHIZOPHRENIA ON FAMILIES

Approximately 1% of the population worldwide will suffer from schizo-phrenia in their lifetime, with the onset of the illness occurring usually in late adolescence or early adulthood. Schizophrenia is characterized by a range of symptoms. Although there are large variations in presentation, it is usually associated with severe disruptions to a sufferer's functioning. First,

Families and Mental Disorders. Edited by Norman Sartorius, Julian Leff, Juan José López-Ibor, Mario Maj and Ahmed Okasha. © 2005 John Wiley & Sons Ltd. ISBN 0-470-02382-1

disturbed behaviour may be associated with delusional thinking, thought disorder and hallucinations. Although these symptoms may be controlled by medication, the course of the illness is often marked by relapses or exacerbations of these psychotic phenomena and approximately one third of sufferers continue to have persistent positive symptoms despite optimum medication [4]. There are also long-term impairments in functioning known as negative symptoms. These include underactivity, lethargy, poor motivation, general mental slowing, restricted emotions and marked interpersonal difficulties. Due to the wide-ranging problems, the illness makes considerable emotional, practical and financial demands on those close to the sufferer—typically the parents or the spouse or partner. These demands are likely to persist over a prolonged period, and advice, help and support may not be readily available.

Under these circumstances, the coping resources of family members may be severely challenged and hence it is unsurprising that the impact of the illness results in negative outcomes in terms of personal distress and burden for many carers. Studies examining the impact of the illness on family members are described below.

Distress and Burden in Families of Schizophrenic Patients

One of the ways in which the impact of psychiatric illness on families has been investigated is in terms of "burden". This concept is described as having two dimensions: objective and subjective [5]. Objective burden can be observed by others and consists of measurable effects on the household, whereas subjective burden is the relative's own perception of the impact of caring. Schene and colleagues [6] refined the concept and suggested that objective burden is the additional caregiving demands imposed on relatives (such as helping, supervising, financial aid) and the loss of their own activities (such as work and social or leisure roles), whereas subjective burden refers to the experiences and emotional responses of a caregiver.

Many surveys have demonstrated that distress and burden associated with caring for a mentally ill family member are very high [6]. However, Chakrabarti and Kulhara [7] report that, in comparative studies across a range of disorders (schizophrenia, affective disorders, anxiety disorders), mean scores of objective burden were greatest among families of schizophrenia patients. A number of studies have assessed the negative impact of schizophrenia on families. Findings indicate that 30–60% of carers suffer significant distress as measured by self-report scales such as the General Health Questionnaire (e.g., 8–12). These levels are above what one would expect in the general population and it is assumed that these elevated levels of distress are associated with the demands of the caring role.

Studies have investigated what patient symptom factors predict high levels of burden in relatives, but there are inconsistencies in findings. Some studies report that positive symptoms are problematic [13,14], while others have found that both positive and negative symptoms are related to burden [15]. Clearly, differences in findings are likely to result from sample and measurement differences [16]. A further complication is that the distinction between subjective and objective burden becomes blurred when relatives' reports are used to assess objective burden [17]. However, there is considerable support for burden and distress being associated with non-psychotic symptoms such as underactivity [18] and negative symptoms [19–21], inappropriate and antisocial behaviour [21,22] and mood disturbance [22,23]. Fadden et al. [20] suggest that, although the positive, florid symptoms such as delusions and hallucinations can also cause problems, they do not tend to be present most of the time, unlike the negative symptoms. Hence, the major proportion of burdensome behaviours seems to come from the negative symptoms, while Provencher and Mueser [22,24] suggest that positive symptoms "interfere only minimally with role functioning in the family".

Although some symptoms may be more likely to cause difficulties for family members, the inconsistencies in findings between studies may also reflect the idiosyncratic nature of difficulties in the context of complex coping situations. Certainly, the lack of a straightforward relationship between symptom severity and relatives' distress [25–27] suggests that distress may be influenced by the family members' response, and a number of studies have looked at coping responses in relation to relatives' outcomes. For example, a study by Birchwood and Cochrane [8] described different coping styles in relatives of schizophrenic patients and found that broad styles of coping were applied with consistency across different patient behaviours. An "ignore/accept style" was associated with lower burden and a "disorganized" (many strategies without consistency or clear style) with higher distress, although the authors note that to some extent the coping style was related to the level of functioning of the patient. A number of studies have found that emotion-focused coping, particularly avoidance, is associated with more distress in relatives (e.g., 25,28,29).

Appraisal Processes and Coping in Families

One of the dominant coping theories is Lazarus and Folkman's [30] transactional model. This theory has gained support from researchers studying dementia caregiving (e.g., 31). The model emphasizes the individual's appraisals of demanding situations as mediators of affective and behavioural responses. Appraisals here refer to people's evaluative judgements about the stressor and may be understood as primary (how threatening the person perceives the situation to be, how much concern the situation elicits for him) and secondary (a person's assessment of his coping resources). Hence, according to Lazarus and Folkman's theory, where a relative appraises situations associated with the mental illness to be problematic or threatening and feels he does not have the resources to cope, then he is more likely to be distressed. Recent research applying the transactional model framework to relatives of schizophrenic patients does suggest that appraisal processes mediate the relationship between illness factors and carer responses [11,21,25]. These studies have employed independent measures of patient symptoms and have demonstrated that the burden and distress experienced by relatives are more dependent on their *appraisal* of the patient's problems than the problems themselves. However, it may well be that some types of problems associated with schizophrenia—for example, the negative symptoms referred to earlier—may elicit particularly challenging appraisals, or that the measurement of clinical symptoms may not correspond to the patient's behaviour in non-clinical settings [32].

Several studies have focused on one particular type of appraisal—the kind of explanations or causal attributions that relatives make about problematic behaviours associated with schizophrenia—in understanding relatives' responses to schizophrenia (see 33 for a review of studies). Although these appraisals seem to be important mainly in terms of how the relative responds to the patient (see later sections on expressed emotion for a fuller description), one study found that self-blaming attributions were predictive of distress in relatives [34]. There may be some merit in increasing the scope of the study of relatives' cognitions about mental illness as a means of understanding variability in how people respond to close relatives with a severe mental illness. In the area of physical health, it is widely accepted that cognitive processes mediate people's adaptation to their own health problems, and the most notable theoretical framework adopted in this work is the self-regulation model of Leventhal and colleagues [35,36]. It has been demonstrated that patients' illness representations or models of illness are based on distinct components—identity, cause, time line and illness consequences, as well as controllability (see 37 for review). These representations have been shown to carry emotional, behavioural and coping implications and are related to health outcomes. It has been suggested [37–39] that illness representations may also have important implications for people's responses to individuals who are ill, particularly in mental illness [40]. A preliminary study by Barrowclough *et al.* [26] supported the utility of this model in the context of relatives of schizophrenia patients using the Illness Perception Questionnaire (IPQ)

[41]. As with previous studies, there was little association between the measures of carer functioning (using measures of distress and burden) and patient functioning. However, where relatives perceived there to be greater negative consequences for the patient from the illness, they showed greater distress and subjective burden.

The transactional model predicts that appraisals of problems will also be influenced by perceptions of the number and efficacy of one's resources to manage the problems. In a longitudinal European study of family burden and coping over time [29], a reduction in family burden was found in relatives who adopted less emotion-focused strategies and received more practical support from their social network. Theory and evidence would suggest then that there are multiple routes to helping relatives to reduce distress and burden. These include modifying threatening appraisals of the illness experience (which may include helping to improve the patient's condition) and increasing relatives' confidence in managing its troublesome aspects, either through their own strategies or with support from others. However, later sections of the chapter show that there have been few attempts to date to develop family interventions directed at improving carer outcomes, and that the little research which is available has produced disappointing results. Despite a good deal of research, it would seem that we are in the early stages of understanding how best to help relatives to safeguard their own well-being.

IMPACT OF FAMILY ENVIRONMENT ON SCHIZOPHRENIA

It is clear that many families of patients with schizophrenia are likely to experience significant stress associated with the caring role. Although writers have acknowledged that such stress affects the well-being of relatives as well as compromising their ability to care for the patient, most family research in schizophrenia has focused on the latter aspect—that is, the impact of the family on the psychosis.

There is a long history of theories that hypothesize an association between the family environment and the development of schizophrenia. In the 1950s and 1960s, writers such as Bateson, Lidz and Laing described various patterns of family structure, interactions and communications which they proposed were responsible for causing schizophrenia [42]. These theories of family pathology failed to withstand empirical investigation and have now been largely discredited. However, some of the ramifications are still felt today, and Hatfield et al. [43] discuss the distress to families that these messages of family blame can cause.

Expressed Emotion Research

In the past thirty years or so, research on the effects of the family environment on the course of schizophrenia has become almost synonymous with the work on expressed emotion (EE). EE refers to a construct encompassing several key aspects of close interpersonal relationships. It reflects critical, hostile or emotionally overinvolved attitudes on the part of a family member toward a relative with a disorder or impairment. Originally developed to assess the emotional climate of households containing a person diagnosed with schizophrenia [44], EE is now a well-validated predictor of poor clinical outcome for this disorder as well as for other psychiatric conditions [45]. Although its name might suggest otherwise, EE is not a measure of emotional expressiveness. Rather, it is a measure of the extent to which an individual family member talks about another family member in a critical or hostile manner or in a way that indicates marked emotional overinvolvement (EOI). These attitudes are assessed using a semi-structured interview called the Camberwell Family Interview (CFI) [46]. The CFI generally takes between one and two hours to complete. The interview is audiotaped and later rated on a number of dimensions using operationalized guidelines.

Criticisms are defined as comments about the behaviour or characteristics of the person (patient) that the respondent clearly resents or finds annoying. Hostility is rated categorically on the basis of whether or not the respondent makes generalized criticisms or expresses attitudes that are rejecting of the patient. The EOI score is a composite measure of factors such as an exaggerated emotional response, over-intrusive or self-sacrificing behaviour, and over-identification with the patient. Positive aspects of the relationship may also be measured in the form of positive comments (a frequency count) and warmth (a scaled score taking into account attitudes and comments evidenced throughout the interview). However, it is the dimensions of criticism, hostility and EOI that are used to determine high and low levels of EE. Relatives scoring above threshold on one or more of these dimensions are assigned "high EE" status. The importance of the EE concept to schizophrenia lies in the predictive validity of the dichotomized EE measure. In a meta-analysis of 26 studies, Butzlaff and Hooley [45] demonstrated that living in a high EE home environment more than doubled the baseline relapse rate for schizophrenia patients 9 to 12 months after hospitalization. Over the years, EE methodology has been applied to other conditions, both psychiatric and medical. EE has been found to be predictive of illness course in other psychiatric conditions, most notably in depression (see 45). There are associations between high EE and childhood psychological disorders, and there are also indications that it may have predictive utility for some chronic medical conditions, including asthma and epilepsy (see 47 for a comprehensive review of EE research in health care).

Although the initial studies by Brown and colleagues [48] suggested that behavioural disturbance and work history were related to EE and relapse, multiple studies have demonstrated that the association of EE with relapse is independent of patient factors such as severity of illness. Even when potentially important patient variables are controlled statistically, EE still makes a significant and independent contribution to relapse [49]. The general findings contained in the literature also provide no strong support for the assumption that the link between EE and relapse results from their shared association with an unmeasured third variable (see 50).

Understanding the EE Concept

Although the predictive validity of EE is no longer in question, research studies continue to attempt to better understand the EE concept and its mechanism in relapse. It is generally understood to have its action within a vulnerability–stress model of schizophrenia (see 51 for a review of the models). In essence, such models conceptualize the psychosis as the result of environmental stress reacting with an underlying predisposition or biological vulnerability to develop the disorder. The models can be applied either to the genesis of the psychosis or to subsequent episodes and postulate a powerful role for environmental stress. Within this framework, EE is seen as one possible source of such stress, capable of triggering or exacerbating symptoms once vulnerability is established through the onset of the illness.

The measure of EE has also been applied to professional carers. Although this line of research is much less well developed than with families, there is accumulating evidence that high EE responses in professionals are associated with negative outcomes [52]. In a prospective study of case managers, Tattan and Tarrier [53] found that the absence of a positive relationship between case manager and patient measured 3 months after engagement was associated with poorer clinical outcome 9 months later independently of initial severity of illness. A positive relationship was also significantly associated with a greater improvement in the patient's quality of life and a negative relationship with the least. Barrowclough et al. [26] investigated staff–patient relationships on a low security inpatient facility. They found that staff viewed the behaviour of patients they felt less positively disposed toward as more the product of the patients' own volition, which is consistent with the associations found in the family caregiver research of less benign interpretation of behaviour and critical attitudes [33]. Patients were sensitive to staff feelings towards them; patients' ratings of perceived thoughts and feelings from staff about them were significantly correlated with those expressed by staff members about the patient. The more negatively perceived patients were significantly more likely to have behavioural disturbances in the 7 months subsequent to the ratings being made.

The extension of EE research to professional carers suggests that people with schizophrenia are sensitive to the effects of interpersonal relationships in general. However, their restricted social networks and lower levels of social functioning may increase the impact of stressful interactions with key formal and informal carers. The studies which have demonstrated that EE is not just of relevance to families provide support for Hatfield's contention that "patients . . . are also influenced by other powerful environments, such as hospital wards, treating physicians, rehabilitation centres, and the like . . . .Whatever is useful in expressed emotion theory needs to be applied to community workers" [54].

Mechanisms of EE in Relapse

There are a number of lines of evidence indicating that high EE in families represents a significant stressor for patients with schizophrenia, and as such may precipitate relapse. First, a series of physiological studies (see 55 for a review) demonstrated that patients' arousal levels differ in response to high and low EE relatives. The presence of a high EE relative is associated with arousal maintenance or increase, and that of a low EE relative with arousal decrease. Second, studies of relative–patient interactions in laboratory settings have supported the view that differences in high and low EE relatives assessed in the CFI translate to differences in real-life situations, with high EE relatives demonstrating more critical and/or more intrusive behaviours. As would be expected, the interactions are dynamic, with patient behaviours contributing to negative interactions, but high EE relatives seem less able to change tack, with their responses more likely to contribute to the escalation of negative exchanges [56]. Further support for high EE as a stressor comes from studies demonstrating that high EE relatives themselves report greater levels of persistent personal distress [11]. Third, a particularly fruitful recent avenue of understanding the variability in how people respond to close relatives with a severe mental illness is represented by studies focusing on the role of attributions. Evidence has accumulated that high and low EE relatives may differ in the beliefs they hold about patients and the problematic behaviours associated with the patient's illness. In particular, there is consistent evidence from several studies that critical relatives are more likely than non-critical ones to hold patients responsible for their difficulties [33]. In reviewing the relationship of EE and attributions to patient relapse, these authors conclude that carers' beliefs may play a role in the relapse process in a variety of ways, e.g. by mediating controlling behaviour which increases patient stress or by decreasing the patient's sense of self-worth, which may serve to reinforce negative self-focused delusions and hallucinations.

Finally, the strongest evidence that EE may act as a causal stressor in relapse comes from family intervention research in schizophrenia, which is reviewed below.

FAMILY INTERVENTIONS AND SCHIZOPHRENIA

The development of multifactorial models of the processes determining risk and relapse in schizophrenia briefly described in previous sections provided the general rationale for the development of family interventions. Their emphasis on the contribution of psychological and socio-environmental stressors to the illness course opened up the way to psychological interventions. Within the context of stress–vulnerability models, an individual's home might be viewed as an environment capable of influencing the illness for better or worse. The reasoning was that if attributes of certain households are responsible for precipitating relapse, then these attributes might be identified and modified, with a resulting reduction in relapse rates. Throughout the past two decades, a series of studies testing this theory have been reported.

There have been several descriptive reviews of the schizophrenia family intervention studies (e.g., 57–61). Typically, the controlled trials recruited families at the point of a patient's hospitalization for an acute episode of schizophrenia and commenced the family intervention when the patient was discharged back to the home. The intervention period lasted from 6 to 12 months, at the end of which relapse rates were compared between patients who received the family intervention as an adjunct to routine care and those who received routine care only. Routine care included the use of prophylactic medication. Table 1.1 presents a summary of studies that have compared family intervention with routine or standard care for patients with schizophrenia.

Although the table selects only studies where the intervention lasted at least for 10 sessions, the variety of programmes delivered is apparent. Interventions developed by the various research groups differed on some important dimensions, including the location of the family sessions (home versus hospital base), the number of sessions offered, the extent of the patient's involvement, whether families were seen individually or in groups, and the precise content of the sessions and the mode of delivery. Since the researchers did not have a clear understanding of the mechanisms of patient relapse in the home environment, determining the content

TABLE 1.1 Controlled studies comparing family intervention with standard treatment for patients with schizophrenia (modified from 61)

Study	Treatment conditions	N	Type of family intervention	Frequency and duration of treatment	Results
Kottgen et al. [62]	Family intervention, high EE Customary care, high EE Customary care, low EE	49	Psychodynamic: separate groups for patients and relatives	Weekly or monthly up to 2 years	2 years: family intervention equal to customary care for families with either high or low EE
Falloon et al. [63,64]	Behavioural family therapy Individual management	36	Home-based behavioural family therapy	Weekly for 3 months Biweekly for 6 months Monthly for 15 months	2 years: behavioural family therapy better than individual management
Leff et al. [65,66]	Family intervention Customary care	24	Psychoeducation to help relatives with high EE Model coping in low EE relatives	Biweekly for relatives' groups for 9 months	2 years: family intervention better than customary care
Tarrier et al. [67–69]	Behavioural family therapy, enactive Behavioural family therapy symbolic Education only Customary care	77	Behavioural family therapy comprising stress management and training in goal setting	3 stress management and 8 goal-setting sessions over 9 months	2 years: behavioural family therapy better than education or customary care; education and customary care equal
Vaughan et al. [70]	Single-family psycho-education and support Customary care	36	Psychoeducation	10 weekly sessions	9 months: single-family education and support equal to customary care

Study	Intervention	N	Type of intervention	Frequency/duration	Results
Mingyuan et al. [71]	Multiple-family psycho-education and support / Customary care	2076 / 1016	Clinic-based lectures and discussions	10 lectures and 3 discussion groups over 12 months	1 year: multiple family education and support better than customary care
Randolph et al. [72]	Behavioural family therapy / Customary care	39	Clinic-based behavioural family therapy	Weekly for 3 months Biweekly for 3 months Biweekly for 6 months	2 years: behavioural family therapy better than customary care
Xiong et al. [73]	Behavioural family therapy / Customary care	63	Clinic-based psychoeducation, skills training, medication/ symptom management	Bimonthly for 3 months Family sessions for 2 years (plus individual sessions with family members and patients): maintenance sessions every 2–3 months	18 months: behavioural family therapy better than customary care
Zhang et al. [74]	Multiple and single family psychoeducation and support / Customary care	78	Multiple-family clinic-based psycho-education counselling, medication/symptom management	Individual and group counselling sessions every 1–3 months for 18 months	18 months: family education and support better than customary care
Buchkremer et al. [75]	"Therapeutic" relatives' group / Customary care	68	"Therapeutic" relatives' groups and initiated relatives	Fortnightly for 2 years	No differences between groups at 1 year or 2 years
Telles et al. [76]	Behavioural family management / Individual case management	– / –	Clinic-based behavioural family management	Weekly for 6 months, every 2 weeks for 3 months, monthly for 3 months	12 months: for total group conditions equal; for "poorly acculturated" patients, individual management better; for "highly acculturated" patients, conditions equal

continued

TABLE 1.1 (*Continued*)

Study	Treatment conditions	N	Type of family intervention	Frequency and duration of treatment	Results
Leff *et al.* [77]	Multiple-family psycho-education and support Single-family psycho-education and support	23	Multiple-family groups in the clinic; single family sessions at home	Biweekly for 9 months, varying amounts afterward	2 years: conditions equal
Zastowny *et al.* [78]	Behavioural family therapy Single-family psycho-education and support	30	Hospital-based behavioural family therapy; hospital based single-family psychoeducation and advice on handling common problems	Weekly for 4 months, monthly for 12 months	16 months: conditions equal
McFarlane *et al.* [79]	Multiple-family psycho-education and support Single-family psycho-education and support	83 89	Multiple-family groups or single family sessions in the clinic	Biweekly sessions for 2 years	2 years: multiple family conditions better than single family condition
Schooler *et al.* [80]	Applied family management Supportive family management	157 156	Applied management comprising home-based behavioural family therapy sessions plus supportive family management; supportive family management comprising clinic-based multiple family groups	Applied family manage-ment: behavioural family therapy weekly for 3 months, biweekly for 6 months, and monthly for 3–6 months plus concurrent monthly supportive family management for 24–28 months; supportive family management monthly for 24–28 months	2 years: conditions equal

involved making certain assumptions about the kinds of problems associated with families which might contribute to stress, and hence deciding what issues needed to be targeted. In practice, all the studies assumed families had inadequate knowledge or misunderstandings regarding the illness and placed an emphasis on educating relatives about schizophrenia, to the extent that some reviewers have subsumed all family intervention under the category "psychoeducation". The other common area targeted was helping the family members in coping with symptom-related difficulties, either by a specific problem-solving approach [81] or through assessment of individual problems and application of appropriate cognitive–behavioural techniques [82]. Despite differences in approaches, Mari and Streiner [83] have provided a useful summary of the common "ingredients" or "overall principles" of the treatments: to build up an alliance with relatives who care for the schizophrenic member; to reduce adverse family atmosphere; to enhance the problem-solving capacity of relatives; to decrease expressions of anger and guilt; to maintain reasonable expectations of patient performance; to set limits safeguarding relatives' own well-being; and to achieve changes in relatives' behaviour and beliefs.

A number of meta-analytic reviews (83, updated by 84 and 85; 86,87) of the family intervention studies have been published. These reviews include family intervention studies where the patient has a diagnosis of schizophrenia or schizoaffective disorder; where there is some form of control or comparison group against which to evaluate any benefits from the experimental treatment; and where patient relapse or hospitalization is examined as the main outcome. The Pharoah et al. [85] analysis adopted fairly stringent inclusion criteria (excluding studies with non-random assignment, those restricted to an inpatient intervention; those not restricted to schizophrenia; and when the intervention took place over less than 5 sessions) and included 13 studies. The review confirms the findings of the earlier descriptive accounts of the studies. It concludes that family intervention as an adjunct to routine care decreases the frequency of relapse and hospitalization; and that these findings hold across the wide age ranges, sex differences and variability in the length of illness found in the different studies. Moreover, the analysis suggests that these results generalize across care cultures where health systems are very different—trials from the UK, Australia, Europe, the People's Republic of China and the USA were included. The more inclusive review [86] examined 25 studies spanning 20 years (1977–1997). Again, it confirmed the lower relapse rate of family-treated patients compared with control groups, finding an effect size of 0.20, corresponding to a decrease in relapse rate of 20%. Although this treatment effect may seem relatively low, one must bear in mind that this analysis includes studies where the intervention was extremely brief and with little resemblance to the intensive programmes in the original studies. For example, the studies of Falloon *et al.* [63], Leff *et al.* [65] and Tarrier *et al.* [67] (see Table 1.1) demonstrated decreased relapse rates for family-treated patients of approximately 40%.

Unfortunately, the absence of treatment fidelity measures makes it very difficult to judge quality control within or between studies. Further comparison analyses within the Pitschel-Walz *et al.* review [86] draw attention to some of the wide variations in the content and duration of programmes in recent years. It would seem that there has been considerable dilution of the potency of the family interventions in the large meta-analyses where there is no quality control. Categorizing studies into those lasting more or less than 10 weeks, they found that longer-term interventions were more successful than short-term interventions; and that more intensive family treatments were superior to a more limited approach (for example, where relatives were offered little more than brief education sessions about schizophrenia). When families were provided with an effective "dose" in terms of duration and intensity of intervention, the Pitschel-Walz *et al.* review [86] suggests there is some evidence of long-lasting effects from family treatment. Several studies found a significant difference remaining between the intervention and control groups at 2 years. The 5- and 8-year follow-up data of Tarrier *et al.* [69] demonstrated how durable are these effects. However, it must be emphasized that all the studies show that relapses increase with the number of years from termination of the intervention.

The most recent meta-analysis by Pilling *et al.* [87] included 18 studies and its conclusions were in line with previous reviews in confirming the efficacy of family intervention for reducing relapse. It included a comparison of single family and group family treatments, and found group treatments to have poorer outcomes in terms of the re-emergence of psychotic symptoms or readmission to hospital. They agree with previous reviewers [83] that the effects from family interventions have decreased over the years, and they suggest that this might in part be explained by the increased use of family group approaches (e.g., 75,79,80,88). However, they add that this may not be due to the group format per se, but rather due to other factors: the variable content of the group treatments; the fact that group treatments may have benefits unmeasured by the studies (e.g. on carer burden); or the fact that group treatments may have particular benefit for sub-populations.

One of the criticisms of the family intervention studies has been their narrow focus on the end results of reductions in patient relapse and hospitalizations [83]. The inclusion of other outcome measures has been variable, and consequently there is usually inadequate systematic data such that can be subjected to meta-analytic review. The Pitschel-Walz *et al.* review [86] is more optimistic than the Pilling *et al.* review [87] in the conclusions that can be drawn about wider patient and family outcomes. As regards patient outcomes, both reviews agree that there is some evidence of better medication compliance. The Pitschel-Walz *et al.* review [86] also asserts that there are indications of improved quality of life and better patient social adjustment in family-treated patients. Several studies have demonstrated that these improved outcomes are achieved with reduced costs to society (e.g., 63,69,73).

As noted by Pilling *et al.* [87], the potential benefit for family members themselves from the interventions has received relatively little attention. It has to be remembered that, although the trials sought to reduce intrafamilial stress, improvement in patient outcomes and not family outcomes was the prime target. Where family burden was assessed as a secondary outcome, the results appear to be inconsistent. For example, among studies which have employed a similar intervention format—behavioural family therapy (BFT)—some (e.g., 64,89) reported reductions in family burden, while a later much larger one [90] found that BFT did not influence family burden. Szmukler *et al.* [91] identify three randomized controlled trials aimed specifically at carers [88,92,93], although with very brief interventions. These studies showed some advantages, although in terms of outcomes that are only indirectly related to distress and burden, such as knowledge and attitudes. The use of different measures makes comparisons between studies assessing carer outcomes problematic. A recent trial with a longer duration of intervention which did focus primarily on improving carer outcomes did not produce encouraging results [91]. A two-phased intervention with 6 family sessions followed by 12 relatives' groups was compared with standard care. Engagement into the trial was poor, and the authors report that the carers' programme did not offer any significant advantage on any of the outcome measures: psychological morbidity, negative appraisal, coping or support. Szmukler *et al.* [91] conclude that there is still uncertainty about the most effective interventions for carers of patients with psychotic disorders.

Dissemination of Family Interventions in Routine Care

In the UK and elsewhere, in recent years, there have been attempts to disseminate the benefits of family intervention in schizophrenia into routine service delivery. This has been largely through training programmes designed to provide clinicians, mainly community psychiatric nurses, with the knowledge and skills required to implement the family work (see 94 for a review of dissemination programmes). Despite the solid evidence base for the efficacy of family-based psychological treatment programmes in schizophrenia, and the efforts of the training programmes, the implementation of family work in routine mental health services has been at best patchy. The consensus view in the literature is that family intervention implementation faces complex organizational and attitudinal difficulties (e.g., 95–97), and insufficient attention has been paid to these in dissemination programmes. In discussing the factors which might make the transference from research to practice difficult, Mari and Streiner [83] suggested that the requirements of durable service-oriented interventions may differ from those based on time-limited research models. In an attempt to demonstrate the effectiveness of family interventions in standard psychiatric settings which take account of these differences, a randomized controlled pragmatic trial was carried out [98]. The family intervention was based on the formal assessment of carer needs, and the programme was carried out by a clinical psychologist in conjunction with the patient's key worker—thus, training was *in situ*. The fact that the intervention was found to be effective in reducing carer needs and in reducing patient relapse at 12 months post-treatment [99] suggests that there are advantages in developing dissemination models based within services. The need for changing the clinical practice of the whole service rather than training individuals is underlined in the work of Corrigan and colleagues [100–102]. However, difficulties arise not only from staff but also from carer reluctance to engage in family work. Several studies of community samples (e.g., 91,98,103) have shown that carer participation in family intervention is relatively low, with only 50% or so of carers taking up the offer of either a support service or family intervention [98], with possibly higher rates when help is offered at a time of crisis [104].

CONCLUSIONS

This chapter has attempted to encompass the main themes and findings from research into families of schizophrenic patients that has taken place in the past 20 years or so. While a number of conclusions can be drawn, some areas are clearly in need of further research and development.

It is now acknowledged that having a close relative who has a severe mental illness very often results in high levels of stress and perceived burden. The consequences of the caring role for relatives would seem to be influenced by a number of factors, including available support and the nature of the patient's problems, but also by the relatives' appraisals of the experience—the sense they make of the illness and the ways in which they perceive the symptoms and their own coping efforts. Despite the problems that relatives experience and the volume of research that has documented their difficulties, few studies have had the primary goal of helping these carers to reduce their distress, and those that have been conducted have by and large shown disappointing results. On the other hand, most of the family intervention work has been targeted at improving patient outcomes, and studies have demonstrated clear gains for patients in terms of reductions in relapses and hospitalizations, such that there is now robust evidence for the efficacy of family interventions in schizophrenia. However, the content of family intervention in evaluated studies has varied widely and there have been problems in the dissemination of the work into routine care. It would seem that successful family interventions require considerable investment in time, skill and commitment, and since for many patients the effect is to delay rather than to prevent relapse, many patients and families will need long-term and continuing intervention. There are also strong indications that the adverse effects of stressful interpersonal interactions in schizophrenia are not confined to family relationships. It would seem that much that has been learned from EE research and family interventions might usefully be transferred to work in improving therapeutic relationships with informal carers.

Future work with families and staff might usefully focus on recent-onset patients. Work with relatives of recently diagnosed schizophrenia patients indicates that help needs to begin from the first onset of the psychosis [104]. It has been suggested that the issues facing a first-episode patient and family are different from those facing someone with a long-term illness [105]. For example, there is often more diagnostic uncertainty, which means that education about the condition needs to be more flexible. Family intervention work in early psychosis programmes has been recognized to be important but has received little evaluation.

Dissemination and engagement issues in family work also need to continue to be addressed. Although many patients and families benefit greatly from the intervention programmes, a substantial number of families are hard to engage, and the implementation of family programmes within services presents many challenges. Finally, further work needs to be done to identify optimum techniques for changing family attitudes where problems are particularly complex, for example in schizophrenia and comorbid substance misuse. To date only one recent trial has evaluated a family-based component for this client group [107,108].

REFERENCES

1. Bengtsson-Tops A., Hansson L. (2001) Quantitative and qualitative aspects of the social network in schizophrenic patients living in the community. Relationship to sociodemographic characteristics and clinical factors and subjective quality of life. *Int. J. Soc. Psychiatry*, **47**, 67–77.
2. Macmillan J.F., Gold A., Crow T.J., Johnson A.L., Johnstone E.C. (1986) The Northwick Park Study of first episodes of schizophrenia: IV Expressed emotion and relapse. *Br. J. Psychiatry*, **148**, 133–143.

3. Gibbons J.S., Horn S.H., Powell J.M., Gibbons J.L. (1984) Schizophrenia patients and their families. A survey in a psychiatric service based on a district general hospital. *Br. J. Psychiatry*, **144**, 70–77.
4. Kane J.M. (1996) Treatment resistant schizophrenic patients. *J. Clin. Psychiatry*, **57**(Suppl. 9), 35–40.
5. Hoenig J., Hamilton M.W. (1967) The burden on the household in an extra-mural psychiatric service. In: Freeman H. (ed.) *New Aspects in the Mental Health Services*. Pergamon, London, pp. 612–635.
6. Schene A.H., Tessler R.C., Gamache G.M. (1994) Instruments measuring family or caregiver burden in severe mental illness. *Soc. Psychiatry Psychiatr. Epidemiol.*, **24**, 228–240.
7. Chakrabarti S., Kulhara P. (1999) Family burden of caring for people with mental illness. *Br. J. Psychiatry*, **174**, 463.
8. Birchwood M., Cochrane R. (1990) Families coping with schizophrenia: coping styles, their origins and correlates. *Psychol. Med.*, **20**, 857–865.
9. Oldridge M.L., Hughes I.C.T. (1992) Psychological well-being in families with a member suffering from schizophrenia: an investigation into longstanding problems. *Br. J. Psychiatry*, **161**, 249–251.
10. Winefield H.R., Harvey E.J. (1993) Determinants of psychological distress in relatives of people with chronic schizophrenia. *Schizophr. Bull.*, **19**, 619–625.
11. Barrowclough C., Parle M. (1997) Appraisal, psychological adjustment and expressed emotion in relatives of patients suffering from schizophrenia. *Br. J. Psychiatry*, **171**, 26–30.
12. McGilloway S., Donnelly M., Mays N. (1997) The experience of caring for former long-stay psychiatric patients. *Br. J. Clin. Psychol.*, **36**, 149–151.
13. Grad J., Sainsbury P. (1963) Mental illness and the family. *Lancet*, **8**, 544–547.
14. Ral L., Kulhara P., Avashti A. (1991) Social burden of positive and negative schizophrenia. *Int. J. Soc. Psychiatry*, **37**, 242–250.
15. Webb C., Pfeiffer M., Mueser K.T., Gladis M., Mensch E., DeGirolama J., Levinson D.F. (1998) Burden and well being of caregivers for the severely mentally ill: the role of coping style and social support. *Schizophr. Res.*, **34**, 169–180.
16. Magliano L., Fadden G., Madianos M., Caldas de Almeida J.M., Held T., Guarneri M., Marasco C., Tosini P., Maj M. (1998) Burden on the families of patients with schizophrenia: results of the BIOMED I study. *Soc. Psychiatry Psychiatr. Epidemiol.*, **33**, 405–412.
17. Halford W.K. (1992) Assessment of family interaction with a schizophrenic member. In: Kavanagh D.J. (ed.) *Schizophrenia: An Overview and Practical Handbook*. Chapman & Hall, Melbourne, pp. 254–274.
18. Platt S., Weyman A., Hirsch S.R. (1983) *Social Behaviour Assessment Schedule*, 3rd edn. NFER-Nelson, Windsor.
19. Creer C., Wing J.K. (1974) *Schizophrenia in the Home*. National Schizophrenia Fellowship, Surbiton.
20. Fadden G., Bebbington P., Kuipers L. (1987) The burden of care: the impact of functional psychiatric illness on the patient's family. *Br. J. Psychiatry*, **150**, 285–292.
21. Quinn J., Barrowclough C., Tarrier N. (2003) The Family Questionnaire (FQ): a scale for measuring symptom appraisal in relatives of schizophrenia patients. *Acta Psychiatr. Scand.*, **108**, 290–296.
22. Provencher H.L. (1996) Objective burden among primary caregivers of persons with chronic schizophrenia. *J. Psychiatry Ment. Health Nurs.*, **3**, 181–187.

23. Jenkins J.H., Schumacher J.G. (1999) Family burden of schizophrenia and depressive illness. Specifying the effects of ethnicity, gender and social ecology. *Br. J. Psychiatry*, **174**, 31–38.
24. Provencher H., Meuser K. (1997) Positive and negative symptom behaviours and caregiver burden in the relatives of persons with schizophrenia. *Schizophr. Res.*, **26**, 71–80.
25. Scazufca M., Kuipers E. (1999) Coping strategies in relatives of people with schizophrenia before and after psychiatric admission. *Br. J. Psychiatry*, **174**, 154–158.
26. Barrowclough C., Lobban F., Hatton C., Quinn J. (2001) An investigation of models of illness in carers of schizophrenic patients using the Illness Perception Questionnaire. *Br. J. Clin. Psychol.*, **40**, 371–385.
27. Boye B., Bentson H., Ulstein I., Notland T.H., Lersbryggen A., Lingjaerde O., Malt U.F. (2001) Relatives' distress and patients' symptoms and behaviours: a prospective study of patients with schizophrenia and their relatives. *Acta Psychiatr. Scand.*, **104**, 42–50.
28. Magliano L., Veltro F., Guarneri M., Marasco C. (1995) Clinical and socio-demographic correlates of coping strategies in relatives of schizophrenic patients. *Eur. Psychiatry*, **10**, 155–158.
29. Magliano L., Fadden G., Economou M., Held T., Xavier M., Guarneri M., Malangone C., Maj M. (2000) Family burden and coping strategies in schizophrenia: 1 year follow-up data from the BIOMED I study. *Soc. Psychiatry Psychiatr. Epidemiol.*, **35**, 109–115.
30. Lazarus R., Folkman S. (1984) *Stress, Appraisal and Coping*. Springer-Verlag, New York.
31. Haley W.E., Levine E.G., Brown S.L. (1987) Stress, appraisal, coping and social support as predictors of adaptational outcome among dementia caregivers. *Psychol. Aging*, **2**, 323–330.
32. Scazufca M., Kuipers E. (1996) Links between expressed emotion and burden of care in relatives of patients with schizophrenia. *Br. J. Psychiatry*, **168**, 580–587.
33. Barrowclough C., Hooley J.M. (2003) Attributions and expressed emotion: a review. *Clin. Psychol. Rev.*, **23**, 849–880.
34. Barrowclough C., Tarrier N., Johnston M. (1996) Distress, expressed emotion and attributions in relatives of schizophrenic patients. *Schizophr. Bull.*, **22**, 691–701.
35. Leventhal H., Diefenbach M., Leventhal E.A. (1992) Illness cognition: using common sense to understand treatment adherence and affect cognition interactions. *Cogn. Ther. Res.*, **16**, 143–163.
36. Leventhal H., Nerenz D.R., Steele D.F. (1984) Illness representations and coping with health threats. In: Baum A., Singer J. (eds) *A Handbook of Psychology and Health*. Lawrence Erlbaum Associates, Hillsdale, NJ, pp. 219–252.
37. Skelton J.A. (1991) Laypersons' judgements of patient credibility and the study of illness representations. In: Skelton J.R., Croyle R.T. (eds) *Mental Representation in Health and Illness*. Springer-Verlag, New York, pp. 247–272.
38. Bishop G.D. (1991) Understanding the understanding of illness. In: Skelton J.R., Croyle R.T. (eds) *Mental Representation in Health and Illness*. Springer-Verlag, New York, pp. 32–59.
39. Croyle R.T., Barger S.D. (1993) Illness cognition. In Maes S., Leventhal H., Johnston M. (eds) *International Review of Health Psychology*, vol. 2. John Wiley & Sons, Chichester, pp. 29–49.

40. Lobban F., Barrowclough C., Jones S. (2003) A review of models of illness for severe mental illness. *Clin. Psychol. Rev.*, **23**, 171–196.
41. Weinman J., Petrie K., Moss-Morris R., Horne R. (1996) The Illness Perception Questionnaire: a new method for assessing the cognitive representation of illness. *Psychol. Health*, **11**, 431–445.
42. Hirsch S.R., Leff J. (1975) *Abnormalities in Parents of Schizophrenics*. Maudsley monographs no. 22. Oxford University Press, London.
43. Hatfield A.B., Spaniol L., Zipple A.M. (1987) Expressed emotion: a family perspective. *Schizophr. Bull.*, **13**, 221–235.
44. Brown G.W., Rutter M. (1966) The measurement of family activities and relationships: a methodological study. *Human Relations*, **19**, 241–263.
45. Butzlaff R.L., Hooley J.M. (1998) Expressed emotion and psychiatric relapse: a meta-analysis. *Arch. Gen. Psychiatry*, **55**, 547–552.
46. Vaughn C., Leff J. (1976) The measurement of expressed emotion in the families of psychiatric patients. *Br. J. Soc. Clin. Psychol.*, **15**, 157–165.
47. Wearden A.J., Tarrier N., Barrowclough C., Zastowney T.R., Rahill A.A. (2000) A review of expressed emotion research in health care. *Clin. Psychol. Rev.*, **20**, 633–666.
48. Brown G.W., Birley J.L.T., Wing J.K. (1972) Influence of family life on the course of schizophrenic disorders: a replication. *Br. J. Psychiatry*, **121**, 241–248.
49. Nuechterlein K.H., Snyder K.S., Minz J. (1992) Paths to relapse: possible transactional processes connecting patient illness onset, expressed emotion and psychotic relapse. *Br. J. Psychiatry*, **161**(Suppl. 18), 88–96.
50. Hooley J.M., Rosen L.R., Richters J.E. (1995) Expressed emotion: toward clarification of a critical construct. In: Miller G. (ed.) *The Behavioral High Risk Paradigm in Psychopathology*. Springer-Verlag, New York, pp. 88–120.
51. Clements K., Turpin G. (1992) *Innovations in the Psychological Management of Schizophrenia*. John Wiley & Sons, Chichester.
52. Kuipers E. (1998) Working with carers: interventions for relative and staff carers of those who have psychosis. In: Wykes T., Tarrier N., Lewis S.J. (eds) *Outcome and Innovation in Psychological Treatment of Schizophrenia*. John Wiley & Sons, Chichester, pp. 201–214.
53. Tattan T., Tarrier N. (2000) The expressed emotion of case managers of the seriously mentally ill: the influence of expressed emotion on clinical outcomes. *Psychol. Med.*, **30**, 195–204.
54. Hatfield A.B. (1987) The expressed emotion theory: why families object. *Hosp. Commun. Psychiatry*, **38**, 341.
55. Tarrier N., Turpin G. (1992) Psychosocial factors, arousal and schizophrenic relapse: a review of the psychophysiological data. *Br. J. Psychiatry*, **161**, 3–11.
56. Hahlweg W.K., Goldstein M.J., Nuechterlein K.H. (1989) Expressed emotion and patient relative interaction in families of recent onset schizophrenics. *J. Consult. Clin. Psychol.*, **57**, 11–18.
57. Barrowclough C., Tarrier N. (1984) Psychosocial interventions with families and their effects on the course of schizophrenia: a review. *Psychol. Med.*, **14**, 629–642.
58. Lam D.H. (1991) Psychosocial family intervention in schizophrenia: a review of empirical studies. *Psychol. Med.*, **21**, 423–441.
59. Kavenagh D. (1992) Family interventions for schizophrenia. In: Kavenagh D.J. (ed.) *Schizophrenia: An Overview and Practical Handbook*. Chapman & Hall, London, pp. 407–423.

60. Dixon L.B., Lehman A.F. (1995) Family interventions for schizophrenia. *Schizophr. Bull.*, **21**, 631–643.
61. Penn D.L., Mueser K.T. (1996) Research update on the psychosocial treatment of schizophrenia. *Am. J. Psychiatry*, **153**, 607–617.
62. Kottgen C., Soinnichesen I., Mollenhauer K., Jurth R. (1984) Results of the Hamburg Camberwell Family Interview study, I–III. *Int. J. Fam. Psychiatry*, **5**, 61–94.
63. Falloon I.R.H., Boyd J.L., McGill C.W., Razani J., Moss H.B., Gilderman A.M. (1982) Family management in the prevention of exacerbations of schizophrenia. *N. Engl. J. Med.*, **306**, 1437–1440.
64. Falloon I.R.H., Boyd J.L., McGill C.W., Williamson M., Razani J., Moss H.B., Gilderman A.M., Simson G.M. (1985) Family management in the prevention of morbidity in schizophrenia: clinical outcome of a 2 year longitudinal study. *Arch. Gen. Psychiatry*, **42**, 887–896.
65. Leff J.P., Kuipers L., Berkowitz R., Eberlein-Fries R., Sturgeon D. (1982) A controlled trial of intervention with families of schizophrenic patients. *Br. J. Psychiatry*, **141**, 121–134.
66. Leff J.P., Kuipers L., Sturgeon D. (1985) A controlled trial of social intervention in the families of schizophrenic patients. *Br. J. Psychiatry*, **146**, 594–600.
67. Tarrier N., Barrowclough C., Vaughn C.E., Bamrah J.S., Proceddu K., Watts S., Freeman H. (1988) Community management of schizophrenia: a controlled trial of a behavioural intervention with families to reduce relapse. *Br. J. Psychiatry*, **153**, 532–542.
68. Tarrier N., Barrowclough C., Vaughn C.E., Bamrah J.S., Proceddu K., Watts S., Freeman H. (1989) The community management of schizophrenia: a controlled trial of a behavioural intervention with families to reduce relapse: a 2 year follow-up. *Br. J. Psychiatry*, **154**, 625–628.
69. Tarrier N., Barrowclough C., Porceddu K., Fitzpatrick E. (1994) The Salford Family Intervention Project for schizophrenic relapse prevention: five and eight year accumulating relapses. *Br. J. Psychiatry*, **165**, 829–832.
70. Vaughan K., Doyle M., McConaghy N., Blaszczynski A., Fox A., Tarrier N. (1992) The Sydney Intervention trial: a controlled trial of relatives' counselling to reduce schizophrenic relapse. *Soc. Psychiatry Psychiatr. Epidemiol.*, **27**, 16–21.
71. Mingyuan Z., Heqin Y., Chengde Y., Jianlin Y., Qingfeng Y., Peijun C., Lianfang G., Jizhong Y., Guangya Q., Zhen W., *et al.* (1993) Effectiveness of psycho-education of relatives of schizophrenic patients: a prospective cohort study in five cities of China. *Int. J. Ment. Health*, **22**, 47–59.
72. Randolph E.T., Eth S., Glynn S.M., Paz G.G., Shaner A.L., Strachan A., Van Vort W., Escobar J.I., Liberman R.P. (1994) Behavioural family management in schizophrenia: outcome of a clinic based intervention. *Br. J. Psychiatry*, **164**, 501–506.
73. Xiong W., Phillips M.R., Hu X., Wang R., Dai Q., Kleinman A. (1994) Family based intervention for schizophrenic patients in China: a randomised controlled trial. *Br. J. Psychiatry*, **165**, 239–247.
74. Zhang M., Wang M., Li J., Phillips M.R. (1994) Randomised control trial family intervention for 78 first episode male schizophrenic patients: an 18 month study in Suzhou, Japan. *Br. J. Psychiatry*, **65**(Suppl. 24), 96–102.
75. Buchkremer G., Klinberg S., Holle R., Schulze-Mönking H., Hornung P. (1997) Psychoeducational psychotherapy for schizophrenic patients and their key relatives: results of a two year follow up. *Acta Psychiatr. Scand.*, **96**, 483–491.

76. Telles C., Karno M., Mintz J., Paz G., Arias M., Tucker D., Lopez S. (1995) Immigrant families coping with schizophrenia—behavioural family intervention v. case management with low income Spanish-speaking population. *Br. J. Psychiatry*, **167**, 473–479.
77. Leff J.P., Berkowitz R., Shavit A., Strachan A., Glass I., Vaughn C.E. (1990) A trial of family therapy versus relatives' groups for schizophrenia. *Br. J. Psychiatry*, **157**, 571–577.
78. Zastowny R.R., Lehman A.F., Cole R.E., Kane C. (1992) Family management of schizophrenia: a comparison of behavioural and supportive family treatment. *Psychiatry Q.*, **63**, 159–186.
79. McFarlane W.R., Lukens E., Link B., Dushay R., Deakins S.A., Newmark M., Dunne E.J., Horen B., Toran J. (1995) Multiple family groups and psychoeducation in the treatment of schizophrenia. *Arch. Gen. Psychiatry*, **52**, 679–687.
80. Schooler N.R., Keith S.J., Severe J.B., Matthews S.M., Bellack A.S., Glick I.D., Hargreaves W.A., Kane J.M., Ninan P.T., Frances A., *et al.* (1997) Relapse and rehospitalisation during maintenance treatment of schizophrenia. The effects of dose reduction and family treatment. *Arch. Gen. Psychiatry*, **54**, 453–463.
81. Falloon I., Boyd J., McGill C. (1984) *Family Care of Schizophrenia*. Guilford, London.
82. Barrowclough C., Tarrier N. (1992) *Families of Schizophrenic Patients: Cognitive Behavioural Intervention*. Chapman & Hall, London.
83. Mari J.J., Streiner D.L. (1994) An overview of family interventions and relapse in schizophrenia: meta-analysis of research findings. *Psychol. Med.*, **24**, 565–578.
84. Mari J.J., Streiner D.L. (1996) Family intervention for people with schizophrenia (Cochrane Review). In: *The Cochrane Library*, 1. Update Software, Oxford.
85. Pharoah F.M., Mari J.J., Streiner D.L. (1999) Family intervention for people with schizophrenia (Cochrane Review). In: *The Cochrane Library*, 4. Update Software, Oxford.
86. Pitschel-Walz G., Leucht S., Bauml J., Kissling W., Engel R.R. (2001) The effect of family interventions on relapse and rehospitalisation in schizophrenia—a meta-analysis. *Schizophr. Bull.*, **27**, 73–92.
87. Pilling S., Bebbington P., Kuipers E., Garety P., Geddes J., Orbach G., Morgan C. (2002) Psychological treatments in schizophrenia: I. Meta-analysis of family intervention and cognitive behaviour therapy. *Psychol. Med.*, **32**, 763–782.
88. Berglund N., Vahhlne J.O., Edman A. (2003) Family intervention in schizophrenia: impact on family burden and attitude. *Soc. Psychiatry Psychiatr. Epidemiol.*, **38**, 116–121.
89. Posner C.M., Wilson K.G., Kral M.J., Lander S., McIllwraith R.D. (1992) Family psychoeducational support groups in schizophrenia. *Am. J. Orthopsychiatry*, **62**, 206–218.
90. Mueser K.T., Sengupta A., Schooler N.R., Bellack A.S., Xie H., Glick I.D., Keith S.J. (2001) Family treatment and medication dosage reduction in schizophrenia: effects on patient social functioning, family attitudes, and burden. *J. Consult. Clin. Psychol.*, **69**, 3–12.
91. Szmukler G., Kuipers E., Joyce J., Harris T., Leese M., Maphosa W., Staples E. (2003) An exploratory randomised controlled trial of a support programme for carers of patients with a psychosis. *Soc. Psychiatry Psychiatr. Epidemiol.*, **38**, 411–418.

92. Solomon P., Draine J., Mannion E., Meisel M. (1997) Effectiveness of two models of brief family intervention: retention of gains by family members of adults with serious mental illness. *Am. J. Orthopsychiatry*, **67**, 177–186.
93. Szmukler G.I., Herrman H., Colusa S., Benson A., Bloch S. (1996) A controlled trial of a counselling intervention for caregivers of relatives with schizophrenia. *Soc. Psychiatry Psychiatr. Epidemiol.*, **31**, 149–155.
94. Tarrier N., Barrowclough C., Haddock G., McGovern J. (1999) The dissemination of innovative cognitive-behavioural psychosocial treatments for schizophrenia. *J. Ment. Health*, **8**, 569–582.
95. Kavenagh D.J., Piatkowska O.M., Clark D., O'Holloran P., Manicavasagar V., Rosen A., Tennant C. (1993) Application of cognitive behavioural family intervention for schizophrenia to multidisciplinary teams: what can the matter be? *Aust. Psychol.*, **28**, 181–188.
96. Hughs I., Hailwood R., Abbati-Yeoman J., Budd R. (1996) Developing a family intervention service for serious mental illness: clinical observations and experiences. *J. Ment. Health*, **5**, 145–159.
97. Fadden G. (1997) Implementation of family interventions in routine clinical practice following staff training programmes: a major cause for concern. *J. Ment. Health*, **6**, 599–612.
98. Barrowclough C., Tarrier N., Lewis S., Sellwood W., Mainwaring J., Quinn J., Hamlin C. (1999) Randomised controlled effectiveness trial of a needs-based psychosocial intervention service for carers of people with schizophrenia. *Br. J. Psychiatry*, **174**, 505–511.
99. Sellwood W., Barrowclough C., Tarrier N., Quinn J., Mainwaring J., Lewis S. (2001) Needs based cognitive behavioural family intervention for carers of patients suffering from schizophrenia: 12 month follow up. *Acta Psychiatr. Scand.*, **104**, 346–355.
100. Corrigan V.A., McCracken S.G. (1995) Psychiatric rehabilitation and staff development: educational and organisational models. *Clin. Psychol. Rev.*, **15**, 1172–1177.
101. Corrigan V.A., McCracken S.G. (1995) Refocussing the training of psychiatric rehabilitation staff. *Psychiatr. Serv.*, **46**, 1172–1177.
102. Corrigan V.A., McCracken S.G., Edwards M., Brunner J., Garman A., Nelson D., Leary M. (1997) Collegial support and barriers to behavioural programs for severely mentally ill. *J. Behav. Ther. Exp. Psychiatry*, **28**, 193–202.
103. McCreadie R.G., Phillips K., Harvey J.A., Waldron G., Stewart M., Baird D. (1991) The Nithscale schizophrenia surveys. VIII. Do relatives want family intervention—and does it help? *Br. J. Psychiatry*, **158**, 110–113.
104. Tarrier N. (1991) Some aspects of family interventions in schizophrenia. I. Adherence with family intervention programmes. *Br. J. Psychiatry*, **159**, 475–480.
105. Kuipers E., Raune D. (2000) The early development of expressed emotion and burden in the families of first-onset psychosis. In: Birchwood M., Fowler D., Jackson C. (eds) *Early Intervention in Psychosis: A Guide to Concepts, Evidence and Interventions*. John Wiley & Sons, Chichester, pp. 128–140.
106. Addington J., Addington D., Jones B., Ko T. (2001) Family intervention in an early psychosis program. *Psychiatr. Rehabil. Skills*, **5**, 272–286.
107. Barrowclough C., Haddock G., Tarrier N., Lewis S., Moring J., O'Brien R., Schofield N., McGovern J. (2001) Randomised controlled trial of cognitive behavioral therapy plus motivational intervention for schizophrenia and substance use. *Am. J. Psychiatry*, **158**, 1706–1713.

108. Haddock G., Barrowclough C., Tarrier N., Moring J., O'Brien R., Schofield N., Quinn J., Palmer S., Davies L., Lowens I., *et al.* (2003) Cognitive–behavioural therapy and motivational intervention for schizophrenia and substance misuse. 18 month outcomes of a randomised controlled trial. *Br. J. Psychiatry*, **183**, 418–427.

2

Familes of People with Dementia

Henry Brodaty

School of Psychiatry, University of New South Wales; and
Prince of Wales Hospital, Sydney, Australia

INTRODUCTION

Populations are ageing—there are proportionately more old people, and average life span is increasing. Improved standards of living through sanitation, nutrition and basic health care as well as advances in medicine, such as in cardiovascular disease, have resulted in the population living to an older age. Concurrently, falling fertility rates over the past century have resulted in a higher proportion of older people in the community.

The consequences of these demographic changes are that there are more older people experiencing diseases of late life and disproportionately fewer younger people to care for them. In Australia, the dementias, of which Alzheimer's disease (AD) is the most common type, are set to become the leading cause of disease burden among women within the next dozen years and the fifth leading cause in men. Unless a cure or prevention is found, there will be a massive increase in the numbers and percentage of the population with dementia over the next 50 years [1].

When a person is diagnosed with dementia, it is rarely just one person's illness. The effects are felt throughout families, friends and the community. This chapter focuses on the impact of dementia on informal caregivers, usually family, sometimes friends.

DEMENTIA

Definition

Dementia is defined as loss of memory and at least one other cognitive function leading to impairment in occupational and/or social functioning

Families and Mental Disorders. Edited by Norman Sartorius, Julian Leff, Juan José López-Ibor, Mario Maj and Ahmed Okasha. © 2005 John Wiley & Sons Ltd. ISBN 0-470-02382-1

which represents a decline from previous levels of function [2]. More succinctly, it can be defined as a global impairment of memory, intellect, behaviour and personality [3].

There are well over 100 causes of dementia, but the breakdown of causes is uncertain. Rates vary according to region, diagnostic method, population studied and definitions used. Also definitive diagnosis, which depends on post-mortem examination, is limited by small sample sizes in autopsy surveys. AD accounts for 55–70% of cases of dementia in developed countries. About half of those with AD pathology have concomitant cerebrovascular disease or have cortical Lewy bodies. Pure vascular dementia (VaD) may account for 10%, mixed AD and VaD for 15%, Lewy body dementia for about 15%, fronto-temporal dementias for about 5%, and other causes are less common [4]. In some Asian countries, such as Japan, the proportion with VaD is higher.

This chapter will focus on AD as the prototype for dementia. As the experiences of caring for a person with AD and caring for other forms of dementia are broadly similar, AD provides a convenient prototype for considering the effects of dementia on families. Differences specific to different dementias will be highlighted in the chapter. Studies specific to AD are indicated as such; otherwise research includes a heterogeneous mix of different types of dementia.

Prevalence

Dementia affects 6% of those 65 or older and 20% of those aged 80 years. There were estimated to be 25 million people with dementia worldwide in 2000. This number is projected to increase to 63 million in 2030 and to 114 million in 2050, with 41 million in less developed regions [5]. AD accounts for approximately 50% of those with a dementing illness, though mixed forms of dementia, e.g. AD plus VaD, may increase this to 70%. Symptoms of AD are frequently confused with other forms of dementia, age-related changes, depressive illnesses, stroke and Parkinson's disease, leading to delayed diagnosis or misdiagnosis [1]. As a consequence, the incidence and prevalence of AD may be even higher.

Clinical Course of AD

AD has an insidious onset and gradual progression, typically over 8–12 years from onset of symptoms to death. The inevitable progression of the disease tends to be gradual, but variable between and within individual patients [6]. As people are living longer and healthier, as pharmacological treatments have become available, and as public awareness has increased, people are presenting earlier with symptoms of memory loss, and dementia is being diagnosed earlier [7]. An understanding of the predicted course of AD and realistic expectations of effects of treatment [8] can assist families to plan more effectively for the increasing demands which lie ahead. It is convenient to consider the clinical progression of AD as occurring over three stages.

Early Stage

In the early stages of AD, persons with the disease experience difficulties with short-term memory, learning and language (such as word finding). Personality changes, which can be subtle, such as increasing rigidity or coarsening, are often recognized in retrospect as early signs. Working memory, remote memory and implicit memory functions are initially affected, although to a lesser extent than new learning and recent declarative memory. Complex concepts may be difficult to understand. Patients with AD can usually express themselves quite well in the early stages of the disease; however, closer examination may disclose object naming and semantic difficulties as well as reduced vocabulary, fluency and expressive language. Spatial disorientation can lead to driving difficulties and constructional apraxia may be evident on drawing tasks. Depressive symptoms may present in the earlier stages of dementia as the patient typically has some awareness of the functional losses associated with these changes. The progression of AD is associated with the loss of the abilities to understand concepts, make informed judgements, calculate, read, write and, eventually, sign one's name. Remote memory is comparatively preserved, but will be affected in time. Judgement and abstraction often show signs of impairment early in AD whereas interpersonal skills and social behaviours can remain relatively intact well into the disease process.

Middle Stages

As the dementia progresses, there is a gradual decline in memory and other cognitive functions. The gradual loss of competency in instrumental activities of daily living, such as the abilities to operate machinery or a telephone, to manage finances or to be compliant with medication, requires the family caregiver to take on a greater role in daily supervision. Patients appear to live in the past, as the impairment of recent memory becomes increasingly significant. Deterioration in the areas of communication, logical reasoning, planning and organizational abilities is substantial. Insight into the condition and the ability to recognize familiar faces are lost during this stage in the disease process [9]. Behavioural changes (aggression, catastrophic reaction, wandering) and psychiatric complications (delusions, hallucinations and misidentification syndromes) typically come at this stage.

Late Stages

The person with AD requires assistance with basic activities of daily living such as bathing, dressing, toileting and eating, as almost all cognitive functions are seriously impaired. Paradoxically, family caregivers often find this stage somewhat easier as the demands become increasingly physical in nature and the emotional strain lessens. Patients may misunderstand aspects of their environment or nursing interventions and this can lead to increased aggression and agitation. Ultimately motor disturbances, double incontinence, immobility and physical wasting occur. The primary causes of death in AD are pneumonia, myocardial infarction and septicaemia [9].

FAMILY AS CAREGIVERS

There is a maxim that when a person is diagnosed with dementia, there is (almost) always a second patient. This is the family caregiver.

Who Are the Family Caregivers?

The terms *caregiver*, *carer* and *caretaker* are variously used to describe the person providing the day-to-day instrumental and emotional care of the person with dementia. *Caregiver* is the term most commonly used in the USA; in the UK and Australia *carer* is more the norm. Some authors, in order to distinguish professional or formal caregivers from family caregivers, call the former group *carers*. We will use the term caregivers to refer to family caregivers, who are the focus of this chapter. The care recipients, or *patients* for the purposes of this chapter, are dependent, disabled and mentally impaired persons with dementia, most commonly AD. Much of the literature on caregivers does not distinguish between caring for a person with dementia in general and AD in particular.

Many family caregivers of people with dementia are spouses, with reports ranging from 30% to 60% [10,11], with about 75% of these being wives [10,12]. Other family caregivers include adult children and their partners, who make up about a third of caregivers, although this proportion is higher in countries such as China, Hong Kong and India [13–15].

Daughters are far more likely to be primary caregivers than sons [16], outnumbering them in a ratio of about 4:1 [17]. Similarly, caregiving often falls to daughters-in-law, particularly in countries such as Korea, Hong Kong, Japan and India [13,15,18,19].

Patterns of Care

In one survey, primary caregivers caring for persons with dementia at home had been doing so for an average of 3.7 years, and those caring for institutionalized patients had been doing so for an average of 6.3 years [20]. The length of time that a person with AD is cared for at home will potentially increase with improved education for family caregivers, pharmacotherapy and community services, and with more stringent criteria for nursing home admission. Families provide almost 10 hours per day of care or 286 hours per month for those persons with dementia still living at home, but slightly more than 1 hour per day or 36 hours per month after the person has entered nursing home care [20].

Approximately 4% of persons with dementia live alone [11]. Persons living alone are less likely to have a caregiver, and are more inclined to earlier institutionalization [21,22]. The caregiving role varies considerably if the family caregiver is providing care remotely rather than living with the person with dementia. Caregivers who are spouses almost always live with the patient, whereas adult children tend to live separately.

The concepts of *care providers* and *care managers* [23] are useful when considering the role of families in the care of the patient with AD. The former provide daily supervision, including hands-on care such as personal hygiene, financial management and housework tasks, as well as super-vision of medication and diet. In contrast, care managers arrange for others to provide care. This can include domiciliary nursing care to assist with medications and personal hygiene, community services to provide companionship and outings, daily meal delivery, transport to appoint-ments, and an accountant to provide financial management. Spouses tend to be care providers, whereas adult children, friends and other relatives tend to be care managers. As a rule, care managers are more likely to set realistic limits, delegate tasks and take an objective approach to the role [24]. Consequently, care managers tend to be less personally involved and experience less psychological distress. Care providers, despite experiencing greater distress, will generally continue caring for much longer.

Cultural and Ethnic Variations in Caregiving

Cultural differences are evident as to which of the family members assume the caring role. In the USA adult children are less likely to be close at hand to provide care when a parent develops AD, due to the mobile nature of that society. Moving the person with dementia away from his or her long-term home to live with the adult child, however, often has a detrimental effect on orientation and overall functioning. In the USA there is evidence that Caucasian, African American and Hispanic caregivers differ in the manner in which they cope with the caring role [25–31]. In Japan, the wife of the eldest son is traditionally responsible for the care of ageing parents.

In developing countries and in many rural settings, an extended family network typically provides care. Older parents may be left stranded when harsher economic conditions in rural economies lead to adult children migrating internally to larger cities or when professional adult children go abroad to further their economic and career prospects. Additionally, older people may incur financial hardship when confronting the need to care for a spouse with AD. Although they may have adequate capital assets in the family home, they may have limited income.

Cultural or ethnic affiliations also influence the manner in which family caregivers approach and view the caring role and the ensuing responsibilities. As an example, the extended family typically takes on the care of persons with dementia in African American communities [25,26,30] and American Hispanic communities [27,31], especially in lower socio-economic groups. In some cultural groups, such as African American and Asian American communities, placing an elderly relative in residential care is considered abandonment and therefore unthinkable, in spite of the extreme burden on the family caregiver [25,28,29]. Although minority group caregivers were found not to have greater support than whites in the USA [32], the caregiver's role was perceived more positively, caregiving tasks were regarded as less subjectively stressful and their effectiveness as caregivers was rated more highly by African American caregivers when compared to Caucasian caregivers [33,34]. Lower levels of depression and subjective burden, as well as greater acceptance of the restrictions on recreational activities, were reported by African American caregivers than Caucasian caregivers [35–37]. Additionally, African American caregivers tend to use religion and prayer as coping strategies, and view God as an essential part of their support system [25,38].

In developing countries, levels of caregiver strain appear at least as high as in the developed world, despite the extended family care structure [39]. There is less co-resident caregiver burden where there are more family members residing in the same household [39].

The beliefs and values of different minority groups can furthermore affect the way family members appraise and understand dementia, and therefore manage it. Some cultures hold the belief that behaviours associated with dementia are consistent with ageing, rather than a disease process, and therefore may evoke little concern until symptoms are quite advanced [31]. In other cultures, symptoms such as confusion, disorientation and memory loss may be viewed as signs of "craziness" [28]. A cross-national European study found that 2.0% of caregiver burden was explained by perceived negative social reactions [40]. Even recently, Mittelman *et al.* [41] reported that 5% of caregivers considered aberrant behaviours could be avoided if the patient "put his mind to it"; 4% believed the patient was doing it deliberately to get his own way; 7% believed the patient was always like that; and 12% believed it was a normal part of ageing. Only 71% saw it as part of the dementia.

As well as ethnic and racial minorities, other groups deserving of special considerations include rural families providing care in service-poor regions, long-distance caregivers, and gay and lesbian caregivers who are navigating discriminatory care arenas [42].

Power of Attorney, Guardianship and Living Wills

Caregivers play a critical role in the financial and legal affairs of the person with dementia. The person with AD will typically lose competency during the middle stages of the disease process. Financial management, enduring or durable power of attorney, enduring (or durable) guardianship, advance directives (also called living wills) and wills should be considered while the patient retains competency. If these matters are ignored in the early stage of the disease, more complex legal arrangements become necessary once the dementia is at an advanced stage. The possibility that the primary caregiver may suddenly take ill or even pre-decease the patient with AD should be canvassed. For example, many couples have mirror wills and, should the caregiver die suddenly, the patient may be unable to act in the capacity of executor. Obtaining enduring power of attorney earlier can avoid subsequent lengthy court proceedings required to obtain legal guardianship. In many jurisdictions it is possible to arrange enduring guardianship and to provide for advance directives which only come into effect when the person with AD loses capacity. Preparations enacted prior to this stage in the disease process can prevent future problems. These important topics should be discussed with the patient and family, both separately and together, to facilitate harmonious decisions.

Informed consent requires a person to understand the treatment offered in respect to its likely benefits and adverse effects, to be told about alternative treatments and to be able to convey a decision to the treating doctor. The level of understanding required varies with the complexity and potential danger of the treatment, e.g. antibiotics for an infection versus cardiac transplantation. As dementia progresses, treatment interventions and the use of medication will require proxy informed consent from the *person responsible*, usually the family caregiver. Legal requirements for consent to medical treatment vary according to jurisdiction. Often there is a hierarchy, with the person closest in the caregiving role deemed to be the person who can give informed consent. In many jurisdictions, if the person with dementia refuses a treatment, only a judicial body such as a Guardianship Tribunal can provide consent.

Rules for testamentary capacity are fairly similar in most Anglophonic countries, namely that the person must know the extent of his or her estate, know who are the potential beneficiaries, be able to judge and weigh up the relative benefits to be conferred, be free of undue influence and not have his or her judgement poisoned by delusions or hallucinations. Reliable and independent assurance is required where a person's capacity is questionable. A legal duty of care may exist to protect the patient with dementia from the influence of those who could exploit them [43]. No such duty, however, affords the potential family beneficiaries protection from unreasonable decisions that the patient may make when affected by strong beliefs and emotions. Although capacity should be questioned when the person's attitude appears to be based on impaired thinking, professional judgement dictates the extent to which lawyers, doctors and/or accountants might examine the convictions that are prompting a decision. It is possible for professionals inexperienced in dealing with those with dementia to be inadvertently misled by their credible presentation and seemingly reasonable justification for any lapses. The patient's genuine lack of insight makes the situation all the more plausible.

EFFECTS OF CAREGIVING

Positive Aspects of Caregiving

Family caregiving has been associated with altruistic and spiritual benefits, as well as positive emotions such as feelings of satisfaction, a sense of meaning, and the pleasure of having been of service to the person with dementia [44–48].

Psychological Stress

There has been a great deal of research into the well-being of caregivers for the patient with AD. As with caregivers of other groups of those with a mental illness, caregivers of people with dementia have increased psychological morbidity [10,49–53] and levels and rates of depression [33,52,54–57].

Rates of major depression and minor depression meeting Research Diagnostic Criteria among caregivers seeking help have been reported at 26% and 18%, respectively, with lower rates among non-help-seekers (10% and 8%, respectively) [58]. Other studies have reported casenesses for depression in dementia caregivers at 29.4% using the Geriatric Mental State (GMS) AGECAT [59], and 41.7% using the Geriatric Depression Scale [56].

Physical Health

Caregivers of people with dementia have poorer physical health [54,60–62] and decreased immunological competence [63,64] than non-caregiver controls. A meta-analysis of 23 studies found a slightly greater risk of health problems in dementia caregivers [61]. Pre-existing conditions, such as hypertension, are more likely to be exacerbated by the caregiving role, and these psychological and physical morbidities ultimately result in increased use of health services [65]. Caregiving has also been associated with a higher mortality rate [66].

Social Effects

Dementia caring is doubly isolating, as friends and some family members withdraw when they feel unsure as to how they should approach the forbidden subject of AD, become uncomfortable with the patient's failing communication and feel embarrassed by the person's behaviours. As the disease inevitably progresses, a greater focus on the caregiving role is required and subsequently restrictions for the caregiver increase in the areas of employment, leisure, friendships and socialization [67].

Financial Costs

Because the majority of patients with AD are cared for in the community by family members, the greatest cost is that associated with informal care provision. Significant financial costs to families arise, both directly and indirectly, in caring for the person with AD. Direct costs are incurred through the need for medical consultations, investigations and pharmaceuticals, as well as personal, nursing and/or residential care. Indirect costs arise out of the loss of the patient's and/or family caregiver's earning potential [1]. The total indirect and direct costs of caring for a person with dementia at home and in residential care have been estimated as similar [68], although direct residential care costs are significantly higher. The majority of the expenses for patients living at home, however, are borne by their families [68], whereas in many countries the cost of residential care is paid in part by the government. An Australian report estimated the cost of informal care at 32% of the total care cost [69].

According to a study of US families caring for a person with dementia, the equivalent of $18 200 was spent annually [70]. Of the families surveyed, 80% reported average out-of-pocket expenditure at $2088 (14% of total) with the greater share (US $11 560 or 59%) attributed to the primary caregiver's time spent in providing care. The US National Longitudinal Caregiver Study examined informal caregiving costs for elderly community-dwelling veterans with dementia. An annual cost was estimated in relation to the value of caregiving time, caregivers' lost income, caregivers' out-of-pocket expenses and caregivers' excess health costs, indicating a total of US$18 385 in 1998 dollars. According to Moore et al. [71], the greater part of this cost was due to caregiving time, excluding typical household tasks ($6295), and caregivers' lost earnings ($10 709).

Predictors of Stress in Caregivers

Predictors of stress can be divided into dementia, caregiver, relationship and environmental variables, which all interact. Thus, the cognitive and functional decline and behavioural disturbances that accompany dementia impose an objective burden on the caregiver. Some caregivers may handle this burden relatively easily; others experience subjective burden or strain which may manifest itself psychologically, physically, socially or financially, as has been described earlier. Exacerbating and protective factors mediate the level of strain experienced by the caregiver. For example, a person with dementia becomes incontinent of urine, i.e. an objective burden. One caregiver regards this as a catastrophe, becomes exasperated and despondent, i.e. experiences great subjective burden and psychological strain, and arranges institutional care. Another caregiver, knowing that this was a likely development, has sought advice, devised strategies to minimize the incontinence such as regular toileting and use of pads, and is little bothered by it.

Dementia Variables

The most consistent finding in relation to caregiver stress is the strong association between disruptive behaviours and caregiver distress. Despite differences in outcome measures, methods of assessing behavioural disturbances, populations and participating countries, robust findings consistently indicate that behavioural disturbances account for approximately 25% of the variance in caregiver psychological distress [12,72–74]. Behaviours associated with caregiver distress include incontinence, immobility, nocturnal wandering, proneness to fall, inability to engage in meaningful activities, communication difficulties, sleep disturbance, loss of companionship, disruptiveness, constant demands and aggression [10,49,52,75].

Functional decline is significantly correlated with restricted caregiver activity and increased caregiver burden [76] but not with depressive symptoms [62,76]. Haley *et al.* [62] found that the patient's ability to perform instrumental activities of daily living was highly correlated with the caregiver's depression score, but not with life satisfaction or self-rated health problems. Interpreting the association between patient functional status and caregiver health is confounded in that patients who have declined functionally are more likely to exhibit behavioural disturbances. Caregiver stress or burden appears unrelated to duration of dementia or to level of cognitive decline once allowance is made for behavioural disturbances. Reported analyses have not always made allowance for the strong effect of behavioural disturbances on caregiver health [10,12,49,52,72–75].

Little evidence exists that any one type of dementia is associated with more psychological stress in family caregivers than another. Similar levels have been reported in caregivers of patients with AD and VaD [77,78] and AD and Lewy body dementia [79]. However, given the higher rate of behavioural disturbances in fronto-temporal dementias and Lewy body dementia, caregivers of patients with these conditions may well have higher levels of stress. Where VaD has had a sudden onset, e.g. after a stroke, the lack of warning and abrupt change in circumstances may have an even more devastating effect on caregivers [80].

Caregiver Variables

Spouses, females and care providers experience greater levels of subjective burden than their counterparts [54,81,82]. The spouses of younger patients may have even higher levels of stress [83].

How the caregiver appraises the situation and deals with it will influence the outcome for the caregiver (see 84 for a review). Effective coping techniques can help to moderate caregiver distress [85] and possibly enhance the quality of life for the person with AD. Problem-focused strategies such as reframing, problem solving and expanding the social network have been associated with improved life satisfaction, decreased caregiver burden and lower depression levels [85]. By contrast, emotion-based responses such as wishfulness, acceptance and fantasy are associated with greater caregiver distress [86]. Immature coping strategies and neurotic personality style tend to be associated with increased caregiver burden, decreased life satisfaction and higher levels of depression [87]. It is proposed that depression in caregivers possibly leads to the adoption of less effective coping styles, which may then further perpetuate the depressive illness.

Relationship Variables

Unsatisfactory premorbid relationships are more often associated with distress in caregivers of those with AD [10]. This may accompany the breakdown in communication between family members, the increase in tension, the loss of companionship, the loss of a confidant(e), the increase in economic and household responsibilities, and the loss of sexual intimacy [81,88,89]. Marital satisfaction reportedly deteriorates significantly with the increasing demands of the caregiving role [10]. An association has been found between expressed emotion and distress in the daughters of people with dementia [90].

Continuing cognitive and physical dependence necessitates the restructuring of family relationships, often with the loss of reciprocity on the patient's part. For the primary caregiver, providing care and supervision ultimately prevails over most aspects of the relationship. Such changes in the premorbid relationship between family caregivers and the person with AD can further exacerbate a stressful situation. The shift in the relationship between caregiver and patient can lead to role conflict. For example, cast in the role of surrogate mother, the wife feels trapped and resentful, but suppresses her negative thoughts, guiltily chastising herself. Sexual intimacy may be lost as the person with dementia loses interest or initiative, while the caregiver feels too stressed or no longer views the patient as a sexual partner. Sometimes the reverse holds and the patient becomes disinhibited and makes excessive demands on his wife. Caregivers who are children of the person with dementia can struggle emotionally with the ultimate role reversal imposed by the advancing disease process. Secondary role strain may occur, where the caregiver, usually a daughter, "the woman in the middle", finds herself caught between the demands of caring for a dementing parent and satisfying the needs of her husband, children and work.

Environmental Variables

The proximity, or the amount of contact that caregivers have, with the patient influences the effects on them. Propinquity increases the level of caregiver burden—those caregivers who live with the person with dementia have higher levels than those who live apart or where the care recipient is in residential care. These caregivers in turn have higher levels of psychological morbidity than caregivers whose care recipients have died [10,91].

Support plays a complex role. Informal supports, i.e. from family and friends, are more likely to be helpful than support from professionals. Measurement of support is not straightforward—merely counting the number of contacts is too crude. For example, other family may be visiting but, far from being supportive, offer criticism, uninformed advice and even negative comments, all of which can be extremely hurtful to a family caregiver struggling to cope. Correlations between levels of support and psychological morbidity can be negative if the support is effective, positive if stressed caregivers are calling for help or neutral if both effects are in operation.

Families with Special Problems

Additional isolation, beyond that usually experienced by others in this role, tends to impact on specific caregiver groups [8]. Migrants with AD may be doubly isolated by culture and language and are less likely to access services, particularly in relation to mental health [92]. A person with AD tends to lose acquired languages first. Reliance on a first language poses significant difficulties when and if integration into mainstream care becomes necessary. Also, migrant groups may seek medical attention only once complications develop or when the disease is more advanced. For example, patients from non-English-speaking backgrounds attending a memory clinic in Australia were more severely demented and had increased rates of psychiatric disorders than comparison patients [93].

Indigenous people also tend to have poorer health, inferior health services and more difficulty accessing services. Within their cultural context, dementia may not be recognized as an illness [94].

Younger people with dementia encounter special problems, as they are more likely to be still working, to have school-age children at home, to have heavier financial commitments, to have greater concern about heritability, to have more difficulty obtaining a diagnosis and to have greater difficulty integrating with mainstream services [83,95].

Patients with AD who are professionals or prominent citizens often find it difficult to accept community and residential services. Persuading such patients that they are no longer able to continue working can be a particular problem. Where couples dement, problems are more than doubled, because of the lack of an informant to obtain a history, a caregiver to assist in management or anyone to compensate for the patient's cognitive losses.

Feelings of obligation and reciprocity in a relationship are not as well developed in second marriages. Resentment and disagreement can arise when children from a previous marriage hold different views on care management, particularly with regard to financial decisions. Some service providers may be challenged by the need to provide services to same-sex partners where one is dementing [42].

The behavioural manifestations and resultant caregiver stress associated with advancing dementia can potentially lead to elder abuse in families. The risk of a physically abusive episode occurring in relation to individuals with AD may be as high as 225% greater than in other people living in the community [96]. Abuse can encompass infliction of mental anguish, use of physical force, financial exploitation and/or deprivation of basic necessities. Contributing factors are caregiver stress, caregiver depression, poor premorbid relationship between caregiver and patient, vulnerability and disempowerment of both patients and caregivers, as well as lack of dementia education, professional supports and respite [97,98]. Recognition of stressors related to dementia caregiving, recognition of the caregiving role in the delivery of services, greater flexibility in service provision, improved access to information about services and powers of attorney, government lobbying, dementia education, and increased public awareness are important in the prevention of abuse [98]. Sometimes the abuse occurs in the reverse direction, with the patient abusing the family caregiver, usually in conjunction with psychiatric complications or interpersonal conflicts.

HELPING FAMILIES CARE THROUGH THE STAGES OF DEMENTIA

Strategies by Stages

The management provided for caregivers of the person with AD should be structured according to the current stage of the disease and tailored to their individual circumstances and needs. When assessment is sought initially and a diagnosis provided, the family require time, information and support to adjust to the news. The manner in which the family and the patient are informed and the information provided, at the initial and progressive stages of the disease process, can impact significantly on their capacity to adjust to the diagnosis [7]. Planning is necessary at this stage in light of the potential practical, financial and legal consequences to follow.

In the middle stages spousal caregivers, in particular, describe the loss of a companion and the absence of a partner with whom to share communication and decision making. Decreasing cognitive abilities with the subsequent increasing dependency and need for supervision place significant demands on family caregivers at this point. Aberrant behaviours start to appear more commonly and with greater severity, further distressing the caregiver.

As the person with AD becomes progressively unable to articulate his or her needs or indicate a source of discomfort, the caregiver assumes greater responsibility for the patient's general health and well-being. In the later stages, the maintenance of nutritional status, medication compliance, hydration, exercise, regular elimination, personal hygiene, mobility status and medical review become increasingly dependent on the caregiver. The high level of nursing care required in the terminal stage of the disease is often beyond the capacity of family caregivers and nursing home admission is typically necessary, although the financial costs of residential care can be a strong disincentive to seek placement.

Behavioural and Psychological Symptoms and the Effect on Families

Patients with AD may present with many different types of behavioural and psychological signs and symptoms. Effective management of AD requires an understanding of the non-cognitive manifestations of the illness as these will generally cause greater caregiver distress than the loss of memory and other cognitive functions [67]. Behavioural and psychological symptoms of dementia (BPSD) can also contribute to a poorer prognosis through earlier institutionalization and reduced functioning than that which is due to the disease alone. BPSD can include depression, delusions, hallucinations, misidentification syndrome, aggression, wandering, screaming, sleep disturbance, agitation, apathy, disinhibition and eating disturbances. The association between BPSD and elder abuse is an obvious concern.

Approximately one third of patients with AD will experience delusions at some point during the disease process, with the most common being related to theft or infidelity on the caregiver's part [99]. Hallucinations are typically auditory or visual in nature and are likely to occur in one quarter of those diagnosed with AD. Misidentification of environmental information tends to present in approximately one third of patients. Characteristic presentations of misidentification syndrome include believing that a familiar person is an imposter, believing that the face in the mirror is a stranger, misidentifying television events as real, and believing that a boarder is staying in the home [100].

Aggressive behaviours are considered to be the most severe non-cognitive symptoms of AD and other dementias, as they cause significant distress for the caregiver, family members and the patient [101]. Management of the aggression through behavioural and socio-economic strategies should be considered initially. Identification of environmental triggers can potentially avoid precipitants for the behaviour. Where indicated, pharmacological intervention in combination with behavioural/environmental methods can reduce aggressive behaviours.

Residential Care and the Family

Patients with dementia who have a co-resident caregiver reportedly have a 20-fold protective effect against permanent admission to residential care [102]. Caregiver psychological distress, financial difficulties and family problems have been consistently associated with institutionalization [24,103–105]. While older family caregivers have a greater tendency to institutionalize the person with dementia [105], spouses who are caregivers are less likely to institutionalize partners with dementia than children. Research indicates that behavioural disturbances, as well as the severity and rate of progression of the illness, are significantly associated with the probability of residential care admission [104,106,107].

Family caregivers can continue to play an important role in the care of the person with AD after admission to residential care, particularly during the initial period of transition. Family members are often well placed to inform staff of the patient's specific care needs, previous routine, social history, support network and any potentially disruptive behaviours, as well as proven strategies to assist in the management of the disease manifestations. Encouraging caregivers to do so may assist them in dealing with their own response to the admission of their relative into residential care, as making this decision frequently induces severe guilt. Institutionalization of a person with dementia may lead to feelings of failure on the caregiver's part and a high prevalence of depression [108]. Open discussion and consultation with family members to facilitate a joint decision can help to moderate strong emotions in the primary caregiver. Equally, the decision to institutionalize the person with AD can produce conflict between family members.

Family caregivers may also need encouragement to gradually re-engage in activities that they have previously forgone due to the increasing demands of the primary caring role. The health of former caregivers showed significant improvement following the cessation of caring for a person with dementia at home [109,110]. Former caregivers also attended medical appointments more often after they ceased caring, possibly because they had more time to attend to their own needs [110].

Death of the Patient and the Effects on Family

Families are often required to make ethical decisions with regard to terminal care in the patient's final stages of AD. Families may need to consult about end-of-life decisions such as whether to initiate enteric feeding devices or active antibiotic treatment for inevitable infections. Some caregivers report considerable relief at the death of the person with dementia, as they felt that death finally provided a release from suffering for the patient [108]. This is not the case, however, for others, particularly if the caring role has dominated their life for some years.

Bereavement support is very important for those caring for individuals with dementia and not often available in long-term care facilities [111]. Family members may need to make decisions regarding post-mortem examination prior to the patient's death and these should be considered in advance to facilitate expeditious arrangements and minimise exacerbation of the family's grief.

Hospital Admission/Acute Care and the Family

People with dementia admitted to hospital often have a marked increase in their confusion because of the change of their routine and their environment, excessive stimulation, and the appearance of many busy strangers. Furthermore, delirium is very common, usually resulting from the illness which has precipitated admission. The family caregiver has a critical role in mediating between the hospital system and the patient. A collaborative approach to treatment and discharge planning can lead to a more satisfactory outcome and the reduced likelihood of readmission.

Caregivers and Research

Caregivers often initiate participation in drug trials and usually patients turn to their caregivers for advice. Occasionally family enthusiasm to participate in research is met by patients' reluctance, which can generate conflict between them and their caregivers. Caregivers play an important and necessary role in the informed consent procedures, providing substitute (or proxy) consent, and in monitoring drug efficacy and adverse effects. Finally, there is growing recognition of the importance of measuring the effects of anti-dementia drugs on the caregivers themselves as secondary beneficiaries of intervention [112].

CAREGIVERS AND INTERVENTIONS FOR AD

Psychosocial Interventions

While it is generally recognized that for pharmacological treatment there are indications and contraindications, side effects, latency periods for onset of action, limited duration of need and the necessity for review, these same important considerations are not always applied to psychosocial interventions [67]. Psychosocial interventions are cost effective in that they have the capacity to reduce caregiver distress and delay nursing home admission [112]. Such interventions can include education, legal and financial information, counselling, family support, medical and allied health care as well as respite care. The same attention and individualized assessment are indicated in the prescription of psychosocial interventions as in the prescription of drug therapies.

Information provision, education and support groups alone have limited efficacy in reducing dementia caregiver stress [113], but other caregiver interventions such as counselling, skills training and cognitive–behavioural therapy have been shown to reduce caregiver stress or burden [41,56,114–119], improve physical activity levels [120] and increase immune response [63]. A sustained reduction in depression for more than three years has also been observed in caregivers receiving an enhanced counselling and support intervention [121].

A meta-analysis of 30 studies of psychosocial interventions with dementia caregivers found that there were significant benefits in caregiver psychological distress, caregiver knowledge, any main caregiver outcome measure and patient mood, but not caregiver burden [101]. Four of these studies demonstrated that interventions delayed nursing home admission. Common elements of successful programmes were involvement of the patient as well as the dementia caregiver; involvement of the whole family, not just the primary caregiver; intervention of sufficient duration and intensity and, anecdotally, having consistency and flexibility when helping the caregiver [101]. Other reviews have confirmed the efficacy of caregiver interventions, though it may be that caregivers of the elderly with stroke, mental illness or physical disability demonstrate a greater benefit from interventions than dementia caregivers [122].

Caregivers' reactions to problem behaviours associated with advancing dementia have also been shown to influence their distress significantly. Compared to caregivers in a control condition, caregivers receiving a multi-component counselling and support intervention reacted less negatively to problem behaviours over time despite the actual frequency of behaviours increasing. Interventions designed to increase caregivers' coping strategies may effectively change their appraisal of the stressors associated with caring for a person with dementia [41].

Such interventions also offer beneficial effects for the person with dementia. For example, behavioural management training provided to caregivers of people with AD and comorbid depression, in a randomized controlled trial, led to a reduction in depression in both the caregiver and the person with dementia [123]. Additionally, Teri et al. [124] found that home-based exercise training for patients, in combination with training in behavioural management techniques for the caregiver, resulted in improved physical health and depression in patients with AD over a 2-year period.

Support Services

National AD associations or societies advocate on behalf of those with dementia and their caregivers throughout most developed countries and in many developing countries of the world (link through Alzheimer's Disease International, www.alz.co.uk). Alzheimer's associations are consumer organizations that offer information, training and support for caregivers of people with AD and other dementias. The role of the associations may also include lobbying for government funding, local awareness campaigns and securing funding for research. The substantial growth of these organizations has helped to highlight the impact of the disease on families, along with the ensuing economic and social implications [112]. Local Alzheimer's associations can also provide library services, Internet access, confidential counselling and specific training courses.

Alzheimer's associations run local support groups for caregivers of people with AD and other forms of dementia. A professional leader and/or a peer caregiver typically facilitates the support group, while computer and telephone networks can offer support to isolated caregivers in rural and remote areas. As patients are diagnosed earlier, services are becoming available for the person with dementia in tandem with those for the caregiver. The Dementia Advocacy and Support Network (www. dasinternational.org) offers an international computer-based support group for people with early-stage dementia [125].

Although support groups and self-help groups are not appropriate for all caregivers, families should be provided with the information to enable them to try this avenue of support as part of their management plan. Failure to seek support and/or access services is commonly due to a lack of knowledge or non-referral by health professionals, rather than insufficient need [112,118,126]. Support groups are able to offer caregivers a sense of belonging, power and purpose [112].

A review of Dutch dementia support groups concluded that participation offered caregivers significant positive effects in their coping and emotional strategies. However, some categories of participants, particularly those with higher caregiver burden, were found to benefit more than others [127]. Another study of dementia caregiver support group participants reported that caregiver distress and perceived quality of life improved [128]. The most common reason that caregivers do not attend support groups is that they have not been informed about them. Cuijpers *et al.* [127] reported that there were three main reasons that affected carers' decision to attend support groups: information, need for help with dealing with problems, and need for help dealing with their feelings of severe burden. Molinari *et al.* [126] reported that the reason given by 80% of carers who did not attend support groups was that they had not received advice encouraging them to attend. Enabling variables such as knowledge of services, cost and access were more important in explaining service use than predisposing and need variables such as demographics, patient behaviour and caregiver burden [129].

Support groups have generally been found to be more effective for caregivers who are isolated from family, friends or other carers, are in more stressful situations, experience greater dissatisfaction, are still in paid employment, contribute a small cost ($5–$20) for group participation, and care for an apathetic and/or institutionalized person with dementia [127,130].

Pharmacotherapy

Cholinesterase inhibitor treatments for people with dementia have been shown to decrease time spent caring and reduce caregiver burden and distress [131]. The beneficial effect on caregivers may be through better management of symptoms, less functional dependence and the subsequent reduction in behavioural disturbance [132–135]. There may also be social and financial benefits of delaying institutionalization in persons with AD [133,136,137].

Although the need to supervise the patient's medication compliance imposes an additional responsibility on the dementia caregiver, pharmacotherapy provides families with hope that something is being done against a disease which was thought to be unremitting and untreatable. That said, caregivers need to be provided with appropriate information and encouraged to maintain realistic expectations of the potential benefits of pharmaceutical treatments [8]. The caregiver of a person with AD may be required to make decisions with regard to participation in clinical drug trial research. The caregiver plays a crucial role in the planning, consent, medication supervision, monitoring of adverse effects, appointments and reporting necessary for such participation. Family caregivers may ultimately gain from a reduction in care hours and stress levels if treatment benefits the person with AD. However, if no benefit to the patient is evident, caregivers will possibly experience disappointment and anger [112]. Although the effects on both the patient with AD and the caregiver should be carefully considered with regard to enrolling in clinical trials, there may be positive effects for caregivers due to an increase in available medical services [138]. Likewise, in a study which looked at participation in an AD clinical drug trial, caregivers perceived it to be a positive experience in spite of the effort required and a lack of patient improvement [139].

CONCLUSIONS

The effective management of family caregivers clearly plays a crucial part in the care of a person with AD. Caregivers are essential partners with health professionals for the long haul. While the physical and cognitive decline of AD are inevitable, the management of AD and other forms of dementia provides challenges and rewards for those involved. Much can be done to maintain and/or improve the quality of life for the patient and the caregiver. Good management of the complexities of the disease process requires not only knowledge of the neurobiology and neuropsychology of dementia, but also a sound understanding of the social implications, the psychodynamics of individual and family changes, and the need to liaise with the patient's support network.

ACKNOWLEDGEMENTS

Lee-Fay Low, Kim Burns and Louisa Gibson provided assistance with the manuscript.

REFERENCES

1. Sadik K., Wilcock G. (2003) The increasing burden of Alzheimer disease. *Alz. Dis. Assoc. Disord.*, **17**, S75–S79.
2. American Psychiatric Association (1997) *Diagnostic and Statistical Manual of Mental Disorders*, 4th edn. American Psychiatric Association, Washington, DC.
3. Lishman W.A. (1987) *Organic Psychiatry: The Psychological Consequences of Cerebral Disorder*, 2nd edn. Blackwell, Oxford.
4. Mendez M.F., Cummings J.L. (2003) *Dementia—A Clinical Approach*, 3rd edn. Butterworth Heinemann, Philadelphia, PA.
5. Wimo A., Winblad B., Aguero-Torres H., von Strauss E. (2003) The magnitude of dementia occurrence in the world. *Alz. Dis. Assoc. Disord.*, **17**, 63–67.
6. Corey-Bloom J. (2000) The natural history of Alzheimer's disease. In: O'Brien J., Ames D., Burns A. (eds) *Dementia*. Arnold, London, pp. 405–416.
7. Wald C., Fahy M., Walker Z., Livingston G. (2003) What to tell dementia caregivers—the rule of threes. *Int. J. Geriatr. Psychiatry*, **18**, 313–317.
8. Brodaty H. (1999) Realistic expectations for the management of Alzheimer's disease. *Eur. Neuropsychopharmacol.*, **9**, S43–S52.
9. Forstl H. (2000) What is Alzheimer's disease? In: O'Brien J., Ames D., Burns A. (eds) *Dementia*. Arnold, London, pp. 371–382.

10. Brodaty H., Hadzi-Pavlovic D. (1990) Psychosocial effects on carers of living with persons with dementia. *Aust. N. Zeal. J. Psychiatry*, **24**, 351–361.

11. US Congress Office of Technology Assessment (1987) *Losing a Million Minds: Confronting the Tragedy of Alzheimer's Disease and Other Dementias*. US Government Printing Office, Washington, DC.

12. Coen R.F., Swanwick G.R., O'Boyle C.A., Coakley D. (1997) Behaviour disturbance and other predictors of carer burden in Alzheimer's disease. *Int. J. Geriatr. Psychiatry*, **12**, 331–336.

13. Shaji K.S., Smitha K., Lal K.P., Prince M.J. (2003) Caregivers of people with Alzheimer's disease: a qualitative study from the Indian 10/66 Dementia Research Network. *Int. J. Geriatr. Psychiatry*, **18**, 1–6.

14. Patterson T.L., Semple S.J., Shaw W.S., Yu E., He Y., Zhang M.Y., Wu W., Grant I. (1998) The cultural context of caregiving: a comparison of Alzheimer's caregivers in Shanghai, China and San Diego, California. *Psychol. Med.*, **28**, 1071–1084.

15. Tsien T.B.K., Cheng W. (1999) Caregiving impacts and needs of Chinese demented elderly families in Hong Kong. Presented at the Asia Pacific Regional Conference for the International Year of Older Persons. Hong Kong, 26–29 April.

16. Lee G.R., Dwyer J.W., Coward R.T. (1993) Gender differences in parent care: demographic factors and same-gender preferences. *J. Gerontol.*, **48**, S9–S16.

17. Brody E.M. (1990) *Their Parent-Care Years*. Springer-Verlag, New York.

18. Lee Y.R., Sung K.T. (1998) Cultural influences on caregiving burden: cases of Koreans and Americans. *Int. J. Aging Hum. Dev.*, **46**, 125–141.

19. Yamamoto-Mitani, N., Ishigaki K., Kuniyoshi M., Kawahara-Maekawa N., Hayashi K., Hasegawa K., Sugishita C. (2004) Subjective quality of life and positive appraisal of care among Japanese family caregivers of older adults. *Qual. Life Res.*, **13**, 207–221.

20. Max W., Webber P., Fox P. (1995) Alzheimer's disease. The unpaid burden of caring. *J. Aging Health*, **7**, 179–199.

21. Mace N.L., Rabins P.V. (1982) Areas of stress on families of dementia patients: a two year follow up. Presented at the Meeting of the Gerontological Society of America, Boston, MA, 21 November.

22. Brody E.M. (1981) "Women in the middle" and family help to older people. *Gerontologist*, **21**, 471–480.

23. Archbold P.G. (1981) Impact of parent caring on women. Presented at the 12th International Congress of Gerontology, Hamburg, 12–17 July.

24. Colerick E.J., George L.K. (1986) Predictors of institutionalization among caregivers of patients with Alzheimer's disease. *J. Am. Geriatr. Soc.*, **34**, 493–498.

25. Wood J.B., Parham I.A. (1990) Coping with perceived burden: ethnic and cultural issues in Alzheimer's family caregiving. *J. Appl. Gerontol.*, **9**, 325–339.

26. Cantor M.H. (1983) Strain among caregivers: a study of experience in the United States. *Gerontologist*, **23**, 597–604.

27. Mintzer J.E., Rubert M.P., Loewenstein D., Gamez E., Millor A., Quinteros R., Flores L., Miller M., Rainerman A., Eisdorfer C. (1992) Daughters' caregiving for Hispanic and non-Hispanic Alzheimer patients: does ethnicity make a difference? *Commun. Ment. Health J.*, **28**, 293–303.

28. Yeo G. (1996) Background. In: Yeo G, Gallagher-Thompson D. (eds) *Ethnicity and the Dementias*. Taylor & Francis, Bristol, pp. 3–7.

29. Wallsten S.M. (1997) Elderly caregivers and care receivers. Facts and gaps in the literature. In: Nussbaum P.D. (ed.) *Handbook of Neuropsychology*. Plenum Press, New York, pp. 467–482.
30. Gelfand D. (1982) *Aging: The Ethnic Factor*. Little & Brown, Boston, MA.
31. Valle R. (1988) Outreach to ethnic minorities with Alzheimer's disease: the challenge to the community. *Health Matrix*, **6**, 13–27.
32. Janevic M.R., Connell C.M. (2001) Racial, ethnic, and cultural differences in the dementia caregiving experience: recent findings. *Gerontologist*, **41**, 334–347.
33. Haley W.E., Roth D.L., Coleton M.I., Ford G.R., West C.A., Collins R.P., Isobe T.L. (1996) Appraisal, coping, and social support as mediators of well-being in black and white family caregivers of patients with Alzheimer's disease. *J. Consult. Clin. Psychiatry*, **64**, 121–129.
34. Smith A. (1996) Cross-cultural research on Alzheimer's disease: a critical review. *Transcult. Psychiatry Res. Rev.*, **33**, 247–276.
35. Gibson R.C. (1982) Blacks in middle and late life: resources and coping. *Ann. Am. Acad. Polit. Soc. Sci.*, **464**, 79–90.
36. Lawton, M.P., Rajagopal D., Brody E., Kleban M.H. (1992) The dynamics of caregiving for a demented elder among black and white families. *J. Gerontol.*, **47**, S156–S164.
37. Roth D.L., Haley W.E., Owen J.E., Clay O.J., Goode K.T. (2001) Latent growth models of the longitudinal effects of dementia caregiving: a comparison of African American and White family caregivers. *Psychol. Aging*, **16**, 427–436.
38. Connell C.M., Gibson G.D. (1997) Racial, ethnic, and cultural differences in dementia caregiving: review and analysis. *Gerontologist*, **37**, 355–364.
39. Prince M., Graham N., Brodaty H., Rimmer E., Varghese M., Chiu H., Acosta D., Scazufca M. (2004) Alzheimer Disease International's 10/66 Dementia Research Group—one model for action research in developing countries. *Int. J. Geriatr. Psychiatry*, **19**, 178–181.
40. Schneider J., Murray J., Banerjee S., Mann A. (1999) EUROCARE: a cross-national study of co-resident spouse carers for people with Alzheimer's disease: I. Factors associated with carer burden. *Int. J. Geriatr. Psychiatry*, **14**, 651–661.
41. Mittelman, M.S., Roth D.L., Haley W.E., Zarit S.H. (2004) Effects of a caregiver intervention on negative caregiver appraisals of behavior problems in patients with Alzheimer's disease: results of a randomized trial. *J. Gerontol. B Psychol. Sci. Soc. Sci.*, **59**, P27–P34.
42. Coon D.W., Ory M.G., Schulz R. (2003) Family caregivers: enduring and emergent themes. In: Gallagher-Thompson D., Thompson L.W. (eds) *Innovative Interventions to Reduce Dementia Caregiver Distress: A Clinical Guide*. Springer-Verlag, New York, pp. 3–27.
43. Dickens B. (2000) Moral, ethical and legal aspects of dementia: a) Legal issues. In: O'Brien J., Ames D., Burns A. (eds) *Dementia*. Arnold, London, pp. 274–278.
44. Sheehan N.W., Nuttall P. (1988) Conflict, emotion, and personal strain among family caregivers. *Fam. Relat. J. Appl. Fam. Child Stud.*, **37**, 92–98.
45. Cohen C.A., Colantonio A., Vernich L. (2002) Positive aspects of caregiving: rounding out the caregiver experience. *Int. J. Geriatr. Psychiatry*, **17**, 184–188.
46. Nolan M., Lundh U. (1999) Satisfactions and coping strategies of family caregivers. *Br. J. Com. Nurs.*, **4**, 470–475.
47. Walker A.J., Jones L.L., Martin S.K. (1989) Relationship quality and the benefits and costs of caregiving. Presented at the Meeting of the National Council on Family Relations, New Orleans, 5–8 November.

48. Archbold P.G. (1983) Impact of parent-caring on women. *Fam. Relat. J. Appl. Fam. Child Stud.*, **32**, 39–45.
49. Gilleard C.J., Boyd W.D., Watt G. (1982) Problems in caring for the elderly mentally infirm at home. *Arch. Gerontol. Geriatr.*, **1**, 151–158.
50. Poulshock S.W., Deimling G.T. (1984) Families caring for elders in residence: issues in the measurement of burden. *J. Gerontol.*, **39**, 230–239.
51. George L.K., Gwyther L.P. (1986) Caregiver well-being: a multidimensional examination of family caregivers of demented adults. *Gerontologist*, **26**, 253–259.
52. Morris R.G., Morris L.W., Britton P.G. (1988) Factors affecting the emotional wellbeing of the caregivers of dementia sufferers. *Br. J. Psychiatry*, **153**, 147–156.
53. Grafstrom M., Winblad B. (1995) Family burden in the care of the demented and nondemented elderly—a longitudinal study. *Alz. Dis. Assoc. Disord.*, **9**, 78–86.
54. Baumgarten M., Battista R.N., Infante-Rivard C., Hanley J.A., Becker R., Gauthier S. (1992) The psychological and physical health of family members caring for an elderly person with dementia. *J. Clin. Epidemiol.*, **45**, 61–70.
55. Schulz R., Williamson G.M. (1991) A 2-year longitudinal study of depression among Alzheimer's caregivers. *Psychol. Aging*, **6**, 569–578.
56. Mittelman M.S., Ferris S.H., Shulman E., Steinberg G., Ambinder A., Mackell J.A., Cohen J. (1995) A comprehensive support program: effect on depression in spouse-caregivers of AD patients. *Gerontologist*, **35**, 792–802.
57. Pinquart M., Sorensen S. (2003) Differences between caregivers and noncaregivers in psychological health and physical health: a meta-analysis. *Psychol. Aging*, **18**, 250–267.
58. Gallagher D., Rose J., Rivera P., Lovett S., Thompson L.W. (1989) Prevalence of depression in family caregivers. *Gerontologist*, **29**, 449–456.
59. Coope B., Ballard C., Saad K., Patel A. (1995) The prevalence of depression in the carers of dementia sufferers. *Int. J. Geriatr. Psychiatry*, **10**, 237–242.
60. Schulz R., Visintainer P., Williamson G.M. (1990) Psychiatric and physical morbidity effects of caregiving. *J. Gerontol.*, **45**, 181–191.
61. Vitaliano P.P., Zhang J., Scanlan J.M. (2003) Is caregiving hazardous to one's physical health? A meta-analysis. *Psychol. Bull.*, **129**, 946–972.
62. Haley W.E., Levine E.G., Brown S.L., Bartolucci A.A. (1987) Stress, appraisal, coping, and social support as predictors of adaptational outcome among dementia caregivers. *Psychol. Aging*, **2**, 323–330.
63. Vedhara K., Bennett P.D., Clark S., Lightman S.L., Shaw S., Perks P., Hunt M.A., Philip J.M., Tallon D., Murphy P.J., *et al.* (2003) Enhancement of antibody responses to influenza vaccination in the elderly following a cognitive–behavioural stress management intervention. *Psychother. Psychosom.*, **72**, 245–252.
64. Kiecolt-Glaser J.K., Glaser R., Shuttleworth E.C., Dyer C.S., Ogrocki P., Speicher C.E. (1987) Chronic stress and immunity in family caregivers of Alzheimer's disease victims. *Psychosom. Med.*, **49**, 523–535.
65. Schulz R., Williamson G.M. (1997) The measurement of caregiver outcomes in Alzheimer disease research. *Alz. Dis. Assoc. Disord.*, **11**, 117–124.
66. Schulz R., Beach S.R. (1999) Caregiving as a risk factor for mortality: the Caregiver Health Effects Study. *JAMA*, **282**, 2215–2219.
67. Brodaty H. (1998) The family and drug treatments for Alzheimer's disease. In: Gauthier S. (ed.) *Pharmacotherapy of Alzheimer's Disease.* Dunitz, London, pp. 123–139.

68. Rice D.P., Fox P.J., Max W., Webber P.A., Lindeman D.A., Hauck W.W., Segura E. (1993) The economic burden of Alzheimer's disease care. *Health Affairs*, **12**, 164–176.

69. Access Economics (2003) *The Dementia Epidemic: Economic Impact and Positive Solutions for Australia*. Alzheimer's Australia, Canberra.

70. Stommel M., Collins C.E., Given B.A. (1994) The costs of family contributions to the care of persons with dementia. *Gerontologist*, **34**, 199–205.

71. Moore M.J., Zhu C.W., Clipp E.C. (2001) Informal costs of dementia care: estimates from the National Longitudinal Caregiver Study. *J. Gerontol. B Psychol. Sci. Soc. Sci.*, **56**, S219–S228.

72. Brodaty H. (1996) Caregivers and behavioral disturbances: effects and interventions. *Int. Psychogeriatr.*, **8**, 455–458.

73. Mangone C.A., Sanguinetti R.M., Baumann P.D., Gonzalez R.C., Pereyra S., Bozzola F.G., Gorelick P.B., Sica R.E. (1993) Influence of feelings of burden on the caregiver's perception of the patient's functional status. *Dementia*, **4**, 287–293.

74. Bond J., Buck D. (1998) Long-term psychological distress among informal caregivers of frail older people in England: a longitudinal study. Presented at the 51st Annual Meeting of the Gerontological Society of America, Philadelphia, PA, 20–24 November.

75. Greene J.G., Smith R., Gardiner M., Timbury G.C. (1982) Measuring behavioural disturbance of elderly demented patients in the community and its effects on relatives: a factor analytic study. *Age Ageing*, **11**, 121–126.

76. Deimling G.T., Bass D.M. (1986) Symptoms of mental impairment among elderly adults and their effects on family caregivers. *J. Gerontol.*, **41**, 778–784.

77. Draper B.M., Poulos C.J., Cole A.M., Poulos R.G., Ehrlich F. (1992) A comparison of caregivers for elderly stroke and dementia victims. *J. Am. Geriatr. Soc.*, **40**, 896–901.

78. Draper B.M., Poulos R.G., Poulos C.J., Ehrlich F. (1996) Risk factors for stress in elderly caregivers. *Int. J. Geriatr. Psychiatry*, **11**, 227–231.

79. Lowery K., Mynt P., Aisbett J., Dixon T., O'Brien J., Ballard C. (2000) Depression in the carers of dementia sufferers: a comparison of the carers of patients suffering from dementia with Lewy bodies and the carers of patients with Alzheimer's disease. *J. Affect. Disord.*, **59**, 61–65.

80. Brodaty H., Green A. (2004) Vascular dementia: consequences for family carers and implications for management. In: Chiu E. (ed.) *Cerebrovascular Disease and Dementia: Pathology, Neuropsychiatry and Management*. Dunitz, Trowbridge, pp. 363–378.

81. Fitting M., Rabins P., Lucas M.J., Eastham J. (1986) Caregivers for dementia patients: a comparison of husbands and wives. *Gerontologist*, **26**, 248–252.

82. Collins C. (1992) Carers: gender and caring for dementia. In: Arie T (ed.) *Recent Advances in Psychogeriatrics 2*. Churchill Livingstone, Singapore, pp. 153–161.

83. Luscombe G., Brodaty H., Freeth S. (1998) Younger people with dementia: diagnostic issues, effects on carers and use of services. *Int. J. Geriatr. Psychiatry*, **13**, 323–330.

84. Schulz R., Gallagher-Thompson D., Haley Q., Czaja S. (2000) Understanding the intervention process: a theoretical/conceptual framework for intervention approaches to caregiving. In: Schulz R. (ed.) *Handbook on Dementia Caregiving. Evidence Based Interventions for Family Caregivers*. Springer-Verlag, New York, pp. 44–45.

85. Pruchno R.A., Resch N.L. (1989) Aberrant behaviors and Alzheimer's disease: mental health effects on spouse caregivers. *J. Gerontol.*, **44**, S177–182.
86. Lazarus R.S., Folkman S. (1984) *Stress, Appraisal and Coping.* Springer-Verlag, New York.
87. Gallant M.P., Connell C.M. (2003) Neuroticism and depressive symptoms among spouse caregivers: do health behaviors mediate this relationship? *Psychol. Aging*, **18**, 587–592.
88. Chenoweth B., Spencer B. (1986) Dementia: the experience of family caregivers. *Gerontologist*, **26**, 267–272.
89. Wright L.K. (1991) The impact of Alzheimer's disease on the marital relationship. *Gerontologist*, **31**, 224–237.
90. Bledin K.D., MacCarthy B., Kuipers L., Woods R.T. (1990) Daughters of people with dementia. Expressed emotion, strain and coping. *Br. J. Psychiatry*, **157**, 221–227.
91. Colvez A., Joel M.E., Ponton-Sanchez A., Royer A.C. (2002) Health status and work burden of Alzheimer patients' informal caregivers: comparisons of five different care programs in the European Union. *Health Policy*, **60**, 219–233.
92. Knox S.A., Britt H. (2002) A comparison of general practice encounters with patients from English-speaking and non-English-speaking backgrounds. *Med. J. Australia*, **177**, 98–101.
93. LoGiudice D., Hassett A., Cook R., Flicker L., Ames D. (2001) Equity of access to a memory clinic in Melbourne? Non-English speaking background attenders are more severely demented and have increased rates of psychiatric disorders. *Int. J. Geriatr. Psychiatry*, **16**, 327–334.
94. Pollitt P.A. (1997) The problem of dementia in Australian aboriginal and Torres Strait Islander communities: an overview. *Int. J. Geriatr. Psychiatry*, **12**, 155–163.
95. Harvey R., Roques P.K., Fox N.C., Rossor M.N. (1998) CANDID—Counselling and Diagnosis in Dementia: a national telemedicine service supporting the care of younger patients with dementia. *Int. J. Geriatr. Psychiatry*, **13**, 381–388.
96. Paveza G.J., Cohen D., Eisdorfer C., Freels S., Semla T., Ashford J.W., Gorelick P., Hirschman R., Luchins D., Levy P. (1992) Severe family violence and Alzheimer's disease: prevalence and risk factors. *Gerontologist*, **32**, 493–497.
97. Williamson G.M., Shaffer D.R. (2001) Relationship quality and potentially harmful behaviors by spousal caregivers: how we were then, how we are now. The Family Relationships in Late Life Project. *Psychol. Aging*, **16**, 217–226.
98. Koch S., Nay R. (2003) Reducing abuse of older people with dementia and their carers. *Australas. J. Ageing*, **22**, 191–195.
99. Burns A., Jacoby R., Levy R. (1990) Psychiatric phenomena in Alzheimer's disease. I: Disorders of thought content. *Br. J. Psychiatry*, **157**, 72–76, 92–94.
100. Burns A., Jacoby R., Levy R. (1990) Behavioral abnormalities and psychiatric symptoms in Alzheimer's disease: preliminary findings. *Int. Psychogeriatr.*, **2**, 25–36.
101. Brodaty H., Green A., Koschera A. (2003) Meta-analysis of psychosocial interventions for caregivers of people with dementia. *J. Am. Geriatr. Soc.*, **51**, 657–664.
102. Banerjee S., Murray J., Foley B., Atkins L., Schneider J., Mann A. (2003) Predictors of institutionalisation in people with dementia. *J. Neurol. Neurosurg. Psychiatry*, **74**, 1315–1316.
103. Lieberman M.A., Kramer J.H. (1991) Factors affecting decisions to institutionalize demented elderly. *Gerontologist*, **31**, 371–374.

104. Brodaty H., McGilchrist C., Harris L., Peters K.E. (1993) Time until institutionalization and death in patients with dementia. Role of caregiver training and risk factors. *Arch. Neurol.*, **50**, 643–650.

105. Yaffe K., Fox P., Newcomer R., Sands L., Lindquist K., Dane K., Covinsky K.E. (2002) Patient and caregiver characteristics and nursing home placement in patients with dementia. *JAMA*, **287**, 2090–2097.

106. Brodaty H. (1999) *Managing Alzheimer's Disease in Primary Care*, rev. edn. Science Press, London.

107. Drachman D.A., O'Donnell B.F., Lew R.A., Swearer J.M. (1990) The prognosis in Alzheimer's disease. "How far" rather than "how fast" best predicts the course. *Arch. Neurol.*, **47**, 851–856.

108. Schulz R., Mendelsohn A.B., Haley W.E., Mahoney D., Allen R.S., Zhang S., Thompson L., Belle S.H., Resources for Enhancing Alzheimer's Caregiver Health Investigations (2003) End-of-life care and the effects of bereavement on family caregivers of persons with dementia. *N. Engl. J. Med.*, **349**, 1936–1942.

109. Grant I., Adler K.A., Patterson T.L., Dimsdale J.E., Ziegler M.G., Irwin M.R. (2002) Health consequences of Alzheimer's caregiving transitions: effects of placement and bereavement. *Psychosom. Med.*, **64**, 477–486.

110. Grasel E. (2002) When home care ends—changes in the physical health of informal caregivers caring for dementia patients: a longitudinal study. *J. Am. Geriatr. Soc.*, **50**, 843–849.

111. Volicer L. (2004) End-of-life care and bereavement: effect on family carers. *Lancet Neurol.*, **3**, 144.

112. Brodaty H., Green A., Low L., Graham N. (2000) Family carers for people with dementia. In: O'Brien J., Ames D., Burns A. (eds) *Dementia*. Arnold, London, pp. 193–205.

113. Brodaty H. (1992) Carers: training informal carers. In: Arie T. (ed.) *Recent Advances in Psychogeriatrics 2*. Churchill Livingstone, Singapore, pp. 163–171.

114. Zarit S.H., Anthony C.R., Boutselis M. (1987) Interventions with care givers of dementia patients: comparison of two approaches. *Psychol. Aging*, **2**, 225–232.

115. Mittelman M.S., Ferris S.H., Shulman E., Steinberg G., Levin B. (1996) A family intervention to delay nursing home placement of patients with Alzheimer disease. A randomized controlled trial. *JAMA*, **276**, 1725–1731.

116. Brodaty H., Gresham M. (1989) Effect of a training programme to reduce stress in carers of patients with dementia. *Br. Med. J.*, **299**, 1375–1379.

117. Brodaty H., Peters K.E. (1991) Cost effectiveness of a training program for dementia carers. *Int. Psychogeriatr.*, **3**, 11–22.

118. Thomson C., Fine M., Brodaty H. (1997) *Carers Support Needs Project: Dementia Carers and the Non-Use of Community Services: Report on the Literature Review Commissioned by the Ageing and Disability Department*. University of New South Wales, Social Policy Research Centre, Sydney.

119. Hinchliffe A., Hyman I., Blizard B., Livingston G. (1995) Behavioural complications of dementia: can they be treated? *Int. J. Geriatr. Psychiatry*, **10**, 839–847.

120. Castro C.M., Wilcox S., O'Sullivan P., Baumann K., King A.C. (2002) An exercise program for women who are caring for relatives with dementia. *Psychosom. Med.*, **64**, 458–468.

121. Mittelman M.S., Roth D.L., Coon D.W., Haley W.E. (2004) Sustained benefit of supportive intervention for depressive symptoms in caregivers of patients with Alzheimer's disease. *Am. J. Psychiatry*, **161**, 850–856.

122. Sorensen S., Pinquart M., Duberstein P. (2002) How effective are interventions with caregivers? An updated meta-analysis. *Gerontologist*, **42**, 356–372.

123. Teri L., Logsdon R.G., Uomoto J., McCurry S.M. (1997) Behavioral treatment of depression in dementia patients: a controlled clinical trial. *J. Gerontol. B Psychol. Sci. Soc. Sci.*, **52**, 159–166.

124. Teri L., Gibbons L.E., McCurry S.M., Logsdon R.G., Buchner D.M., Barlow W.E., Kukull W.A., LaCroix A.Z., McCormick W., Larson E.B. (2003) Exercise plus behavioral management in patients with Alzheimer disease: a randomized controlled trial. *JAMA*, **290**, 2015–2022.

125. Yale R. (1995) *Developing Support Groups for Individuals with Early-Stage Alzheimer's Disease: Planning, Implementation, Evaluation.* Health Professions Press, Baltimore, MD.

126. Molinari V., Nelson N., Shekelle S., Crothers M.K. (1994) Family support groups of the Alzheimer's Association: an analysis of attendees and non-attendees. *J. Appl. Gerontol.*, **13**, 86–98.

127. Cuijpers P., Hosman C.M., Munnichs J.M. (1996) Change mechanisms of support groups for caregivers of dementia patients. *Int. Psychogeriatr.*, **8**, 575–587.

128. Fung W.Y., Chien W.T. (2002) The effectiveness of a mutual support group for family caregivers of a relative with dementia. *Arch. Psychiatry Nurs.*, **16**, 134–144.

129. Toseland R.W., McCallion P., Gerber T., Banks S. (2002) Predictors of health and human services use by persons with dementia and their family caregivers. *Soc. Sci. Med.*, **55**, 1255–1266.

130. Pillemer K., Suitor J. (2002) Peer support for Alzheimer's caregivers: is it enough to make a difference? *Res. Aging*, **24**, 171–192.

131. Tariot P.N., Truyen L. (2001) Reminyl (galantamine) reduces caregiver distress. Presented at the 10th Congress of the International Psychogeriatric Association. Nice, 9–14 September.

132. Cummings J.L., Schneider L., Tariot P.N., Kershaw P.R., Yuan W. (2004) Reduction of behavioral disturbances and caregiver distress by galantamine in patients with Alzheimer's disease. *Am. J. Psychiatry*, **161**, 532–538.

133. Fillit H.M., Gutterman E.M., Brooks R.L. (2000) Impact of donepezil on caregiving burden for patients with Alzheimer's disease. *Int. Psychogeriatr.*, **12**, 389–401.

134. Matthews H.P., Korbey J., Wilkinson D.G., Rowden J. (2000) Donepezil in Alzheimer's disease: eighteen month results from Southampton Memory Clinic. *Int. J. Geriatr. Psychiatry*, **15**, 713–720.

135. Feldman H., Gauthier S., Hecker J., Vellas B., Emir B., Mastey V., Subbiah P., Donepezil MSAD Study Investigators Group (2003) Efficacy of donepezil on maintenance of activities of daily living in patients with moderate to severe Alzheimer's disease and the effect on caregiver burden. *J. Am. Geriatr. Soc.*, **51**, 737–744.

136. Lopez O.L., Becker J.T., Wisniewski S., Saxton J., Kaufer D.I., DeKosky S.T. (2002) Cholinesterase inhibitor treatment alters the natural history of Alzheimer's disease. *J. Neurol. Neurosurg. Psychiatry*, **72**, 310–314.

137. Geldmacher D.S., Provenzano G., McRae T., Mastey V., Ieni J.R. (2003) Donepezil is associated with delayed nursing home placement in patients with Alzheimer's disease. *J. Am. Geriatr. Soc.*, **51**, 937–944.

138. Albert S.M., Sano M., Marder K., Jacobs D.M., Brandt J., Albert M., Stern Y. (1997) Participation in clinical trials and long-term outcomes in Alzheimer's disease. *Neurology*, **49**, 38–43.

139. Mastwyk M., Macfarlane S., LoGiudice D., Sullivan K.A. (2003) Why participate in an Alzheimer's disease clinical trial? Is it of benefit to carers and patients? *Int. Psychogeriatr.*, **15**, 149–156.

3

Families of People with Major Depression

Julian Leff

TAPS Research Unit, London, UK

INTRODUCTION

Many people in developed countries who suffer from depression live alone, but those who reside in a family are mostly living with a spouse or partner, and many have children. In developing countries the great majority of depressed people, like the rest of the population, live in a nuclear or extended family, but very little research has been focused on these settings. In the West, studies of major depression have predominantly involved women, largely because they have about twice the risk of becoming depressed as men [1]. However, recent research has also included men in the samples studied. The main focus has been on the emotional relationship within the couple, the effect on the mental health of the well partner of caring for a depressed patient, and the evaluation of interventions aimed at improving the couple's relationship. There is a paucity of work on the coping skills of the well partner. Each of these topics will be dealt with in this chapter.

THE EMOTIONAL RELATIONSHIP

Couples can have an unsatisfactory relationship without either of them developing depression. This observation raises the question of whether there is some specific quality to the relationship of a couple where one partner has developed depression. Beach *et al.* [2] tackled this question by comparing the relationships of couples with a discordant marriage and in

Families and Mental Disorders. Edited by Norman Sartorius, Julian Leff, Juan José López-Ibor, Mario Maj and Ahmed Okasha. © 2005 John Wiley & Sons Ltd. ISBN 0-470-02382-1

which the wife was depressed with discordant couples without depression. They used a measure of cohesion, and found that while the non-depressed couples had low levels of cohesion, the couples in which the wife was depressed were significantly lower on this measure.

Brown and Harris [3] conducted a series of studies of depressed women to identify the interaction of stressful experiences and vulnerability factors. They found that a high proportion of episodes of depression were preceded during a three-month period by an excess of life events which occasioned losses of valued relationships or material losses. However, by no means all women who experienced such a loss went on to become depressed. By comparing the women who developed a depressive illness following a loss event with those who remained mentally healthy, Brown and Harris were able to identify features which rendered the former vulnerable. The three key factors were loss of mother before the age of 12, having three children under the age of 5, and lacking an intimate relationship. While some women were protected from depression by an intimate (non-sexual) relationship with another woman, most of the mentally healthy women had male partners who gave them strong emotional support.

Not only does the relationship with a partner influence the vulnerability to depression, it also affects recovery from a depressive episode. Goering et al. [4] followed up married women who had been hospitalized for major depression and found that only one half recovered over the next six months. They found that women who had high levels of dissatisfaction with the amount or quality of their spouse's communication, affection, or relationship with the children were significantly less likely to recover. This result found confirmation in a study by Keitner et al. [5] of patients hospitalized for major depression, the majority of whom were married women. Recovery over 12 months was significantly more likely when there was good functioning in roles (recurrent patterns of behaviour necessary to fulfil the instrumental and affective needs of family members), affective involvement (amount of interest, care and concern that family members invest in each other) and behaviour control (style of maintaining discipline and standards of behaviour).

A number of researchers have studied the relationship between depressed people and their partners, often using different methods of assessment. Waring and Patton [6] employed a measurement of intimacy in marriage, the Waring Intimacy Questionnaire [7], in a sample of patients who met the Research Diagnostic Criteria (RDC) for non-bipolar major depression. The patients, comprising 40 women and 35 men, completed the General Health Questionnaire (GHQ-28) and the Beck Depression Inventory (BDI) in addition to the Intimacy Questionnaire. In addition, 25 spouses were available to fill in all three questionnaires. For male patients the total intimacy score was correlated with age (+0.33), number of children (+0.34) and occupation (+0.46), while for females, only income was positively correlated (+0.46). For both men and women, the total intimacy score was negatively correlated with depressive symptoms, but the relationship was much stronger for women (BDI -0.74, GHQ-28 depression score -0.49) than for men (BDI -0.29, GHQ-28 depression score -0.29). This suggests that women are more reliant on a high level of intimacy to maintain their mental health than men. There was no difference in total intimacy scores between patients (19.1) and spouses (21.7), indicating that they shared the same perception of this aspect of their relationship, which had not been coloured by the patients' depressed state of mind. The burden of caring for a depressed person was reflected in the high proportion of spouses, 36%, who reported enough symptoms on the GHQ-28 to be classified as probable cases of non-psychotic emotional illness. As we shall see, this is a common finding. Compared to the spouses who did not rate as suffering from an emotional illness, the "cases" reported lower total intimacy scores, less ability to resolve conflict, less affection and much less compatibility. It is not clear whether this is a consequence of both partners being depressed, or whether the poorer quality of the relationship led to emotional distress in the carer.

Some light has been thrown on the direction of cause and effect in the problematic relationships of depressed people by an ingenious study by Coyne [8]. He arranged for 45 female undergraduates to talk for 20 minutes on the telephone to a randomly chosen female subject. The subjects were selected from 30 outpatients attending a mental health centre, 15 of whom were depressed and another 15 non-depressed. In addition there were 15 mentally healthy control subjects. The paired subjects were free to talk about anything they wished and the conversation was audiotaped. After the conversation, subjects and target individuals were asked to complete questionnaires concerning mood, perception of the other person and willingness to interact again under various conditions. The tapes were scored for activity, other–self ratio of speech, approval responses, hope measures and genuineness. The undergraduates were found to be significantly more depressed, anxious and hostile following conversations with the depressed patients than with the other two groups. There were no significant differences in activity, approval responses, hope measures or genuineness. Subjects talked more about the target individual than about themselves when the target was depressed. Subjects were also significantly more rejecting of the depressed patients than the other two groups, and there was a strong correlation between the degree of rejection and the depth of the patients' depressed mood. These results indicate that interaction with a depressed person can induce a variety of negative moods in a healthy individual and can provoke rejection.

Another approach to determining the direction of cause and effect was taken by Barnett and Gottlieb [9]. They conducted an extensive review of the relevant literature to distinguish variables that are observable only during a depressive episode from those that either precede the disorder or persist following recovery. They argue that the former are less likely to play a causal role in depression, and come to a number of conclusions based on this premise. Patients no longer in a depressive episode have greater dependency needs; that is, they desire approval, approach, attention and help from others to a greater extent than do non-depressed controls. On the other hand, they tend to socialize less and participate less in social situations than do controls, thus limiting their access to the support they crave. Barnett and Gottlieb conclude that low social integration may be characteristic of people prone to depression, since it predicts the onset of depression and the course of existing symptoms, and distinguishes remitted depressives from control subjects. They also found that disturbances in interpersonal functioning preceded episodes of depression and persisted after their resolution. In an unpublished study reported in their paper, Gottlieb discovered a significant difference between men and women carers in their relationship with the depressed person. Following recovery of a depressed woman, the couple reported no significant change in their marital satisfaction. By contrast, couples in which the husband had been depressed reported a significant improvement in their satisfaction. This suggests that women may be more tolerant than men of the interpersonal behaviours associated with depression. Alternatively, men and women who have recovered from depression may differ in their behaviour towards their spouse.

THE IMPACT ON THE PARTNER

The effect on the partner of living with a depressed person was relatively neglected for many years in favour of studying the relatives of people with schizophrenia or dementia. Even today, the literature on the carers of depressed people is tiny compared with studies on the carers of people developing either of the above conditions. One of the first pieces of research on this topic was conducted by Fadden et al. [10]. They amalgamated items from several questionnaires to create a schedule, which they used to interview the spouses of 25 people with depression. They included patients with unipolar depression, bipolar depression and depressive neurosis, which were chronic or recurrent. A much higher percentage of male relatives (83%) than female (42%) worked. For 41% of carers the financial situation had become much worse since the patient's illness, mostly due to loss of the patient's earnings. A reduction in social activities was experienced by 71% of spouses, half of whom reported that they never went out with the patient socially. This was particularly marked when the patient was male. An additional deprivation was that fewer friends visited the home. The problem was compounded by the fact that many spouses were embarrassed and reluctant to tell people about the patient's depression. This effect of stigma is identical to that seen in the families of people with schizophrenia. It not only leads to the social isolation of the carers and patients, but the failure to be open about the illness also serves to maintain the stigma.

Nearly half the spouses mentioned difficulties in their marital relationship, wives being more likely than husbands to perceive a deterioration. One third reported that sexual relations had ceased as a result of the depression. Almost half the spouses had no idea what practical steps they could take to deal with the patient's mood disturbance, and only two felt they had been given sufficient information by professionals to fully understand the patient's difficulties. One third of spouses sometimes felt they could not cope with the situation any longer and would have to find a way out. This sense of desperation was reported by more wives than husbands. Wives also more commonly than husbands experienced grief over the loss of the person they related to before the illness: 58% compared with only 8%. Once again, this is common to relatives of people with schizophrenia. Spouses lost the facility of confiding in their partner and commonly had to take decisions on their own. Not surprisingly, these burdens on the carer unrelieved by help from professionals led to mental ill-health, and 38% would have been identified as in need of treatment according to their psychiatric symptoms. The findings of this pioneering study are echoed in subsequent research, in particular the greater vulnerability of women carers to the strain of the caring role.

A study by Jacob *et al.* [11], published in the same year as the research described above, complements the findings of Fadden *et al.* They developed a Family Distress Scale for Depression composed of 25 items, and applied it to 112 family members or friends of patients suffering from recurrent episodes of major depression. Of the 112 subjects, 80 lived with the patients and 68 of these were spouses. A total of 60 respondents (54%) scored above the half-way point of the scale, indicating that a majority often or almost always experienced strain. The most distressing behaviour, rated by 62% as often or almost always upsetting, was hearing the patient express feelings of worthlessness, inadequacy and low self-esteem. Nearly half reported that the patient's low mood made them feel depressed or low. Subjects living with the patient expressed significantly greater annoyance from the problems occasioned by the patient's illness and were more burdened by lack of cooperation than those living elsewhere, a finding that is only to be expected.

One study of this topic has been conducted in a developing country, where extended families are still the norm. Chakrabarti *et al.* [12] studied 90 patients with major affective disorder who were inpatients or outpatients in the city of Chandigarh, in northern India. The patients had been ill for two years or more. The relatives were interviewed with a number of instruments, including the Family Burden Interview Schedule [13], which was developed in an Indian setting. Unlike in Western samples, men constituted the majority of the patients (66%). The patients were mainly professionals, semiprofessionals and housewives, with few farmers or unskilled workers, reflecting the urban nature of Chandigarh. Bipolar affective disorder was the diagnosis for 81% of them, the remainder suffering from major depression. The relatives were divided into 61% spouses, 20% parents, 12% children and 7% others. This difference from Western samples, which are almost exclusively spouses, stems from the different family structure in a developing country. Only a single relative reported no burden, while the other 89 experienced moderate to severe burden. The objective burden was significantly greater for relatives of bipolar patients than for those caring for patients with major depression. The major portion of variation in burden was accounted for by the degree of the patient's dysfunction and the duration of the illness.

The research on carers of people with dementia is vast compared with the similar studies of depression. Wijeratne and Lovestone [14] mounted a pilot study to compare the carers of people suffering from either of these two conditions. All the patients were aged over 65 years and attended a psychogeriatric service in London with a diagnosis of depression or dementia. All the carers of depressed patients were spouses, whereas some of the carers of the dementia patients were children. Carers' scores on the GHQ-28 were significantly higher for dementia patients than for depressed patients; however, this was entirely accounted for by carers who were children. There was no difference in the proportion of cases between spouses of depressed and dementia patients: about one quarter. Scoring above the caseness level of the GHQ-28 was associated with behavioural difficulties in the patient, including apathy, physical disability and social disturbance; unsatisfactory premorbid relationship with the patient; and carers' dissatisfaction with their social contacts. A very similar comparison of the carers of depressed and dementia patients was conducted by Rosenvinge et al. [15] also using the GHQ-28. They found that 44% of carers of the chronically depressed patients reached the threshold for caseness, compared with 85% of carers of dementia patients. However, they did not distinguish between spouses and children of the patients, which almost certainly accounts for the large difference between the two groups of carers. They also found that duration of caring correlated significantly with carer stress in the depressed group, but not in the dementia group. The finding for the carers of depressed patients echoes the results of the study in India.

Another study comparing the spouses of depressed and dementia patients was carried out in Finland [16]. Of the 22 depressed patients, 10 suffered from recurrent depression, 9 had a single episode and 3 had bipolar disorder. The 43 dementia patients were divided into those admitted with psychiatric or behavioural symptoms, and those admitted for memory or diagnostic assessment. Spouses of the former group were significantly more burdened than the spouses of depressed patients, whose burden did not differ from spouses of the latter type of dementia patients. The GHQ-12 was used to determine caseness, and, once again, the group with the highest number of cases was the spouses of dementia patients with behavioural problems, while the spouses of the remaining dementia patients had a similar proportion of cases (45%) as the spouses of the depressed patients (57%). As in the Indian study, the more the patient's function was impaired, the more burdened was the spouse.

A more qualitative approach was taken by Muscroft and Bowl [17], who mailed the questionnaire developed by Fadden et al. [10] to members of the Depression Alliance, a self-help organization. They received responses from 51 carers of depressed people and interviewed 10 of them in depth. They learned that managing the illness was hardest when there were young children, since parents did not know how to explain the illness to them. Spouses did not usually feel guilty for their partner's depression and generally held psychosocial models implicating family history and life events as causal factors. A dominant theme was mourning the loss of the person who had been familiar to them, trying to get him or her back, and clinging on to the little that was available. One husband said: "She's three-quarters dead: but I have the quarter that's still alive". This response, which was also documented by Fadden et al. [10], is commonly encountered in the relatives of people with schizophrenia, who often feel that the person they knew has been replaced by a stranger [18]. Spouses, more than parents or children, felt that their lives had been taken over by the illness. They complained that they never regained their accustomed roles. Caregivers in general wanted professionals to listen to them, to take them seriously and to understand their difficulties.

In the study by Jacob et al. [11], nearly half the carers reported that their own mood was lowered in response to the patient's depression. This effect was the focus of research by Wittmund et al. [19] in Leipzig. They assessed 45 partners of patients with anxiety, 54 of patients with depression, and 52 of patients with schizophrenia. The patients had chronic illnesses with a mean duration of 10 years. The patients had a similar degree of impairment regardless of their diagnosis. The authors found that 41% of spouses met ICD-10 criteria for any mental disorder. A higher proportion of women was affected (52%) than of men (32%), the commonest diagnosis in both sexes being depression. There was no difference in the proportion of spouses affected by depression across the three diagnostic groups of patients. The risk of developing depression was significantly related to the impairment of the patient's functioning as measured by the Global Assessment of Functioning scale, a similar finding to that of the Indian study on burden.

EXPRESSED EMOTIONS

The evidence presented above that close relationships are influential in the origin and maintenance of depression is augmented by the research on relatives' expressed emotion (EE). This measure of a carer's emotional response to a person with a psychiatric illness was developed by Brown and Rutter [20] and employed initially in studies of schizophrenia. Vaughn and Leff [21] conducted one of the earliest replications of the research on EE and the course of schizophrenia, and included a comparison group of patients with depressive neurosis (major depression without psychotic features). The depressed patients differed from those with schizophrenia in that most of the latter lived with parents, whereas all but one of the former lived with a partner. Whereas a cut-off point of six critical comments made by the carer separated patients with schizophrenia with a high risk of relapse from those with a low risk, the best predictive threshold for depressed patients was found to be two critical comments. A recent review of the EE research on schizophrenia and depression by Butzlaff and Hooley [22] indicated that the association between EE and the course of depression was even stronger than that for schizophrenia. This conclusion, taken together with the research findings summarized above, constitutes a strong argument for attempting to improve the outcome of depression by working with the couple's relationship.

COUPLE THERAPY FOR DEPRESSION

The first controlled trial of marital therapy for depression was conducted by Friedman [23]. It was a four-cell design with random assignment to amitriptyline or placebo, and to weekly marital therapy or to minimal contact. The drop-out rate was 15%, leaving 150 subjects who completed the whole course of 12 weeks. For those subjects who completed the trial, marital therapy showed no advantage over minimal contact in alleviating depressed mood. However, patients who had received marital therapy rated their marriage as better than those in the minimal contact group.

Waring et al. [24] mounted a similar trial in which doxepin was compared with a placebo, and patients, all of whom were women, were also randomized to 10 weekly sessions of cognitive marital therapy or to minimal contact. A preliminary report on the first 12 couples to complete the trial showed no difference between cognitive marital therapy and minimal contact conditions. The sample size is too small to draw any definitive conclusions and no further reports appear to have been published.

O'Leary and Beach [25] randomly assigned 36 couples to individual cognitive therapy for the depressed wife, behavioural marital therapy for the couple, or a waiting list control. Both active therapies were given weekly for 16 weeks. The drop-out rate from the active therapies was 25%. Both therapies were effective in reducing depression compared with the controls. However, marital therapy was more effective than the other two conditions in increasing marital satisfaction.

Jacobson et al. [26] recruited 72 married women with depression to a trial in which they were randomly assigned to 20 sessions of behavioural marital therapy, cognitive therapy or a combination of the two. The drop-out rate was 17%, and 60 subjects, none of whom was receiving antidepressants, completed the trial. All three treatments were equally effective in reducing depressive symptoms. However, only behavioural marital therapy increased marital satisfaction in couples who initially scored high on marital distress.

It does not seem sensible to offer marital therapy to couples who are satisfied with their relationship, and Emanuels-Zuurveen and Emmelkamp [27] included in their trial only depressed patients with a high level of marital distress. They randomized 36 patients to 16 weekly sessions of individual cognitive therapy or behavioural marital therapy. No subjects received antidepressants, and 25% dropped out of the trial. Both treatments were equally effective in reducing depressive symptoms, but marital therapy produced more improvement in the relationship than cognitive therapy.

The findings of these trials are relatively consistent in demonstrating that individual cognitive therapy and behavioural marital therapy are equally effective in relieving depressive symptoms, but only marital therapy is able to improve the marital relationship, particularly when it is unsatisfactory. The drop-out rate from these psychosocial interventions was relatively low, ranging from 15% to 25%. No trial continued for more than six months and all were concerned solely with the treatment of depressive episodes. Most treatments, whether pharmacological, psychological or psychosocial, are reasonably effective in reducing depressive symptoms. However, depressive illnesses have a strong tendency to recurrence, and few studies have evaluated the prophylactic value of any treatment. Furthermore, in none of the above studies was marital therapy compared directly with antidepressants, still the commonest form of treatment. A recent trial was conducted which attempted to remedy these deficiencies.

THE LONDON DEPRESSION INTERVENTION TRIAL

This randomized controlled trial [28] developed out of the research on EE and depression. The aim was to ameliorate the emotional atmosphere in the home, as in the trials of family intervention for schizophrenia. The psychosocial treatment chosen was systemic couple therapy, as this approach had been shown to reduce criticism in families with problematic relationships [29]. Systemic couple therapy aims to help the patient and partner to gain new perspectives on the presenting problems, to attach different meanings to depressive types of behaviour, and to experiment with new ways of relating to each other [30]. The term "marital therapy" has been superseded by "couple therapy", since so many people now live in stable partnerships without marrying.

The trial was designed to evaluate the prophylactic value of the treatments as well as their efficacy in reducing depression. The first phase, lasting one year, involved active treatment. Thereafter the treatments in both arms of the trial were discontinued and subjects were followed for a further year.

The majority of patients were referred to the study by primary or secondary services, although one third responded to advertisements in newspapers. There were no differences on salient features between patients coming from these two sources. To enter the trial, they had to have been in a stable relationship for at least a year, and the partner needed to make two or more critical comments in response to the Camberwell Family Interview. In fact, only 5 out of 99 suitable couples were excluded on this basis. Eventually 77 couples were randomly assigned to either antidepressant medication or couple therapy, 40 of whom received the latter.

The antidepressant regime began with desipramine, alongside which two sessions of education about depression and its treatment were given to the patient and partner to improve compliance. Serum levels were checked regularly to monitor compliance. If there was no response after six weeks, desipramine was replaced by fluvoxamine. After six months on a treatment dose, the dose was gradually reduced to a maintenance level. At the end of one year, the antidepressant was tailed off over two weeks, although two patients chose to remain on medication and two others relapsed as soon as it was stopped, so that it had to be resumed.

The total drop-out rate from drug treatment over the course of the treatment year was 56.8%, while that for couple therapy was 15%, a highly significant difference. This indicates that couple therapy was far more acceptable to the subjects in the trial than medication, reflecting a well-known prejudice in the general population against antidepressant drugs [31]. Patients who dropped out differed from those who completed the trial in being significantly younger and having higher scores on the BDI.

The patients' level of depression was assessed with the BDI and the Hamilton Rating Scale for Depression (HRSD) [32] at the start of the trial, and at one-year and two-year follow-ups. The statistical analysis was based on the likelihood approach, since this allows for drop-outs. The analysis was conducted on an intention-to-treat basis and included all patients for whom data were available for at least one of the follow-ups in addition to the initial assessment.

Analysis of the BDI scores revealed that both treatment groups improved during the first year, although patients who received couple therapy showed a greater improvement than those on drugs. On average the BDI scores of patients in couple therapy fell by 6.4 points (95% CI 1.62–11.54) more than those on drugs. The advantage for couple therapy was maintained over the second year after treatments had been discontinued.

It can be concluded that couple therapy is at least as efficacious as antidepressant drugs for both the treatment and prevention of depression, and may even be superior.

CONCLUSIONS

A low level of intimacy and of cohesion in partner relationships is associated with depression, particularly in women. Intimacy is also important to the carer's mental health, and carers are more likely to be identified as cases of psychiatric disorder when intimacy is lacking. Recovery from depression is aided by good communication with the partner, expression of care and concern by the partner, and adequate fulfilment of parental roles. Patients who have recovered from depression desire approval, attention and help from others, but prevent themselves from achieving this by reducing their social activity. Disturbances of interpersonal relationships precede depressive episodes and persist after recovery, suggesting they may play a causal role in the development and maintenance of depression. Depressed patients can induce depression, anxiety, hostility and rejecting attitudes in healthy subjects.

The loss of the spouse's earnings imposes a financial burden on the carer. A reduction in social activity ensues, due partly to the patient's difficulty in facing social situations and partly to a deliberate avoidance of friends and relatives by the carer through shame and embarrassment. Deterioration in the marital relationship affects wives more profoundly than husbands, and sexual activity ceases in one third of couples. Spouses felt that their lives had been taken over by the illness. The experience of burden is largely determined by the duration of the illness and the degree of the patient's dysfunction. It was particularly distressing for carers to hear the patient express feelings of worthlessness, inadequacy and low self-esteem, and nearly half had their own mood lowered by the patient's depression. More than half the carers experience strain and this is reflected in a high proportion qualifying as psychiatric cases: four studies record levels of 38–45%. Psychiatric symptoms in the carer were associated with an unsatisfactory premorbid relationship with the patient, and with the carer's dissatisfaction with their social contacts. A consistent complaint was lack of information from professionals, and the need for professionals to listen to the carers.

The earlier studies suggested that behavioural marital therapy is as efficacious as cognitive therapy in the treatment of depression. There is substantial evidence that cognitive therapy is as efficacious as antidepressants. The London Depression Intervention Trial has shown that systemic couple therapy is at least as efficacious as drugs both for the treatment of depression and for the prevention of relapse. It is much more acceptable to patients with partners than drugs. The challenge now is to make these efficacious psychosocial treatments available at primary care level, where the great majority of depressed patients are treated.

REFERENCES

1. Bebbington P., Hurry J., Tennant C., Sturt E., Wing J.K. (1981) The epidemiology of mental disorders in Camberwell. *Psychol. Med.*, **11**, 561–580.
2. Beach S.R., Nelson G.M., O'Leary K.D. (1988) Cognitive and marital factors in depression. *J. Psychopath. Behav. Assess.*, **10**, 93–105.
3. Brown G.W., Harris T. (1978) *Social Origins of Depression: A Study of Psychiatric Disorders in Women*. Tavistock, London.
4. Goering P.N., Lancee W.J., Freeman S.J.J. (1992) Marital support and recovery from depression. *Br. J. Psychiatry*, **160**, 76–82.
5. Keitner G.I., Ryan C.E., Miller I.W., Kohn R., Bishop D.S., Epstein N.B. (1995) Role of the family in recovery and major depression. *Am. J. Psychiatry*, **152**, 1002–1008.
6. Waring E.M., Patton D. (1984) Marital intimacy and depression. *Br. J. Psychiatry*, **145**, 641–644.
7. Waring E.M., Reddon J.R. (1983) The measurement of intimacy in marriage: the Waring Intimacy Questionnaire. *J. Clin. Psychol.*, **39**, 53–57.
8. Coyne J.C. (1976) Depression and the response of others. *J. Abnorm. Psychol.*, **85**, 186–193.
9. Barnett P.A., Gottlieb I.H. (1988) Psychosocial functioning and depression: distinguishing among antecedents, concomitants and consequences. *Psychol. Bull.*, **104**, 97–126.
10. Fadden G., Bebbington P., Kuipers L. (1987) Caring and its burdens: a study of the spouses of depressed patients. *Br. J. Psychiatry*, **151**, 660–667.
11. Jacob M., Frank E., Kupfer D.J., Carpenter L.L. (1987) Recurrent depression: an assessment of family burden and family attitudes. *J. Clin. Psychiatry*, **48**, 395–400.

12. Chakrabati S., Kulhara P., Verma S.K. (1992) Extent and determinants of burden among families of patients with affective disorders. *Acta Psychiatr. Scand.*, **86**, 247–252.
13. Pai S., Kapur R.L. (1981) The burden on the family of a psychiatric patient: development of an assessment scale. *Br. J. Psychiatry*, **138**, 332–335.
14. Wijeratne C., Lovestone S. (1996) A pilot study comparing psychological and physical morbidity in carers of elderly people with dementia and those with depression. *Int. J. Geriatr. Psychiatry*, **11**, 741–744.
15. Rosenvinge H., Jones D., Judge E., Martin A. (1998) Demented and chronic depressed patients attending a day hospital: stress expressed by carers. *Int. J. Geriatr. Psychiatry*, **13**, 642–643.
16. Leinonen E., Korpisammal L., Pulkkinen L.-M., Pukuri T. (2001) The comparison of burden between caregiving spouses of depressive and demented patients. *Int. J. Geriatr. Psychiatry*, **16**, 387–393.
17. Muscroft J., Bowl R. (2000) The impact of depression on caregivers and other family members: implications for professional support. *Counselling Psychol. Q.*, **13**, 117–134.
18. Kuipers E., Leff J., Lam D. (2002) *Family Work for Schizophrenia: A Practical Guide*. Gaskell, London.
19. Wittmund B., Wilms H.-U., May C., Angermeyer M.C. (2002) Depressive disorders in spouses of mentally ill patients. *Soc. Psychiatry Psychiatr. Epidemiol.*, **37**, 177–182.
20. Brown G.W., Rutter M. (1966) The measurement of family activities and relationships: a methodological study. *Human Relations*, **19**, 241–263.
21. Vaughn C., Leff J.P. (1976) The influence of family and social factors on the course of psychiatric illness. A comparison of schizophrenic and depressed neurotic patients. *Br. J. Psychiatry*, **129**, 125–137.
22. Butzlaff R.L., Hooley J.M. (1998) Expressed emotion and psychiatric relapse: a meta-analysis. *Arch. Gen. Psychiatry*, **55**, 547–552.
23. Friedman A.S. (1975) Interaction of drug therapy with marital therapy in depressive patients. *Arch. Gen. Psychiatry*, **32**, 618–637.
24. Waring G.M., Chamberlaine C.H., McCrank E.W., Stalker C.A., Carver C., Fry R., Barnes S. (1988) Dysthymia: a randomised study of cognitive marital therapy and antidepressants. *Can. J. Psychiatry*, **33**, 96–99.
25. O'Leary K.D., Beach S.R.H. (1990) Marital therapy. A viable treatment for depression and marital discord. *Am. J. Psychiatry*, **147**, 183–186.
26. Jacobson N.S., Dobson K., Fruzzetti A.E., Schmaling D.B., Salusky S. (1991) Marital therapy as a treatment for depression. *J. Consult. Clin. Psychol.*, **59**, 547–557.
27. Emanuels-Zuurveen L., Emmelkamp P.M.G. (1996) Individual behavioural–cognitive therapy v. marital therapy for depression in maritally distressed couples. *Br. J. Psychiatry*, **169**, 181–188.
28. Leff J., Vearnals S., Brewin C.R., Wolff G., Alexander B., Asen A., Dayson D., Jones E., Chisholm D., Everitt B. (2000) The London Depression Intervention Trial. Randomised controlled trial of antidepressants v. couple therapy in the treatment and maintenance of people with depression living with a partner: clinical outcome and costs. *Br. J. Psychiatry*, **177**, 95–100.
29. Asen K., Berkowitz R., Cooklin A., Leff J., Loader P., Piper R., Rein I. (1991) Family therapy outcome research: a trial for families, therapists, and researchers. *Family Process*, **30**, 3–20.

30. Jones E., Asen E. (1999) *Systemic Couple Therapy and Depression*. Karnac, London.
31. Paykel E.S., Hart D., Priest R.G. (1998) Changes in public attitudes to depression during the defeat depression campaign. *Br. J. Psychiatry*, **173**, 519–522.
32. Hamilton M. (1960) A rating scale for depression. *J. Neurol. Neurosurg. Psychiatry*, **23**, 59–61.

Families of People with Bipolar Disorder

Gabor I. Keitner*‡, **Christine E. Ryan***‡
and Alison Heru‡§

*Rhode Island Hospital, Providence, Rhode Island, USA
‡Brown University, Providence, Rhode Island, USA
§Butler Hospital, Providence, Rhode Island, USA

INTRODUCTION

Bipolar disorder is a chronic remitting and relapsing illness that causes significant burden to patients, families and society. It has a lifetime prevalence of approximately 1.0% [1–3] and an annual incidence rate of 0.009–0.015% (i.e. 9–15 new cases per 100 000) for men and 0.007–0.03% (7–30 new cases per 100 000) for women [4]. It has recently been argued that the 1% lifetime prevalence estimate is more likely characteristic of bipolar I disorder only and that 5% is a more accurate estimate if bipolar spectrum disorders are considered [5]. In any one year, the majority of individuals with a lifetime diagnosis of bipolar disorder receive inpatient or outpatient treatment within the mental health service system [6]. Bipolar disorder is a significant source of distress, disability and burden on other family members. In 1990, the World Health Organization identified bipolar disorder as the sixth leading cause of disability-adjusted life years in the world among people aged 15 to 44 years [7]. Ultimately, 19% of bipolar patients will die from suicide [4].

Although pharmacotherapy is available to address acute episodes of the illness, relapse over time is almost inevitable for the bipolar patient. Even if a patient has not relapsed, residual symptoms persist between episodes. Post *et al.* [8] recently reported on 258 bipolar patients followed prospectively for 1 year: 26% were ill most of the year, 41% were

Families and Mental Disorders. Edited by Norman Sartorius, Julian Leff, Juan José López-Ibor, Mario Maj and Ahmed Okasha. © 2005 John Wiley & Sons Ltd. ISBN 0-470-02382-1

intermittently ill and 33% minimally ill. These numbers correspond with our own findings of the course of bipolar illness in patients followed for 28 months as part of a randomized treatment trial [9]: 27% had a poor course, 48% had a fluctuating course and 25% had a good course of illness [10]. In an observational study with a mean follow-up period of 13 years, Judd *et al.* [11] estimated that patients were symptomatic 47% of the time. 10% of these patients reported being symptomatic all of the time [11]. Angst [12] noted that bipolar patients spent approximately 20% of their lifetime in illness. In a recent study by Dore and Romans [13], one third of the bipolar patients had been ill for 10 years or more.

CHRONIC ILLNESS AND EFFECTS ON THE FAMILY

The family has long been recognized as a key factor in caring for medically ill patients [14] as well as patients with severe mental illness [15]. However, because clinicians did not initially understand that mood disorders were chronic conditions or that the family had an impact on a patient's functioning [16], research focused first on relatives of schizophrenic patients, and later on patients with dementia. Studies often centred on burden [17,18], as it was clear that the family had assumed major responsibility for a relative's care, especially when lack of funding limited the amount of available resources in the community [15,19,20]. A number of models were generated that explained the interplay between a patient's course of illness and the family environment. These models emphasized stress-coping processes [21,22], multiple role strain [23,24], expressed emotion (EE) [25,26], social support as a buffer against stressors [27,28] or family systems [29,30].

Family members often struggle with the ambiguity of living with a person with mental illness and make valiant attempts to control the illness and pursue normalcy [31,32]. Although traditionally viewed as burdensome, caring for an ill relative also entails a sense of reward and satisfaction [33]. While one person is usually identified as the primary caregiver, other family members are also involved in caring for the ill relative. Thus, it may be important to include as many members of the family as possible for the assessment of, or intervention for, their caretaking roles.

Family members describe losses pertaining to hopes, dreams and expectations, and grieve for what might have been, experiencing feelings of shock, disbelief, anger, despair, guilt, anxiety and shame [34]. Family members sometimes describe that they feel like they are riding an emotional rollercoaster, with alternating periods of relapse and remission. These cycles create considerable turmoil for family members, who often experience intense distress when renewed hope is shattered by yet another relapse. In spite of these strains, family members often identify family strengths that have developed, such as improved family bonds and commitments, expanded knowledge and skills, and advocacy skills. They also affirm their potential for personal resilience, noting that they become better, stronger and more compassionate people. They cite their contributions to their family, their enhanced coping effectiveness and their healthier perspectives and priorities. Family members also comment positively on the resilience of their relative with mental illness.

Temporary separation because of illness-related difficulties is common. Many family members have to decrease their work hours or take time off during episodes of illness, thereby reducing their income and, possibly, jeopardizing their job security. In a study by Dore and Romans [13], 27% of caregivers experienced a reduction in income, while 29% incurred major financial costs as a result of caring for their relative. Burden is highest when the illness is most severe, during hospitalizations and periods of increased symptom severity [35]; nonetheless, caregivers continue to report significant strain, burden and poor family functioning even after hospitalization [36].

Burden is a loose construct that has been defined in various ways, but usually includes a measure of subjective and objective distress. Objective burden is a measure of the observable and verifiable disruption to the family's life, such as financial difficulties, curtailed social activities and loss of vacations. Subjective burden is a measure of the extent to which relatives feel burdened, and includes worrying, tension, insomnia and resentment. Subjective burden is a more powerful predictor of caregiver distress [37] than objective burden, and some family members will report little subjective burden in the face of high objective burden [38]. The level of subjective burden depends upon many variables, including the relationship between the family member and patient, the expectations and comfort in the role of caregiving, social supports, financial resources, health, gender, age, and other responsibilities of the primary caregiver.

A family that is able to cope with one crisis may be overwhelmed when there is an accumulation of stressors [39]. The ability to cope well with adversity has been described as resilience [40], but early work on resilience focused on the individual and viewed the quality of resilience as an innate characteristic of the person [41]. Recent work on family resilience has focused on how strengths within a family, such as good parenting, can offset family difficulties. Examples of family processes thought to mediate recovery from illness or crisis and allow for successful functioning of the whole family include clear and direct communication, collaborative problem solving, maintaining a strong family structure and establishing good emotional relatedness [29,42]. It is possible that some family strengths may offset difficulties in other areas of family functioning. For example, a warm and supportive attitude towards the patient may offset difficulty with the practical aspects of caring for an ill family member.

Another approach to examining the relationship between family members and an ill relative is the "stress process" model, which describes direct effects, such as increased practical responsibilities, and indirect effects, such as reduced social support. Stress modifiers that are associated with better family health include individual variables, such as a benign appraisal of stressors, positive coping skills and good social support [43]. The quality of the marital relationship is also considered a stress modifier, so that a "good" relationship may moderate the effects of increased stress.

The study of caring for ill relatives has moved from a study of burden to a study of the process of caregiving, including the adaptations that family members make over time.

BIPOLAR ILLNESS AND ITS EFFECTS ON THE FAMILY

The month-to-month symptom change in bipolar illness is striking and different from illnesses characterized by a chronic, deteriorating course. Patients with bipolar disorder may be resistant, hostile, depressed or manic in a relatively short span of time. Family needs may also vary, depending on the polarity of the patient's illness, the role of the patient and family members (e.g. the patient is a child or spouse), and whether it is the first episode (or diagnosis) or represents one of several recurrent episodes.

The specific family experience of caring for relatives with bipolar I disorder has been described by Dore and Romans [13]. Their 2-year study of 41 caregivers reported concerns similar to those reported for all mental illness. In addition, concerns about the acute disruption that occurs with a manic episode—including increased violence, the quality of the marital relationship, and the effect on parenting and children—were more pronounced in families in which one member had a bipolar disorder.

Recent research that views bipolar disorder as a chronic illness has found that the illness imposes a heavy psychosocial burden on family members and contributes to marital/family breakdown [13,44]. Dore and Romans [13] reported that 71% of caregivers of bipolar patients have major stress associated with their caregiving role; 27% felt stress even when the patient was not in episode. Living with uncertainty itself becomes a stressor for family members, who do not know when the patient will become ill again [45]. Studies of families of bipolar patients identified high levels of family burden [16], significant relationship difficulties and increased interpersonal conflict, including the experience or fear of violence [13]. Severity of the burden is associated with prolonged illness and high levels of dysfunction [16]. In a pilot study of family members of patients with chronic, recurring mood disorders (i.e. both unipolar and bipolar patients), 72% of the caregivers reported depressive symptoms [36].

The impact of a relative's illness, however, should not be viewed solely in terms of morbidity or psychiatric symptoms [46]. Outcomes also encompass the family's well-being, functioning or quality of life. Besides marital, parenting and interpersonal problems, other burdens that family members contend with include financial difficulties, social stressors and legal issues [35,47–50]. In addition, many caregivers receive limited information about bipolar disorder and have numerous questions about how they should manage their relative. Common concerns include whether they should accept certain disruptive behaviours or confront these behaviours when they occur, how to separate wilful behaviour from illness-related behaviour, how to deal with noncompliance by the patient, how to recognize prodromal symptoms, and how to get patients to a health facility when they do not want to go.

Bipolar disorder may impact on specific areas of family life. For example, Heru and Ryan [36] reported that family roles and communication were viewed as particularly problematic. Role difficulties can occur when another family member has to assume responsibilities of the patient in addition to meeting his/her own daily tasks or when the patient refuses to relinquish a role that he/she is unable to fulfil. Problems in communication may reflect difficulties with intimacy or closeness when a family member is ill, in addition to the lack of insight and irritability during manic episodes and withdrawal and apathy during depressions, which make it difficult to connect with the patient.

Family members cope better and experience less perceived burden when they understand that their relative's problematic behaviour is caused by illness and not by the patient's wilful misconduct. The concept of burden is also associated with the belief that the patient could control his/her symptoms [35]. Healthier coping strategies for families include problem-focused skill training, positive communication development and increase in social involvement [51].

FAMILY EFFECTS ON THE COURSE OF ILLNESS

Historically, the mental health system has implied that families have somehow "caused" the patient's illness. While the causal association is no longer credible, it is clear that, just as an illness may impact a patient's family, the family environment may affect the course and outcome of a patient's illness [30]. Naturalistic studies of patients hospitalized with major depression provided empirical evidence of an association between family functioning and course of a depressive illness [52] and a significant association between poor family functioning (rated objectively and subjectively) and poorer course of illness [53]. Conversely, better family functioning was one of five factors that increased the odds of a patient recovering from a depressive episode that required hospitalization [54].

Few naturalistic studies have been done with bipolar patients, and fewer include family factors as part of the analysis. An early cross-sectional study comparing families of patients with a variety of psychiatric illnesses found that families with a bipolar relative reported unhealthy functioning in six of seven family dimensions [55]. The EE model, first used with schizophrenic patients, has been applied to bipolar patients as well. EE, a measure of critical, hostile or emotionally overinvolved attitudes towards a psychiatrically ill relative, predicted relapse rates in schizophrenic, unipolar and bipolar patients [56]. Perlick *et al.* [48] argued that family burden had an effect even when patients had relatively low symptom levels and that caregiver/family burden predicted subsequent adverse clinical outcomes among patients with bipolar disorder.

Bipolar illness may be associated with increased interpersonal problems [49] or it may be that practical difficulties and emotional strains experienced by the family may have an adverse effect on both the patient and family members [48]. Families may hinder a patient's recovery by pressuring the patient to resume premorbid responsibilities prematurely, particularly if the patient's illness includes a lengthy hospital stay, convalescence or absence from work. Family members' fear and anxiety may exacerbate the patient's unease, and role, social, marital and sexual functioning may be disrupted [57].

The family may also positively contribute to the patient's outcome by assisting with medication and treatment compliance, monitoring the illness and side effects, and help with logistical issues of transportation and making/keeping appointments, sharing role responsibilities, and promoting better diet and exercise [30,57,58]. In addition, family members, as well as the patient, may be able to identify and recognize prodromal and residual symptoms.

In a collaborative study between two university-affiliated psychiatric hospitals, 74 outpatients with bipolar I disorder were asked to record prodromal and residual symptoms for previous episodes of mania and major depression. An adult family member provided similar information about his/her relative in 45 of these cases [58]. Patients and their family member were able to identify both prodromal and residual symptoms. Agreement between patient and family members on reported symptoms was strong for the prodromal phase of both polarities, but less so for the residual phases. Patients and family members reported more prodromal symptoms than residual symptoms, but more than half of the patients experienced both manic and depressive residual symptoms.

TREATMENT OUTCOME STUDIES

The literature highlighting the important role that social factors, particularly interpersonal and family ones, play in the outcome of bipolar disorder is quite extensive. Studies testing the hypothesis that family interventions may actually modify the social variables in such a way as to positively impact the bipolar illness are much fewer and more recent. There are several reasons for the limited number of treatment outcome studies that are available for review. Family therapy is not currently in fashion, so that few investigators are drawn to test its effectiveness. Family therapists tend not to be oriented towards empirical validation of their treatment methods and researchers tend to be drawn to more manualized psychotherapies.

There are additional problems in studying treatment effects for patients with bipolar disorder. Bipolar disorder is a relapsing, remitting illness with an unpredictable course of episode duration and frequency. Definitions of response to treatment (e.g. low symptom levels for 2 consecutive months) have to be reconsidered, as patients can be doing well for intermittent time periods but still have an unfavourable course over the long term. As in pharmacotherapy, dose and duration of treatment may be important factors that influence outcome. Some family treatments consist of 6–8 sessions over the course of 2–6 months, while others provide 25 or more sessions over a 1-year period. The timing of the adjunctive family interventions also vary. Some therapists start the family treatment during an acute hospitalization, some shortly after discharge but still during the acute episode, while others introduce family meetings only when the patient has been stabilized.

Psychometrically validated measures of family functioning are few, as are family therapy techniques that are operationalized enough so as to be empirically testable. Finally, treatment outcome studies, especially those testing psychotherapies in conjunction with pharmacotherapy, are difficult to design and implement, in addition to being very expensive. Few research groups are able to take on the challenge of surmounting these obstacles in order to provide sound data to test the usefulness of family treatments in bipolar disorder.

While having many commonalities, different family interventions have different features. Some studies use co-therapists, others only one therapist. Some family therapies are provided in a multi-family group format. Some are provided in the patient's home. There is also wide variability in the training and experience of the family therapists conducting the treatments. In spite of these limitations, the studies that have been reported suggest that adjunctive family interventions are useful in modifying family functioning and the course of bipolar disorder.

One of the earliest descriptions of the importance of including other family members in the treatment of manic patients was provided by Fitzgerald

[59]. He described the family dynamics of 25 manic patients, of whom 12 were seen on a regular basis with one or more family members. No systematic data was collected. Fitzgerald's clinical impression was that family therapy was helpful in improving communications within the family and understanding of the illness, with the consequence of promoting compliance with lithium.

Following up on this clinical lead, Davenport et al. [60] compared three groups of bipolar patients discharged after hospitalization at the National Institute of Mental Health and followed for a mean of 3.9 years. Eleven patients (when euthymic) and their spouses received group couples therapy in addition to medication management. They were compared to 11 bipolar patients followed monthly for pharmacotherapy and 42 bipolar patients treated as usual in their community, where they received mainly pharmacotherapy. The patients receiving the additional group couples therapy did not have any rehospitalizations, marital failures or suicides, in contrast to the other groups. They also reported better social and family functioning. The interpretation of these findings, however, was confounded by significant pretreatment differences in the three groups, with the couples therapy group being older and married for a longer time.

The first systematic randomized clinical trial of adjunctive family therapy, conducted by Glick and his colleagues at the Paine Whitney Clinic in New York [61], randomly assigned 169 inpatients and their families to treatment as usual or additional inpatient family intervention (IFI). Of these patients, 21 had a DSM-III diagnosis of bipolar disorder (13 manic, 7 depressed and 1 mixed). The other patients had schizophrenia, unipolar depression or substance abuse. The bipolar patients were predominantly female, white and single, with a mean age of 32; 12 received IFI and 9 the comparison treatment. The family intervention (mean of 8.6 sessions) was undertaken during the patient's inpatient stay (mean 51.1 days). The goals of the IFI were to help the patient/family accept the reality of the illness, identify possible precipitating stresses and likely future stresses, develop coping strategies to manage these stresses and accept the need for continued follow-up treatment [62]. Although there were no differences between the family treatment and comparison groups on length of hospital stay or the amount of medications received, the treatment group did spend more hours with therapists per week.

Outcome measures included symptoms, social role functions, global function and family attitudes at 6- and 18-month follow-up periods. Family treatment was associated with better global symptomatic outcome and role functioning at both 6 and 18 months for female but not male bipolar patients. Bipolar families receiving IFI also reported a more positive attitude towards the patient and less feelings of burden [63]. IFI was beneficial mainly for female bipolar patients and their families. It had a negative effect on unipolar patients and was not particularly helpful to male bipolar patients. The reasons for these differential effects were not clear from the study. Outcome was not associated with medication compliance but was associated with psychosocial treatment compliance and lessened rejection of the patient by other family members. IFI also did not lead to a lower rate of rehospitalization [64].

Retzer et al. [65] conducted an uncontrolled study of adjunctive systemic family therapy for 20 bipolar men and women with a mean age of 31. These outpatients received approximately 6 family sessions over a mean of 14 months. Outcome measures included rehospitalization rates, medication usage and systemic family functioning. They found that family therapy reduced rehospitalization rates by 68% from their historic hospitalization pattern. They also noted that patients were less likely to be prescribed medications or combinations of medications over the course of follow-up. The authors attributed these changes to families learning to change their thinking patterns from "either/or" to "both-and" logic and for the patient from being a "victim" to an "agent" with a greater sense of autonomy. Because there was no control group in this study, it is not possible to know to what the changes noted were related.

Over time family interventions have been modified to include greater amounts of education about bipolar illness as one way to modify attitudes and decrease critical and unaccepting behaviours shown to increase the likelihood of relapse [56].

Van Gent and Zwart [66] provided 5 structured psychoeducational group sessions to the partners of 14 bipolar manic patients and compared them to 12 treatment-as-usual controls. The partners of the patients were randomly assigned to the two groups. The therapy sessions were aimed at increasing the partner's knowledge of the disease, medications and coping strategies. Outcome measures included knowledge of the illness, relationship variables, symptoms and compliance. The intervention did increase knowledge of the illness and its treatment. However, there was no change in patient and partner interactions. The intervention also did not lead to symptomatic change. There was no difference in compliance or in readmission rates between the two groups over the follow-up year.

Honig et al. [67] studied the effects of a 6-session, 2-hour multi-family psychoeducational intervention given at 2-week intervals. Their goal was to modify EE in the families in order to improve the course of bipolar disorder. A total of 19 couples participated in the groups and were compared to 18 couples on a waiting list. Outcome was defined as changes in family EE ratings. They found that EE ratings in families were quite stable and resistant to change: 75% of the EE ratings stayed the same in both groups. Four relatives (21%) in the treatment groups did change from high to low EE status, while none of the relatives in the control group did. Consistent with other studies, high EE status in relatives was associated with more decompensations and rehospitalizations.

Following a similar theme, Clarkin *et al.* [68] evaluated the relative benefit of adding a marital psychoeducational intervention to standard medication treatment for married patients with bipolar disorder. In their study, 46 inpatients, outpatients and their spouses were randomly assigned to adjunctive 25-session marital intervention ($n = 19$) or medications only ($n = 23$) (4 patients dropped out). The polarity at the intake episode was not noted. Outcome measures included symptoms, social functioning and medication adherence at baseline and 11-month follow-up. Medication adherence was good in both groups, but significantly better in the experimental group. There was no effect of the marital treatment on patient symptoms. Social and global functioning did improve significantly more in the experimental group than in the control group.

Based on findings on the effectiveness of family intervention in reducing levels of criticism in families of schizophrenic patients and thereby forestalling relapse of the illness, Miklowitz and colleagues conducted a series of studies to explore if a similar approach would work as well in patients with bipolar disorder. Family focused therapy (FFT) was developed by Miklowitz and Goldstein to provide education about bipolar disorder, communication training and problem-solving skills training, with the expectation that this would positively impact the course of bipolar disorder. In a non-randomized pilot study, they found that acutely ill bipolar patients who received pharmacotherapy and a 9-month outpatient programme of FFT had lower 9-month relapse rates (1 of 9 patients) than historical comparison patients (14 of 23 patients) who received pharmacotherapy alone [69].

Miklowitz *et al.* [70] proceeded to undertake a randomized controlled trial of FFT in 101 inpatients or outpatients with bipolar disorder. Patients were assigned to 21 sessions of FFT ($n = 31$) over 9 months or to a comparison treatment of two family education sessions and crisis management (CM) ($n = 70$). Both groups received similar levels of pharmacotherapy. The family intervention was conducted by two therapists in the families' homes. Outcome measures included relapse status, symptom severity and medication compliance. Patients receiving FFT had a significantly higher one-year survival rate (71%) than those receiving CM (47%). FFT was particularly effective in preventing depressive but not manic relapses. Patients in the FFT group also showed greater improvement in depressive symptoms but not manic symptoms. There was no difference between the groups on treatment compliance. In this study, high EE family attitudes were only noted in patients with parental relatives. The greatest improvement with FFT was in patients with the highest depression scores in high EE families.

In an attempt to understand mediators of change in families receiving FFT, Simoneau et al. [71] assessed changes in face-to-face interactional behaviour in the FFT groups ($n = 22$) and the CM group ($n = 22$). Members of families who received the FFT showed more positive nonverbal (but not verbal) interactional behaviour during a one-year post-treatment problem-solving assessment, without showing a corresponding decrease in negative interactional behaviours.

The results of these FFT trials did not take into account the fact that FFT and CM were not matched on number of therapist contact hours, with the FFT designed to provide more therapy time. In order to correct for this limitation, Rea et al. [50] evaluated the effects of FFT and pharmacotherapy ($n = 28$) against an individually focused patient treatment ($n = 25$) in a randomized design matched for number of therapy contacts. The individual treatment included education, case management and problem-solving training, in addition to standard pharmacotherapy. Outcome measures included relapse and rehospitalization rates over one year and measures of compliance. Subjects were recently hospitalized bipolar manic patients. Compliance rates were high and comparable in both treatment groups. The probability of having a relapse to a mood episode was no different between the two groups over the 1-year treatment and 1-year follow-up. Patients in the FFT (28%), however, had fewer relapses during that time period than those in the CM group (60%). Most significantly, patients in the FFT group had a significantly lower rate of rehospitalization (12%) than the CM group (60%). The family intervention had its greatest impact in assisting patients and their families to avoid the need for rehospitalization during sympto-matic deterioration.

Instead of comparing potentially competing models of family or indivi-dual treatments, Miklowitz et al. [72] presented preliminary data on adjunctive integrated family and individual therapy (IFIT) with mood stabilizing pharmacotherapy in 30 bipolar depressed and manic patients in an open design and in comparison to historical CM treatment. Patients received 25 sessions each of FFT and interpersonal and social rhythm therapy (IPSRT). IPSRT focused on interpersonal problems, identifying triggers for social rhythm disruptions, stabilization of daily routines and relapse pre-vention. Patients receiving IFIT had significantly longer survival intervals (time without relapsing) than those receiving CM (42.5 versus 34.5 weeks). Both treatment groups showed symptomatic improvement, but patients in the IFIT group showed greater reduction in depressive symptoms over 1 year with the treatment than those in the CM group.

A recent randomized study evaluated the effectiveness of a multi-family group (excluding the patient) psychoeducational programme ($n = 30$) on reducing caregiver burden in relatives of bipolar patients. Reinares et al. [73] provided 12 psychoeducational 90-minute weekly group sessions focusing on information about the illness, its management, family interaction and coping skills. The intervention was provided when the patient was in remission. The comparison group ($n = 15$) received treatment as usual. As expected, the relatives in the experimental group improved their knowledge about bipolar disorder. Importantly, caregivers receiving the additional educational groups blamed the patient less for his/her illness and felt less subjective burden in their caretaking role. There were no changes in objective measures of family burden. The intervention did not change the family environment (cohesion, expressiveness and conflict), although, as the study was conducted when the patient was euthymic, there may have been less family dysfunction than if the patient had been in an episode.

Another family therapy system that has been investigated in the treatment of bipolar disorder is the McMaster model of family functioning and the problem centred systems therapy of the family (PCSTF) [74]. The PCSTF [29] emphasizes active collaboration between the therapist and family members, with a focus on the families' responsibility for change, and on problem-solving skills, behavioural change and open and direct communications with and within the family.

A total of 92 bipolar patients (manic, depressed and mixed) were randomly assigned to three treatment conditions: pharmacotherapy alone (P) ($n = 29$), pharmacotherapy plus family therapy (P+FT) ($n = 33$) using the PCSTF, and pharmacotherapy plus a multi-family psychoeducational group intervention (P+MFGT) ($n = 30$). The multi-family group treatment [75] consisted of 4–6 families (including the patient) who met for 6 sessions with co-therapists, focusing on education about the illness and its treatment, coping strategies and mutual support. The mean number of family therapy sessions was 12 and the number of multi-family group sessions was 6. Outcome measures included symptomatic change, recovery status and family functioning. The proportion of subjects within each treatment group who recovered did not differ significantly (P = 55%, P+FT = 48%, P+MFGT = 70%). Time to recovery also did not differ between the groups (7–10 months) [76]. There was no main effect for polarity or severity of the index episode or level of family functioning as risk factors for recovery [77]. Males who were manic and married at intake were more likely to respond than males who were depressed and single. In contrast, there was no difference in response of females by polarity or marital status at index episode.

Family therapy was related to significant improvement in family functioning, while not related to recovery. Bipolar patients with good or poor family functioning at index episode improved their family functioning significantly by the 28th month of follow-up. Improvement in family functioning was not related to symptomatic improvement, but to receiving family treatment [75].

CONCLUSIONS

Bipolar disorder causes significant burden to families. Family needs vary, depending on the polarity of the illness, the role of the patient and family members, and whether it is the first episode or one of several recurrent episodes. Family members cope better and experience less burden when they understand that their relative's problematic behaviour is caused by the disorder and not by his/her wilful misconduct. The family may positively contribute to the patient's outcome by assisting with treatment compliance and help identify and recognize prodromal and residual symptoms.

The research outcome literature on the effectiveness of family interventions in the management of bipolar disorder is at an early stage of development. Significant and meaningful strides have been made. A number of questions, however, still need resolution in future studies. It is still not clear, for instance, whether family interventions are more effective for the manic or depressive phase of the illness. Should family intervention be started during the acute phase of the disorder or should the treatments be delivered once the patient is in remission? Should families be met with singly or in a multi-family group format? Should the patient always be included? Should the family meetings be held in a clinic or in the patient's home? Should there be one or more therapists conducting the family interventions? What is the optimal number of sessions in terms of effectiveness or economic feasibility? These are some of the issues that will hopefully be clarified over time with well-designed studies.

In the interim, it is clear that family interventions, while perhaps not impacting significantly on patient's symptomatic status, do make a significant difference for families. Family interventions clearly improve the families' knowledge and understanding of the illness. They lead to a lack of sense of isolation by the family and a decrease in their perception of illness burden. Family interventions lead to a better connection with the family to the patient's treatment and are helpful in delaying and/or reducing relapses and the need for rehospitalizations.

In spite of some differences in family approaches to the management of bipolar disorder, there are many more commonalities. All family interventions encourage active collaboration between the therapist and the families. They emphasize education about the illness and the available treatments. The interventions focus on improving problem-solving skills and communications and in decreasing levels of criticism within the family. They help to develop and improve coping skills by the family to deal with prodromal and residual symptoms and to develop strategies for dealing with relapses. Finally, they all provide support to buffer the perturbation that patients and families experience with the fluctuating course of bipolar disorder.

REFERENCES

1. Weissman M.M., Bland R.C., Canino G.J. (1996) Cross-national epidemiology of major depression and bipolar disorder. *JAMA*, **276**, 293–299.
2. Woods S.W. (2000) The economic burden of bipolar disease. *J. Clin. Psychiatry*, **61**, 38–41.
3. Newman C.F., Leahy R.L., Beck A.T., Reilly-Harrington N.A., Gyulai L. (2002) *Bipolar Disorder: A Cognitive Therapy Approach*. American Psychological Association, Washington, DC.
4. Goodwin F.K., Jamison K.R. (1990) *Manic–Depressive Illness*. Oxford University Press, New York.
5. Akiskal H.S. (2003) Validating "hard" and "soft" phenotypes within the bipolar spectrum: continuity or discontinuity? *J. Affect. Disord.*, **73**, 1–5.
6. Bourdon K.H., Rae D.S., Narrow W.E., Manderscheid R.W., Regier D.A. (1994) National prevalence and treatment of mental and addictive disorders. In: Manderscheid R.W., Sonnenschein M.A. (eds) *Mental Health Services, United States, 1993*. US Government Printing Office, Washington, DC.
7. Murray C.L., Lopez A.D. (1996) *The Global Burden of Disease*. Harvard University Press, Cambridge, MA.
8. Post R.M., Leverich G.S., Altshuler L.L., Frye M.A., Suppes T.M., Keck J.P.E., Elroy S.L., Kupka R., Nolen W.A., Grunze H., *et al.* (2003) An overview of recent findings of the Stanley Foundation Bipolar Network (Part I). *Bipolar Disord.*, **5**, 310–319.
9. Miller I.W., Keitner G.I., Ryan C.E., Bishop D.S., Keller M.B., Epstein N.B., Stout R., Lavori P. (1997) *Family Treatment of Bipolar Disorder*. National Institute of Mental Health grant R0IMH048171.
10. Ryan C.E., Keitner G.I., Kelley J., Solomon D.A., Miller I.W. (2003) Response to treatment in patients with severe bipolar disorder: gender, polarity, and social support. Presented at the Meeting of the American Psychiatric Association, San Francisco, CA, 17–22 May.
11. Judd L.J., Akiskal H.S., Schettler P.J., Endicott J., Solomon D.A., Lean A.C., Rice J.A., Keller M.B. (2002) The long-term natural history of the weekly symptomatic states of bipolar I disorder. *Arch. Gen. Psychiatry*, **59**, 530–537.
12. Angst J. (1988) Clinical course of affective disorder. In: Helgason T., Daly R.J. (eds) *Depressive Illness: Prediction of Course and Outcome*. Springer-Verlag, New York, pp. 1–44.
13. Dore G., Romans S.E. (2001) Impact of bipolar affective disorder on family and partners. *J. Affect. Disord.*, **67**, 147–158.
14. Robinson B.C. (1983) Validation of a caregiver strain index. *J. Gerontol.*, **38**, 346–348.
15. Lebowitz B.D., Light E. (1996) The aging caregivers of psychiatric patients: healthcare perspectives. *Psychiatr. Ann.*, **26**, 785–791.
16. Chakrabarti S., Kulhara P., Verma S.K. (1992) Extent and determinants of burden among families of patients with affective disorders. *Acta Psychiatr. Scand.*, **86**, 247–252.
17. Hoenig J., Hamilton M.W. (1996) The schizophrenic patient in the community and his effects on the household. *Int. J. Soc. Psychiatry*, **12**, 165–176.
18. Baronet A.M. (1999) Factors associated with caregiver burden in mental illness: a critical review of the research literature. *Clin. Psychol. Rev.*, **19**, 819–841.
19. Lefley H.P. (1996) *Family Caregiving in Mental Illness*. Sage, Thousand Oaks, CA.
20. Johnson E.D. (2000) Differences among families coping with serious mental illness: a qualitative analysis. *Am. J. Orthopsychiatry*, **70**, 126–134.

21. McCubbin H.I., Patterson J.M. (1983) Family stress and adaptation to crisis: a double ABCX model of family behavior. In: Olsen D.H., Miller B.C. (eds) *Family Studies Review Yearbook*. Sage, Beverly Hills, CA, pp. 87–106.

22. Lazarus R.S., Folkman S (1984) *Stress, Appraisal, and Coping*. Springer-Verlag, New York.

23. Pearlin L.I., Schooler C. (1978) The structure of coping. *J. Health Soc. Behav.*, **19**, 2–21.

24. Pearlin L.I., Lieberman M.A., Menaghan E.G., Mullan J.T. (1981) The stress process. *J. Health Soc. Behav.*, **22**, 337–356.

25. Vaughn C.E., Leff J.P. (1976) The influence of family and social factors on the course of psychiatric illness (a comparison of schizophrenic and depressed neurotic patients). *Br. J. Psychiatry*, **129**, 125–137.

26. Brown G.W., Birley J.L.T., Wing J.K. (1972) Influence of family life on the course of schizophrenic disorders: a replication. *Br. J. Psychiatry*, **121**, 241–258.

27. Aneshensel C.S., Stone J.D. (1982) Stress and depression; a test of the buffering model of social support. *Arch. Gen. Psychiatry*, **39**, 1392–1396.

28. Brugha T.S. (1995) Social support and psychiatric disorder: overview of the evidence. In: Brugha T.S. (ed.) *Social Support and Psychiatric Disorder: Research Findings and Guidelines for Clinical Practice*. Cambridge University Press, Cambridge.

29. Epstein N.B., Bishop D.S., Levin S. (1978) The McMaster model of family functioning. *J. Marriage Fam. Counsel.*, **4**, 19–31.

30. Keitner G.I., Miller I.W. (1990) Family functioning and major depression: an overview. *Am. J. Psychiatry*, **147**, 1128–1137.

31. Rose L., Mallinson R.K., Walton-Moss B. (2002) A grounded theory of families responding to mental illness. *Western J. Nurs. Res.*, **24**, 516–536.

32. Karp D.A., Tanarugsachock V. (2000) Mental illness, caregiving, and emotion management. *Qual. Health Res.*, **10**, 6–25.

33. Heru A. (2000) Family functioning, burden and reward in the caregiving for chronic mental illness. *Fam. Syst. Health*, **18**, 91–103.

34. Marsh D.T., Johnson D.L. (1997) The family experience of mental illness: implications for intervention. *Prof. Psychol. Res. Pract.*, **28**, 229–237.

35. Perlick D., Clarkin J.F., Sirey J., Raue P., Greenfield S., Struening E., Rosenheck R. (1999) Burden experienced by caregivers of persons with bipolar affective disorder. *Br. J. Psychiatry*, **174**, 56–62.

36. Heru A., Ryan C.E. (2002) Depressive symptoms and family functioning in the caregivers of recently hospitalized patients with chronic/recurrent mood disorders. *Int. J. Psychosoc. Rehabil.*, **7**, 53–60.

37. Noh S., Avison W.R. (1988) Spouses of discharged patients: factors associated with their experience of burden. *J. Marriage Fam.*, **50**, 377–389.

38. Thompson E., Doll W. (1982) The burden of families coping with the mentally ill: an invisible crisis. *Fam. Relat.*, **31**, 379–388.

39. Patterson T.L., Semple S.J., Shaw W.S. (1990) Researching the caregiver: family members who care for older psychotic patients. *Psychiatr. Ann.*, **12**, 722–784.

40. Luthar S., Cicchetti D., Becker B. (2000) The construct of resilience: a critical evaluation and guidelines for future work. *Child Develop.*, **71**, 543–562.

41. Rutter M. (1987) Psychosocial resilience and protective mechanisms. *Am. J. Orthopsychiatry*, **57**, 316–331.

42. Walsh F. (2003) Family resilience: a framework for clinical practice. *Fam. Process*, **42**, 1–18.

43. Goode K.T., Haley W.E., Roth D.L., Ford G.R. (1998) Predicting longitudinal changes in caregiver physical and mental health. A stress model. *Health Psychol.*, **17**, 190–198.
44. Honig A., Hofman A., Rozendaal N., Dingemans P. (1997) Psychoeducation in bipolar disorder: effects on expressed emotion. *Psychiatry Res.*, **72**, 17–22.
45. Corring D. (2002) Quality of life: perspectives of people with mental illness and family members. *Psychiatr. Rehabil. J.*, **25**, 350–359.
46. Szmukler G.I., Burgess P., Herman H., Benson A., Colusa S., Bloch S. (1996) Caring for relatives with serious mental illness: the development of the experience of caregiving inventory. *Soc. Psychiatry Psychiatr. Epidemiol.*, **31**, 137–168.
47. Schultz R., Visintainer P., Williamson G.M. (1990) Psychiatric and physical morbidity effects of caregiving. *J. Gerontol.*, **45**, 181–191.
48. Perlick D.A., Rosenhack R.R., Clarkin J.F., Rave P., Sirey J. (2001) Impact of family burden and patient symptom status on clinical outcome in bipolar affective disorder. *J. Nerv. Ment. Dis.*, **189**, 31–37.
49. Hirschfield R.M.A., Calabrese J.R., Weissman M.M., Reed M., Davies M.A., Frye M.A., Keck P.E., Lewis L., McElroy S.L., McNulty J.P., et al. (2003) Screening for bipolar disorder in the community. *J. Clin. Psychiatry.*, **64**, 53–59.
50. Rea M.M., Tompson M.C., Miklowitz F.J., Goldstein M.J., Hwang S., Mintz J. (2003) Family-focused treatment versus individual treatment for bipolar disorder: results of a randomized clinical trial. *J. Consult. Clin. Psychol.*, **71**, 482–492.
51. Chakrabarti S., Gill S. (2002) Coping and its correlates among caregivers of patients with bipolar disorder: a preliminary study. *Bipolar Disord.*, **4**, 50–60.
52. Keitner G.I., Miller I.W., Epstein N.B., Bishop D.S., Fruzzetti A.E. (1987) Family functioning and the course of major depression. *Compr. Psychiatry*, **28**, 54–64.
53. Miller I.W., Keitner G.I., Whisman M.A., Ryan C.E., Epstein N.B., Bishop D.S. (1992) Depressed patients with dysfunctional families: description and course of illness. *J. Abnorm. Psychol.*, **101**, 637–646.
54. Keitner G.I., Ryan C.E., Miller I.W., Norman W.H. (1992) Recovery and major depression: factors associated with 12-month outcome. *Am. J. Psychiatry*, **149**, 93–99.
55. Miller I.W., Kabacoff R.I., Keitner G.I., Epstein N.B., Bishop D.S. (1986) Family functioning in the families of psychiatric patients. *Compr. Psychiatry*, **27**, 302–312.
56. Butzlaff R.L., Hooley J. (1998) Expressed emotion and psychiatric relapse. *Arch. Gen. Psychiatry*, **55**, 547–552.
57. Ryan C.E. (2002) Clinical and research issues in the evaluation and treatment of families. *Med. Health R. I.*, **85**, 278–280.
58. Keitner G., Solomon D.A., Ryan C.E., Miller I.W., Mallinger A., Kupfer D.J., Frank E. (1996) Prodromal and residual symptoms in bipolar I disorder. *Compr. Psychiatry*, **37**, 362–367.
59. Fitzgerald R.G. (1972) Mania as a message: treatment with family therapy and lithium carbonate. *Am. J. Psychother.*, **26**, 547–553.
60. Davenport Y., Ebert M., Adland M., Goodwin F. (1977) Couples group therapy: an adjunct to lithium maintenance of the manic patient. *Am. J. Orthopsychiatry*, **47**, 495–502.
61. Glick I.D., Clarkin J.F., Spencer J.H., Haas G.L., Lewis A.B., Peyser J., DeMane N., Good-Ellis M., Harris E., Lestelle V. (1985) A controlled evaluation of inpatient family intervention. *Arch. Gen. Psychiatry*, **42**, 882–886.

62. Haas G., Glick I., Clarkin J., Spencer J., Lewis A., Peyser J., DeMane N., Good-Ellis M., Harris E., Lestelle V. (1988) Inpatient family intervention: a randomized clinical trial, II: Results at hospital discharge. *Arch. Gen. Psychiatry*, **45**, 217–224.

63. Clarkin J.F., Glick I.D., Haas G.L., Spencer J.H., Lewis A.B., Peyser J., DeMane N., Good-Ellis M., Harris E., Lestelle V. (1990) A randomized clinical trial of inpatient family intervention. *J. Affect. Dis.*, **18**, 17–28.

64. Glick I.D., Clarkin J.F., Haas G.L., Spencer J.H., Chen C.L. (1991) A randomized clinical trial of inpatient family intervention: VI. Mediating variables and outcome. *Fam. Process*, **30**, 85–99.

65. Retzer A., Simon F.B., Weber G., Stierlin H., Schmidt G. (1991) A followup study of manic–depressive and schizoaffective psychoses after systemic family therapy. *Fam. Process*, **30**, 139–153.

66. VanGent E.M., Zwart F.M. (1991) Psychoeducation of partners of bipolar–manic patients. *J. Affect. Disord.*, **129**, 125–137.

67. Honig A., Hofman A., Hilwig M., Noorthoorn E., Ponds R. (1995) Psychoeducation and expressed emotion in bipolar disorder: preliminary findings. *Psychiatry Res.*, **56**, 299–301.

68. Clarkin J.F., Carpenter D., Hull J., Wilner P., Glick I. (1998) Effects of psychoeducational intervention for married patients with bipolar and their spouses. *Psychiatr. Serv.*, **49**, 531–533.

69. Miklowitz D., Goldstein M. (1990) Behavioral family treatment for patients with bipolar affective disorder. *Behav. Modif.*, **14**, 457–489.

70. Miklowitz D.J., Simoneau T.L., George E.L., Richards J.A., Kalbag A., Sachs-Ericsson N., Suddath R. (2000) Family-focused treatment of bipolar disorder: 1-year effects of a psychoeducational program in conjunction with pharmacotherapy. *Biol. Psychiatry*, **8**, 582–592.

71. Simoneau T.L., Miklowitz D.J., Richards J.A., Saleem R., George E. (1999) Bipolar disorder and family communication: effects of a psychoeducational treatment program. *J. Abnorm. Psychol.*, **108**, 588–597.

72. Miklowitz D.J., Richards J.A., Frank E., Suddath R.L., Powell K.B., Sacher J.A. (2003) Integrated family and individual therapy for bipolar disorder: results of a treatment development study. *J. Clin. Psychiatry*, **64**, 182–191.

73. Reinares M., Vieta E., Colom F., Martinez-Aran A., Torrent C., Comes M., Goikolea J.M., Benabarre A., Sanchez-Moreno J. (2004) Impact of a psychoeducational family intervention on caregivers of stabilized bipolar patients. *Psychother. Psychosom.*, **73**, 312–319.

74. Ryan C.E., Epstein N.B., Keitner G.I., Miller I.W., Bishop D.S. (in press) *Evaluating and Treating Families. The McMaster Approach.* Brunner/Mazel, New York.

75. Keitner G.I., Ryan C.E., Solomon D.A., Kelley J.E., Miller I.W. (2003) Family therapy and family functioning in patients with mood disorders. Presented at the Meeting of the American Psychiatric Association, San Francisco, CA, 17–22 May.

76. Miller I.W., Canino G.J. (in press) Does adjunctive family therapy enhance recovery from bipolar I mood episodes? *J. Affect. Disord.*

77. Keitner G.I., Solomon D.A., Ryan C.E., Kelley J.E., Miller I.W. (2003) Recovery from acute mood episodes of bipolar I disorder. Presented at the 34th Annual Meeting of the Society for Psychotherapy Research, Weimar, 23–27 June.

5

Families of People with a Severe Anxiety Disorder

Gail Steketee and Jason Fogler

Boston University School of Social Work, Boston, Massachusetts, USA

INTRODUCTION

Anxiety disorders rank among the most prevalent mental illnesses [1,2]. Disorders in this taxon range from the highly circumscribed specific phobias, in which people can lead relatively normal lives by avoiding a single feared object or situation [3], to disorders marked by pervasive and chronic impairment. In this chapter, we discuss the effects on families of two of the most severe anxiety disorders, panic disorder with agoraphobia (PDA) and obsessive–compulsive disorder (OCD). In particular, we describe the family constellations of people with PDA and OCD, focusing on the quality of these patients' marriages, as well as addressing the role of heredity and family environment in the aetiology of these disorders. We then address family factors found to predict treatment outcome for PDA and OCD, especially relatives' expressed emotion and patients' perceived sensitivity to relatives' criticism. We conclude with a discussion of the available family-focused treatments for PDA and OCD and offer recommendations for future directions in research and treatment.

PANIC DISORDER WITH AGORAPHOBIA

PDA is perhaps best characterized as a "fear of fear", in which people worry about the recurrence, and perceived catastrophic consequences, of panic attacks. This leads to avoidance of situations and places "from which escape might be difficult (or embarrassing) or in which help may not be available in the event of having an unexpected or situationally predisposed panic attack or panic-like symptoms" [1]. A panic attack is the sudden and intense experience (i.e. abrupt onset with symptoms peaking within 10 minutes) of

Families and Mental Disorders. Edited by Norman Sartorius, Julian Leff, Juan José López-Ibor, Mario Maj and Ahmed Okasha. © 2005 John Wiley & Sons Ltd. ISBN 0-470-02382-1

four or more of the following symptoms: palpitations, pounding heart or accelerated heart rate; sweating; trembling or shaking; sensations of shortness of breath or smothering; feeling of choking; chest pain or discomfort; nausea or abdominal distress; feeling dizzy, light-headed, unsteady or faint; derealization (feelings of unreality) or depersonalization (being detached from oneself); fear of losing control or going crazy; fear of dying; paraesthesias (numbness or tingling sensations); chills or hot flushes [1]. Panic attacks may be "unexpected" or "situationally predisposed", that is triggered by specific environmental cues.

Avoided activities may include enclosed or wide-open spaces, driving, travelling over bridges, being in crowds, shopping malls, grocery stores, theatres and places of worship. White and Barlow [4] identify a second cluster of avoided activities likely to produce physical sensations similar to panic-like symptoms. Such interoceptive avoidance includes ingesting substances (e.g. caffeine, alcohol), participating in activities (e.g. intense exercise, sexual relations) or entering certain environments (e.g. saunas or hot, stuffy rooms).

One 28-year-old woman had developed panic attacks during her teens and gradually restricted her activities to all but essential travel in order to get to work or engage in other activities she considered essential (e.g. doctor's appointments). She had carefully mapped out her driving routes so she knew where hospital emergency rooms were located in case she needed assistance. She feared having a heart attack or stroke as a result of panic sensations that included racing heart, pressure in her chest and feeling light-headed. She was also concerned that she might be "going crazy" and need to be put in a mental institution, mainly in response to feelings of depersonalization that accompanied feeling faint (most likely due to hyperventilation when she felt these disturbing sensations). She was able to drive for durations of about 1 hour if her boyfriend drove with her, but she could not fly or take public transportation even if he was with her. He often accompanied her on weekend errands or to social events with friends to enable her to attend. Generally, he was supportive, but increasingly frustrated with her restrictions that prevented their taking vacations together or visiting distant friends and family.

OBSESSIVE–COMPULSIVE DISORDER

If PDA is best characterized as a disorder of avoidance, OCD may best be characterized as a disorder of neutralization, the active escape from thoughts or situations that provoke considerable emotional distress. The individual with OCD experiences intrusive thoughts, impulses or images called obsessions. These ideas may be about contamination (e.g. germs, chemicals), making mistakes and causing harm, failure to prevent harm, and having dangerous, immoral or unacceptable thoughts (e.g. image of stabbing someone, idea of being gay, thoughts of molesting children). These unwanted thoughts produce negative emotions such as anxiety, guilt and shame. To stop, prevent or undo these obsessions and relieve the associated discomfort, people enact repetitive behaviours (compulsions), such as washing or checking, or mental acts, such as counting, repeating words or images to oneself or praying. Failing to neutralize the obsession or complete the compulsion brings intense anxiety, often because of imagined disastrous outcomes. Closely related is the concept of thought–action fusion [5], that the consequences of thinking something are the same as actually doing it. Hence, in OCD, imagined dangers lead to a downward spiral of defensive and maladaptive rituals.

This syndrome is illustrated in a woman who initially reported contamination fears regarding germs and dirt, as well as both washing and checking behaviour to clean "infected" areas and verify that no evidence of the problem remained. This problem resolved during her mid-20s following a course of behavioural treatment in which she was exposed to the source of contamination (public rest rooms, floors, grass etc.) and prevented from washing or cleaning until her anxiety and feeling of contamination reduced. Several years later, at age 37, when her mother died after a lengthy illness, she became obsessed with the idea that "my mother might have been buried alive" and a wish to verify that this was not true. This included seeking reassurance from other family caretakers and the undertakers, and checking her memory repeatedly for details of her mother's death (she had been present with other family members at the time of death). She also experienced contamination from "my mother's essence" and avoided handling many of her mother's personal possessions (purse, lipstick, clothing etc.). Not surprisingly, her sisters were increasingly frustrated at the repetitive questions about their mother's death. Although her husband joked about her anxiety, he was upset when she avoided buying a new mattress he wanted because she had "magically" associated the purchase of a mattress with the mattress on which her mother died.

FAMILY CONSTELLATION AND FAMILY PROBLEMS

Families and Panic Disorder with Agoraphobia

The clinical research literature has nearly exclusively focused on a family constellation in which the identified patient with PDA is a married, Caucasian woman [see 6 for review]. This is not entirely unreasonable, given that the incidence of PDA in women is twice as high as in men [7,8]. Interestingly, one study found that, if anything, women with PDA are more likely to be married (84%) and less likely to be divorced/separated (4%) or "never married" (12%) than a control group of women without psychiatric disorders [9]. However, the Epidemiological Catchment Area Study found a bimodal distribution in the age of onset for PDA—15–24 years and 45–54 years [10]—and rare cases of panic attacks and PDA have been reported in prepubescent children [11–13]. The implications of these findings are that the family constellation of a person with PDA can vary widely, including husbands, wives, boyfriends, girlfriends [see 14], parents of adolescent patients, or teenage and adult children of a parent with PDA. Indeed, anecdotal clinical evidence suggests that it is not uncommon for a parent with PDA to rely on his or her children as "safe persons" in anxiety-triggering situations [14]. Further, with the inclusion of conditions such as *ataque de nervios*, a panic-like syndrome found in Caribbean and Latin American populations [15,16], the interdependent nature of these cultures would greatly expand the range of family constellations that could be targeted for clinical research and intervention (e.g. extended families including aunts, uncles, cousins etc.).

Family and genetic studies indicate an extremely high likelihood that panic disorder (and other anxiety disorders) run in families and will be transmitted from parents to their offspring. Hettema *et al.* [17] concluded from their meta-analysis of family and twin studies that the heritability of panic disorder is 43%, with the remaining variance in liability attributable to non-shared environment effects, such as traumatic events, that are specific to the at-risk child. Biederman *et al.* [18] similarly found an association between parental panic disorder, with or without comorbid major depression, and a 5- to 7-fold increased risk for PDA in offspring. They also found an association between parental depression and increased risk for separation anxiety disorder and ≥2 anxiety diagnoses in offspring. Complicating matters further, having separation anxiety disorder as a child may be associated with additive risk for earlier onset of panic disorder and PDA [19, also see 9]. These findings suggest two possible pathways towards PDA: direct heritability from parents and indirect heritability from depression in parents to separation anxiety in childhood and later development of panic and agoraphobic avoidance. Indeed, Barlow [20] posits that what is inherited in mood and anxiety disorders is a more general "proneness to anxiety" and negative affect rather than a specific "panic gene" per se.

Findings about whether PDA negatively influences ratings of marital satisfaction are equivocal, and many authors contend that there is little empirical evidence supporting the assertion that marriages of people with PDA are essentially different from those of non-psychiatrically-disordered individuals [6,21]. As Carter *et al.* [6] noted, the suggestion that the marriages of agoraphobic women were distressed and that the pathogenic source of their disorder was related to their marriages came from a series of uncontrolled studies [e.g. 22,23], that did not use control samples and arbitrarily identified "good" and "poor" marriages. Buglass et al. [24] were the first to contradict these assumptions by suggesting that marital dissatisfaction is a secondary consequence of PDA onset: husbands and wives of PDA patients described their pre-onset marital relationship very similarly to husbands and wives in a control group. Differences only emerged post-onset. Similarly, Arrindell and Emmelkamp [25] found that their sample of 30 agoraphobic women and their husbands reported significantly higher levels of marital maladjustment than 38 non-distressed couples, but significantly less maladjustment than either 14 matrially distressed couples or 14 women with non-phobic psychiatric disorders and their husbands. In another controlled study, McLeod [26] examined perceived marital satisfaction in couples where neither, one or both members had a diagnosis of panic disorder or PDA. Wives of panic-affected husbands reported significantly greater levels of marital distress, but husbands of panic-disordered wives did not report more marital distress. The implication of these findings is that marriages of patients with PDA are not significantly different from marriages in the general population. They could be affected by any number of factors not necessarily related to mental illness, including pre-onset marital functioning and satisfaction and whether the husband or wife is the identified patient. Gender role expectations may play some role here, in that men with agoraphobic wives may be more tolerant of their wives' functional incapacity and their own need to accompany them out of the home. In contrast, wives may have less tolerance of the comparable situation due to cultural and gender role expectations of men.

Families and Obsessive–Compulsive Disorder

In contrast to patients with PDA, a large proportion of OCD sufferers are single. Only 35% of men with OCD have ever married, compared to 60–75% of women [for review see 27,28], and this difference may in part be due to the earlier onset of OCD in males. In women, OCD typically begins in their early 20s, whereas onset for males commonly occurs in middle adolescence. This earlier age of onset in males can have profound developmental effects that disrupt education, socialization, sexual experience and employment. The implications of these findings are that fewer than half of OCD treatment-seekers could benefit from marital interventions, and approximately 25% of OCD adult patients will still be living with their parents. Indeed, many live with or maintain daily contact with parents or other family members [29].

Studies of transmission of OCD within families indicate a modest tendency for OCD to occur among biological family members. The number of probands with OCD who have immediate family members with this disorder or a syndromal variant is approximately 20–25% of cases [e.g. 30–33]. However, other types of mood and anxiety disorders occur at high rates among family members of patients with OCD [30,34,35]. From a clinical standpoint, these findings mean that most adults who present for treatment for PDA or OCD will have grown up living with parents who themselves have some form of anxiety or depression. However, the limited information available indicates that relatives' depression and anxiety symptoms are not significantly related to patients' OCD symptoms or depression [36]. Some patients with OCD will have grown up in households where parents also had this disorder, and a somewhat higher percentage (30–40%) will have parents with obsessive traits [see 37]. However, when OCD does occur in parents and their children, the symptom patterns are often different [33]. For example, parents who have fears of harming and checking rituals may have children with washing rituals. This finding argues against observational learning as a major mode of transmission of OCD symptoms, though it is still possible that some general attitudes are learned in this way, such as excessive avoidance of danger or perfectionistic tendencies. Much remains to be learned about the relationship of these personality patterns and beliefs to OCD symptoms, although some studies have reported that the parents of those with OCD frequently exhibit such traits [38,39].

Much like the findings about the marriages of patients with PDA, a substantial number (32–50%) of married OCD patients and their spouses report having distressed relationships, but average scores on most marital measures fall in the normative range [e.g., 27,40]. Clinical experience and demographic data from several studies of OCD patients suggest a relatively low divorce rate, as low as 3–5%, for married OCD patients [e.g., 34]. Marital distress was not associated with severity of OCD symptoms or negative mood, but patients who endorsed higher levels of marital distress engaged in more avoidance [41]. Referring to both spousal and parental families, 50% of OCD clinic patients scored in the unhealthy range on one or more aspects of family functioning, including affective responsiveness, roles, family problem solving and behaviour control [42]. However, no significant differences were found between communication in families with an OCD member and normative families.

In sum, many studies indicate that families of patients with severe anxiety disorders such as PDA and OCD have some dysfunction, but it is not clear that the degree of difficulty is substantially different from normative families. When family problems are evident, the causal directionality is unclear: does the anxiety disorder worsen family functioning or does poor family functioning exacerbate PDA and OCD symptoms, or is the relationship reciprocal? Among OCD patients, many will be living alone or with families of origin, rather than with spouses, and this may alter the nature of family intervention. Among both groups, some patients will have grown up with parents who themselves have anxiety problems and this may influence treatment outcome when patients are living with or in close contact with affected parents.

FAMILY EFFECTS ON THE DEVELOPMENT OF ANXIETY DISORDERS

A handful of studies [e.g., 9,43] address the question of how the upbringing of PDA patients may have contributed to the onset of their disorder. Using the Parental Bonding Instrument (PBI), which measures care and over-protection, Wilborg and Dahl [43] found that, compared to a non-psychiatric control group, patients with moderate or severe levels of agoraphobia recalled their parents as exercising low levels of care and high levels of protection. Patients with mild or no agoraphobia were no different from the control group in their reporting on the PBI. Laraia et al. [9] found similar but slightly conflicting results using a battery of self-report measures, but not the PBI, in 80 women with PDA and 100 women without a history of psychiatric disorder. The women with PDA recalled their childhood environments as more conflicted and their parents as less warm and supportive than controls, but there were no significant differences in reported rates of other hypothesized risk factors for PDA, such as parental overprotection, parental death, divorce or sexual mistreatment. While provocative, the retrospective nature of these studies makes it difficult to draw definitive conclusions. Are the cited differences in upbringing real or an artefact of the influence of mental disorder on memory and perception?

In a better-controlled study of attachment to parents, Chambless et al. [44] asked 52 adult OCD and 35 PDA patients and their parents to complete the PBI. Interestingly, but perhaps not surprisingly, clients rated parents more negatively than parents rated themselves, especially for maternal over-protection and paternal care. Parents were most likely to describe their parenting as optimal (46% mothers, 42% fathers), whereas the majority of clients reported that their parents exercised affectionless control (41% of mothers and 43% of fathers). Clients rated mothers and fathers quite similarly on care (high correlation), whereas correlations between mothers' and fathers' ratings approached zero. The clients' global view of their parenting experience suggests that the clients' ratings may have more to do with their perceptions than with their parents' actual behaviours. Clients' ratings of their parents were not related to own mood or other pathology, but poor client social adjustment correlated with low parental care and more overprotection.

In the Chambless *et al.* study [44], mothers' parental bonding, but not fathers', was related to personality traits. Clients who reported lower maternal care displayed more avoidant personality traits, whereas those reporting higher maternal overprotection showed more passive-aggressive traits; both groups had more dependent traits. Overall, these findings suggest that poor parental bonding constitutes a general risk factor for both PDA and OCD. The finding that relationships were more apparent for maternal rather than paternal variables (especially maternal care) is not surprising in a country where mothers are overwhelmingly likely to be the primary caregivers. Overcontrolling parents may undermine the confidence of some offspring, who become dependent, whereas others develop indirect ways to resist control and excessive protection. The findings are in keeping with Bowlby's [45] idea that, without a safe base in the bond with the parent, children become fearful of exploration and have difficulty developing appropriate independence.

Panic Disorder with Agoraphobia

In a highly influential article, Goldstein and Chambless [46] distinguished between "simple" and "complex" agoraphobia. Simple agoraphobia was theorized to arise from physical disorders or drug experiences that engendered physical sensations mistaken for threatening cues. In contrast, the complex variant was hypothesized to be rooted in a pervasively fearful temperament, a "hysterical" tendency to misidentify and misattribute the source of anxiety (e.g. anxiety due to interpersonal conflict is misattributed to fear of crowds or traffic), and dependent personality traits that predisposed a person to adopt and benefit from a sick role. People with simple agoraphobia without personality complications were thought to have a better prognosis, whereas those with the complex form had more persistent symptoms because of the dependent role reinforced by significant others. Carter and Schultz [14] offer the example of an agoraphobic wife who becomes very competent at housework and paying bills, such that her husband depends on her to do these tasks. The non-disordered spouse may become dissatisfied with possible changes in this (albeit dysfunctional) equilibrium during treatment and make conscious and unconscious efforts to return the agoraphobic partner to a less autonomous position.

Similarly, Friedman [47] proposed that patients with PDA elicit polarized behaviour from significant others to maintain their dependent role. He suggested that people with panic disorder viewed relatives as safety signals (soothing companions) or as indifferent or even punitive partners, and that relatives responded similarly, in a polarized manner. That is, they either tried to protect the patient, thereby reinforcing pathology, or they pressured the patient prematurely for independent behaviour that led to more phobic avoidance. In some cases, the relative alternated between the two strategies, fostering a circular push–pull pattern that eventually produced resentment and entrenched panic and avoidance symptoms.

Friedman's observations strongly parallel the Goldstein and Chambless interpersonal theory of PDA, as well as the components of the predictive clinical construct known as expressed emotion (EE) [48]. EE consists of criticism (expressed disapproval of behaviour) and hostility (harsh disapproval or rejection of the person) and emotional overinvolvement (EOI, overprotective or overly doting caretaking behaviour). The criticism and hostility aspects seem consistent with Friedman's observations of family members' premature "pushing" of independent behaviour, whereas EOI resonates with Friedman's clinical observation of permitting regressive and dependent behaviour. Friedman used the phrase "critical overinvolvement" to describe what he saw as the polarized reactions of these family members, evident in the case of an elderly woman with PDA and her reluctant caretaker. The latter confided to the therapist: "...I said damn it, I don't feel good, it's just a loaf of bread, go back, go around the corner. (Shouting) And I am trying to tell her to walk down the block slowly, I'll be there on the stoop... Try to fight it, damn it." Emotionally overinvolved overprotection is captured in this caretaking sister's description of how she hovers over her sister to make sure she gets out of bed, even at the expense of her own physical and mental health ("...I get a tightness here in my chest. I have to take Inderal [propranolol] for my nerves"). The influence of EE on the outcome of treatment for PDA and OCD will be discussed later in this chapter.

Obsessive–Compulsive Disorder

Several researchers have commented on the often extensive family involvement in patients' OCD symptoms [e.g., 42,49]. These clinical observations mimic Friedman's [47] reports about the families of patients with PDA. Cooper [50] surveyed 225 family members of adults with OCD and reported that 75% experienced disruption in their lives because of the OCD, including loss of personal relationships, loss of leisure time and financial problems. Indeed, nearly 75% of OCD relatives participated at least minimally in rituals or avoidance or modified their behaviour to accommodate patients' symptoms [51–53]. Accommodations include providing reassurance (>30%), active participation in rituals and/or avoidance at patient's request (33–60%), taking over patient duties (>33%) and modifying family activities and routines (>35%). These efforts were usually intended to reduce patient distress and time spent on rituals. Not surprisingly, greater family participation was significantly related to family distress [36,51], as well as more rejecting attitudes [52]. According to Calvocoressi et al. [51,52], approximately 40% of family members felt responsible for their relatives' OCD. Like Friedman's clinical observations about PDA families, greater accommodation to OCD symptoms was also related to more family dysfunction, suggesting that family interventions may be needed to address these difficulties.

Studying children and adolescents and their parents, Hibbs et al. [54] concluded that family members of patients with OCD show high levels of EE. Among OCD families, 82% were rated high on EE; this was twice the rate found among control families (41%). The children from high EE families also showed more physiological reactivity than those from low EE families [55]. Similar findings were reported in a community study [56] in which parents of children with separation anxiety disorder (a potential precursor of PDA) had significantly elevated rates of EE, particularly EOI, compared to those of children without psychiatric disorders. Hirshfeld et al. [57] found an interaction between maternal panic disorder, child behavioural inhibition (a risk factor for developing anxiety disorders), number of child anxiety disorders and maternal criticism. Compared to a group of psychiatric controls, these anxious mothers expressed higher rates of critical EE towards children who displayed more behavioural inhibition, regardless of the number of psychiatric disorders the child had. Maternal criticism was also associated with a higher frequency of child disorders, suggesting a transactional relationship between maternal panic, child temperament and disorder, and EE.

EFFECTS OF FAMILIES' INTERACTION ON TREATMENT OUTCOME

Although a number of studies of predictors of immediate and long-term treatment outcome of PDA and OCD symptoms have been conducted, only a handful of these have examined family factors. Below we review this research, mainly for behavioural therapy (BT) or cognitive and behavioural treatments (CBT).

Partner Satisfaction, Partner Inclusion and Treatment Outcome

Carter et al. [6] reviewed nine studies examining the relationship of marital satisfaction to the outcome of women with PDA who received BT or CBT.

Overall, although some studies found that greater marital satisfaction predicted better outcome, no clear relationship was observed, especially for more recent better controlled studies. However, including spouses in treatment was associated with better treatment outcomes [58], with effects maintained at 2-year follow-up [59]. Along similar lines, Arnow *et al.* [60] found that adding a communication skills component to exposure therapy increased treatment gains significantly more than adding a relaxation skills component, again suggesting the importance of addressing family and interpersonal factors in treatment for PDA. Interestingly, no difference was found between using friends versus spouses as co-therapists in treatment [61]. Unfortunately, without a control group treated without a co-therapist, it is difficult to determine whether these findings speak to the more general importance of the PDA patient's social support system beyond the marital dyad or to the possibility that treatment for PDA is not significantly improved by the inclusion of co-therapists. The latter possibility is suggested by studies with null findings for spouse inclusion in treatment [62,63]. However, Carter *et al.* [6] noted that these studies researched behavioural rather than CBT methods, and thus their null findings may be an artefact of using different treatments.

Studies of behaviourally treated adults with OCD have yielded similarly conflicting findings regarding family variables as predictors of outcome. Several researchers have proposed that family support is necessary for clients to benefit from behavioural therapy [64,65], but this is contradicted by other studies. For example, OCD patients from distressed marriages did not fare worse than those from non-distressed marriages [40,41,66]. In fact, marital satisfaction improved after treatment regardless of pretreatment satisfaction, especially with regard to patient's demands and dependency on spouses [41; see also 67]. Thus, BT via exposure and response prevention appears to be good for marriages, and initial marital distress does not seem to impede outcomes for anxiety symptoms. However, these studies of marital distress do not address the question of whether parental or other family support is necessary for non-married patients. The EE literature discussed below covers a wider range of family constellations.

Expressed Emotion

In an early effort to examine family predictors of outcome, Steketee [68] assessed self- and family-reported familial interactions in relation to treatment gains an average of 9 months after BT for patients with OCD. Pretreatment general social support was not a predictor of outcome, but poor social and familial functioning and patient-rated negative household interactions (anger, criticism, relatives' beliefs that the OCD patient was malingering) predicted fewer gains at follow-up. Conversely, positive feelings among household members predicted more improvement. These negative family interaction variables resemble those coded for EE in other patient populations, and this study led to further research on the effects of EE for anxiety disordered patients.

Among the family variables examined as predictors of outcome in other mental disorders, EE appears to be the most studied construct. EE consists of five variables (criticism, hostility, EOI, warmth and positive remarks) coded by trained raters from the Camberwell Family Interview (CFI). The CFI is a semi-structured interview designed to elicit open-ended narrative responses about the identified patient by their relative, which can then be rated for each of the 5 coded responses. Numerous studies have indicated that high EE, defined by above-threshold ratings of criticism, hostility and overinvolvement, is a consistent predictor of relapse for schizophrenia and depression, with findings replicated in many countries [69]. Do EE and related constructs predict outcome for PDA and OCD? Chambless and Steketee [66] examined EE variables as predictors of BT outcome in a mixed sample of 60 OCD patients and 41 agoraphobics with moderate to severe symptoms; 11 patients refused to participate in this study, because relatives refused or the patient was unwilling to include them. Patients received 22 sessions of exposure therapy, with no family involvement in treatment except a brief assessment and education about the planned therapy. Interestingly, the number of critical comments by family members recorded during the CFI ranged widely. The overall mean number was rather high compared to other patient samples, but few relatives displayed hostility (global criticism or rejection of the person rather than his/her behaviour). Most criticisms focused on the patient's chronic sick role (lack of motivation, problematic personal habits, burden to the relative) and on his/her anxiety symptoms [70]. Overall outcomes from the BT were quite good, with substantial reductions in target PDA and OCD symptoms after treatment and at 1-year follow-up.

EOI was associated with more dropout, as was hostility: those with hostile relatives were six times more likely to drop out. Hostility also predicted poor outcome after treatment. The patient's perception of more criticism was a significant predictor of poor outcome at post-test, and also tended to predict follow-up benefit. Interestingly, critical comments by relatives tended to predict better, not worse, outcome, a finding also reported by Peter and Hand [71] for panic patients treated with exposure. At follow-up, none of the EE variables predicted outcome, mainly because most patients who were affected by these family variables were no longer included in the follow-up sample, having dropped out or already failed to benefit.

Emmelkamp *et al.* [72] included EE in their model of relapse in OCD. They hypothesized that relapse is likely when patients lack coping skills and social support or when they experience high EE in the face of stressors after treatment. They suggested that problems will be further compounded if relatives attribute OCD symptoms to a disease process over which individuals have little control. This model is similar to a diathesis/stress model proposed for schizophrenics in which patient vulnerability to internal and environmental cues provokes symptoms that upset family members. These family members respond adaptively by engaging in problem solving or maladaptively by becoming overinvolved, frustrated, angry and/or rejecting. Maladaptive reactions are hypothesized to provoke more stress in the patient, leading to more symptoms and eventual relapse. In a partial retrospective test of this relapse model for OCD, Emmelkamp *et al.* [72] found that the combination of EE ratings, avoidant coping style and life events/daily hassles significantly predicted relapse ($r = 0.44$), whereas general social support did not, consistent with previous findings [68]. Among patients who relapsed, high EE ratings (measured only at follow-up rather than before treatment) were evident in three of four relapsers, but not in either of the two partial relapsers, suggesting that EE was partly associated with adverse outcomes. The authors recommended involving spouses or family members in treatment that emphasized empathic listening skills and communications training.

Research findings from these few studies of PDA and OCD outcomes are generally supportive of the need to take family interaction into consideration in planning treatment. With regard to EE, relative's criticism of a patient to an independent observer when the patient is not present does not appear to be problematic, so long as it is not hostile. In fact, criticism of PDA and OCD behaviours may serve as a motivator for patients to obtain therapy and to work on their problem during exposure treatment. This is especially suggested by Peter and Hand's [71] study of PDA patients and their spouses, one of the few studies to account for the effects of both relatives' and patients' CFI-assessed EE. These authors found that treatment outcome was actually better when both patients and spouses were critical of each other ("high EE dyad"), especially at follow-up. They interpreted this finding as a reflection of the couple's willingness to address problems openly and honestly. Whether the same dynamic would prove predictive in non-spousal families has not been studied.

Hostile criticism, however, is a serious problem and appears to make it difficult for patients to continue in treatment and to benefit from it. Chambless *et al.* [44] used structural equation modelling with a sample of 60 patients with OCD and 42 patients with PDA to identify the links between relatives' hostile criticism, patients' perceived criticism, relatives' personality traits, patients' symptoms, and patients' and relatives' observer-rated ability to solve problems constructively. They found that relatives' self-reported angry thoughts and feelings about the patient were directly associated with both their own hostile criticism and with patients' perceived criticism. Low rates of constructive problem solving between patient and relative were also linked to relatives' hostility. Patients' self-reported pathology directly predicted their own perceptions of criticism, but not their relatives' hostility, suggesting a possible disconnection between hostile relatives' and patients' perceptions that may be amenable to family intervention. Indeed, Arnow *et al.*'s [60] finding that treatment for women with PDA was enhanced by including a communication skills training component for patients and their spouses suggests that bridging this disconnection may be an important ingredient to successful treatment outcomes.

Patients' perceptions that their relatives are critical of them interferes with benefits from treatment [66,73]. Perceived criticism has been linked to the relatives' awareness of their own criticism and with a lack of relatives' positive comments, suggesting that patients are at least partly correct in their perceptions. However, perceived criticism is also correlated with negative personality traits in the patient (although not with the severity of their target anxiety problems [73]), indicating that some aspects of this perception may simply reflect the patient's own negative attitudes that also interfere with benefits from therapy. More research is needed to clarify how perceived criticism works and whether it requires change in the patient, the relative or both. While these questions remain to be clarified, a growing body of clinical evidence suggests that problem-solving skills training for both patients and relatives will prove useful in resolving some of the PDA and OCD symptoms. Steketee *et al.* [29] have suggested assessment and intervention strategies for reducing criticism, overinvolvement and hostility during BT for OCD. Their proposed techniques parallel those of Friedman [47] for reducing the polarized responses ("critical overinvolvement") of relatives of PDA patients.

Excessive accommodation on the part of relatives has also proved problematic. In a small sample of 17 OCD patients, Amir *et al.* [36] reported that greater family accommodation and modification of routine correlated with more severe OCD symptoms after treatment. One possible reason is that overinvolvement and accommodation decrease patients' sense of self-efficacy. More research is needed to determine whether EOI is closely linked to relatives' excessive accommodation to patients' wishes with regard to OCD symptoms. So far, the link between these constructs has not been examined and, since both appear to generate problems for the family as a whole, understanding them better will be important in determining how to intervene.

FAMILY-FOCUSED TREATMENT INTERVENTIONS

Research on chronic mental illness suggests that group treatment and multi-family group interventions may have some advantages of efficiency and cost effectiveness over other formats for delivery of behavioural treatment [74,75]. These methods may facilitate stress reduction and problem-solving skills via ventilation and modelling within the group context. In view of the often extensive involvement of family members in the rituals and avoidance of PDA and OCD patients and the apparent predictive capacity of family variables in several studies of PDA and OCD, it is reasonable to hypothesize that treatments that include family members will be beneficial for many PDA and OCD patients and their families. Of interest in evaluating the outcome of such treatments is the determination of the processes by which these methods have their effect. The literature on outcome prediction indicates that fruitful avenues are likely to include assessment of EE, perceived criticism and perceived family functioning.

The family treatments for PDA and OCD outlined below enlist family members as co-therapists and informants in CBT. CBT focuses on reducing patients' behavioural symptoms (avoidance for PDA, rituals and avoidance for OCD) by exposing them to feared situations and changing their dysfunctional thoughts and beliefs. Cognitive and behavioural theories of PDA and OCD [see 4,5] posit that anxious symptoms are maintained by dysfunctional thoughts (e.g. belief in the catastrophic consequences of contamination by germs or being short of breath) and the avoidance of opportunities to test the validity of these beliefs. Over time, people with PDA and OCD have learned that they can reduce their anxiety through symptomatic behaviour and increasingly rely on these dysfunctional strategies to the point where they believe that they cannot function without them. CBT strategies gradually expose patients to feared situations with the strict instruction that they cannot use their compensatory (safety) behaviours. Ideally, patients learn that they can function despite anxiety and that the catastrophic consequences they fear are highly unlikely to occur. Teaching patients cognitive restructuring techniques to question and challenge their dysfunctional beliefs is a useful tool for helping patients engage in the behavioural exercises. Rather than assume that they are imprisoned by their anxiety, questioning the validity of their beliefs gives patients the possibility that they can change their lives for the better.

Family Treatments for PDA

Cognitive–behavioural interpersonal family therapy for PDA [14,76] enlists the patient's spouse as co-therapist in an essentially cognitive–behavioural (i.e. cognitive restructuring and exposure-focused) programme for treating the patient's symptoms. However, time is allotted for both members of the couple to air frustrations, thoughts and concerns about the effects of the symptoms, both positive and negative, on their marital relationship. Gore and Carter [76] offer the example of a woman with PDA whose fear of being abandoned by her spouse for not getting better quickly enough paradoxically inhibited her from working on her homework exercises. Discussing these fears opens the door to learning new communication patterns that are less anxiety triggering, thereby facilitating treatment. The additive benefit of including spouses in CBT for PDA has been demonstrated in a number of small-sample controlled outcome studies [for review, see 6]. Although promising, these findings have yet to be replicated in large-sample, controlled studies.

Friedman [47] reported that his integrated CBT and family systems approach to treating PDA had a low dropout rate (5%), comparable to that of Barlow *et al.*'s [58] controlled study of the additive benefit of including spouses in PDA treatment. Friedman also proposed that only 10–15% of PDA patients have anxiety symptoms severe enough to warrant the additional inclusion of family members in treatment. He suggested that these severe clients are especially likely to drop out or relapse in the event that their family members decline his invitation to become even "minimally involved". Although promising, these anecdotal reports require substantiation via empirical replication in controlled outcome studies.

Family Treatments for OCD

Several researchers have noted advantages for support group involvement of both patients and family members. Marks *et al.* [77] employed an open-ended monthly group for family members and patients who had completed initial individual BT for OCD. Family members discussed the impact of OCD symptoms on the family and plans for coping strategies, and patients rehearsed behavioural exercises in the group. Recently, several reports have outlined psychoeducational foci for time-limited family support groups, including sessions on diagnosis, assessment, theories of OCD, BT including exposure and stopping rituals, medications and prevention of relapse [50,78,79]. Psychoeducational group goals included improving self-esteem, sharing feelings and experiences, accepting patients' realistic limitations, and learning strategies for coping with OCD symptoms. The use of co-leaders to respond adequately to the emotional needs of group members was encouraged. These reports noted high participant satisfaction with educational groups, but provided no outcome data.

As with other anxiety disorders, most quantitative family research in OCD has focused on the effect of including family members in BT. Case studies showed advantages to parental involvement in treatment for children and young adults [80–82]. In a controlled study with a small sample, Emmelkamp and DeLange [83] compared the outcome of Dutch clients treated behaviourally with or without the spouse as co-therapist. Unfortunately, the content of interventions aimed at reducing conflict or enhancing communication was not described. Patients treated with spouse assistance improved more at post-test, but not at follow-up. In a second, larger study of 50 subjects, spouse assistance made no difference in outcome either after treatment or at follow-up, although improvement in marital satisfaction was reported [40]. It is noteworthy that, in these studies, spouses were not specifically trained in communication with the patient regarding their symptoms, but in a later report, Emmelkamp *et al.* [72] encouraged the inclusion of partners and emphasized empathic communication as an important factor in outcome.

Emmelkamp *et al.*'s negative findings regarding spouse involvement in a Dutch sample are contradicted by Mehta's [84] study of family involvement in treatment in India. Involving family members in exposure and response prevention treatment for 30 patients led to significantly greater gains in OCD symptoms, mood state, and social and occupational functioning compared with unassisted treatment. This added benefit was evident at post-test and at follow-up. Unlike Emmelkamp's study of spouses only, Mehta's sample included an equal number of spouses and parents. Non-anxious, firm family members were more successful in providing support and supervision than anxious and inconsistent ones, and especially those who engaged in argument and ridicule. This treatment was also longer and more intense (24 sessions in 12 weeks) than the 8 sessions in 5 weeks of Emmelkamp and colleagues. It is also possible that Mehta's study employed a less confrontational family role, that according to Hafner [85] might help reduce family hostility. The discrepant findings could also reflect cultural differences in the style of family interaction, especially if Indian families were lower on EE, as findings from other studies suggest [86].

Two studies have focused on reducing family accommodation to OCD symptoms. Thornicroft *et al.* [87] reported an uncontrolled effort to reduce relatives' involvement in OCD symptoms. Their inpatient treatment programme in the UK emphasized self-treatment and teaching relatives to assist in the therapy programme. BT included standard exposure and response prevention plus strategies for self-control and social skills training. The family component focused on reducing relatives' involvement in rituals by training them to monitor patient behaviour and encourage self-exposure in a non-critical manner. Relatives practised under the therapist's supervision on the ward. This programme produced decreases in OCD symptoms of about 45% at discharge ($n = 45$) and 60% at a 6-month follow-up ($n = 22$), with concomitant improvement in functioning ranging from 33% (work) to 48% (home) at follow-up. These results were excellent for this severe inpatient population who scored in the extreme range on disability from OCD symptoms.

A more recent and better controlled trial by Grunes *et al.* [88] examined the benefits of relatives' participation in an 8-week psychoeducational group designed to help reduce accommodation to OCD symptoms, in which 28 patients who received individual exposure and response prevention were randomly assigned to have their relative participate in the family group or not. Patients whose family member was involved in the group had greater reduction in OCD symptoms (32% reduction in a standard measure) and in depressed mood compared to those whose relatives did not participate (12% reduction). Benefits were maintained at a 1-month follow-up. The gains in the latter group are quite low compared to usual benefits from outcome trials using BT but, since this group of patients was considered generally treatment refractory, it appears that the family intervention was especially helpful. In addition, relatives who participated in the educational group experienced a reduction in family accommodation as well as depressed and anxious mood. Which aspect of change in relatives' behaviour played a role in improved outcome in the patients is an important question for future research.

In another study of family intervention, Van Noppen *et al.* [75] completed an uncontrolled study of the effects of 10–12 weeks of multi-family behavioural treatment for 19 OCD adults and their family members. Family members and patients together received education about OCD and exposure treatment and were taught family contracting for behaviour change, along with direct exposure during family group sessions. Six monthly follow-up sessions helped families review progress and identify additional needs. OCD symptoms reduced by 26% and gains were maintained at follow-up, with additional benefits evident in family functioning. Poorer family functioning on roles and communication predicted worse outcome. These findings suggest that group interventions that involve family members are beneficial, especially over the long term, but the gains were modest compared to those produced by individual BT programmes. Nonetheless, they argue for the need for further study of this cost-effective multi-family method, which has also proved very useful for treatment of patients with chronic mental illness [74].

An indirect study of family-related interventions is found in Hiss *et al.*'s [89] test of relapse prevention treatment appended to exposure and response prevention. They compared this to a placebo intervention called "associative therapy". The relapse prevention included a session with a significant other in which maladaptive interpersonal problems such as anger and criticism and unrealistic expectations by relatives were addressed, along with other components designed to reduce stress-related exacerbation of symptoms. The addition of the relapse prevention content led to fewer relapses in OCD symptoms and to less depression and anxiety compared to placebo, but whether the intervention with relatives contributed to this is unknown.

Recent reports of family intervention with childhood OCD are particularly promising. Piacentini *et al.* [90] provided data on the use of psychoeducation, disengagement from the child's OCD symptoms (reduced accommodation) and interventions for conflict and family disruption. Nearly 80% of 42 patients responded well (much improved) to this protocol, although not all received all of the family components. Waters *et al.* [91] provided pilot data on the efficacy of a 14-week cognitive–behavioural family treatment for 7 children with OCD. Treatment included components on education, parental participation in childhood relaxation training, reduction of accommodation, parental anxiety management, family support and problem-solving skills training. This treatment package led to considerable benefits for 6 of the 7 children at post-test, with a 59% average reduction in OCD symptoms and scores in the normal range for all at 3-month follow-up, although one child relapsed partially. Family accommodation also improved substantially. These childhood studies are particularly promising and suggest that, when treated early with family involvement, OCD symptoms can be much reduced, if not eliminated, in many children.

The above studies are not yet so definitive that they clearly establish whether relatives' involvement in BT of OCD significantly enhances outcome. However, findings appear promising. Fine-grained analyses have not yet indicated what traits characterize patients and family members who respond to these methods. Findings from the extensive literature on family characteristics of patients with schizophrenia that have predicted outcome of family treatment for this disorder offer some direction for research on OCD in this regard.

CONCLUSIONS

Overall, what is needed is a model for the effects of criticism, hostility and EOI on patient symptoms and on therapy outcome. Such a model must explain the findings and include illness variables and personality features. For example, the patients' personality features and events in their lives are likely to influence their perception of criticism and the degree to which relatives respond to them with hostility. Further, trait anxiety is likely to affect both relatives' and patients' affective reactions (less positive reactions and more negative ones) and coping deficits, especially the lack of problem-solving skills. Family EOI and accommodation to symptoms may further reduce patients' self-efficacy and coping or problem-solving skills, perhaps especially in OCD. These features will undoubtedly contribute to state anxiety, avoidance and rituals in both disorders. The implications of such a model and of the findings reported here are that it will be especially important to reduce relatives' hostility. This requires helping hostile relatives to re-examine their attitudes toward the patient and the disorder and learn better problem-solving skills. This is especially suggested by Chambless *et al.*'s [44] structural equation model linking relatives' poor problem-solving skills to their expressed hostility, which in turn is associated with patients' perceived criticism of their relatives. If these methods fail, therapists may need to help patients distance themselves from these relatives.

Based on the research findings to date, we make the following recommendations for intervention. We suggest psychoeducational interventions for family members who are unfamiliar with PDA and OCD, who accommodate to patients' symptoms and who tend to be critical and/or negative in their attitude. These interventions should include information about the biological, psychological and social aspects of PDA and OCD, and about the adverse effects of family accommodation and strategies for extricating themselves from this type of behaviour. For example, blaming the therapist is one way for family members to resist involvement in rituals such as reassurance seeking. Even more useful may be behavioural contracting in which family members agree aloud on who does what with whom to limit rituals and family involvement and increase exposure and reduction in agoraphobic avoidance or obsessive anxiety. The effects of hostile criticism may best be addressed by determining the source of the hostility and correcting any blaming beliefs and attributions about the causes of the behavioural symptoms when this is feasible. Finally, family education should include information about the treatment procedures and their likely effects and side effects (e.g. patient distress from exposure and response prevention).

Only cooperative family members should be invited to assist in treatment, and instructed in the role of coach, supporter and cheerleader. Desirable traits in relatives for assisting in treatment might be similar to those found helpful for therapists: respectful, understanding, interested, encouraging, challenging, explicit, having a sense of humour, and not being permissive or fostering dependency, which have been found unhelpful. Excessive behavioural and emotional involvement should be discouraged, so that patients are able to undertake therapy decisions independently. Patients must learn for themselves how to tolerate exposure when panic symptoms arise or obsessive thoughts intrude and they need to control their avoidance and rituals. Relatives may need to learn how to avoid arguments about tasks and roles during the therapy process while re-establishing normal family routines.

In addition, family therapy may be needed to support relatives in dealing with frustrating patient behaviours and to encourage more positive communication and reduce anger expression. Communication training has rarely been part of family treatments, except on an informal basis, but, as suggested by Arnow *et al.* [60], may be especially helpful regarding managing the symptoms themselves. This applies particularly to relatives who themselves are affected by anxiety disorders or anxious traits, and may also need help to improve their own functioning. Role playing of conversations, learning to identify and stop hostile comments, correcting faulty beliefs about the patient, finding creative solutions for problems, and engaging in behavioural contracting may prove useful. Such interventions are likely to require longer treatments or perhaps sequential phases of treatment involving family members and working to increase patient skills and self-efficacy and relatives' communication and problem-solving skills. These may prove especially helpful for treatment refractory patients who have not benefited readily from standard cognitive–behavioural and pharmacological methods.

REFERENCES

1. American Psychiatric Association (2000) Anxiety disorders. In: *Diagnostic and Statistical Manual of Mental Disorders*, 4th edn, text revised. American Psychiatric Association, Washington, DC, pp. 429–484.
2. Barlow D.H. (2002) The experience of anxiety: shadow of intelligence or specter of death? In: Barlow D.H. (ed.) *Anxiety and its Disorders: The Nature and Treatment of Anxiety and Panic*, 2nd edn. Guilford Press, New York, pp. 1–36.
3. Antony M.M., Barlow D.H. (2002) Specific phobias. In: Barlow D.H. (ed.) *Anxiety and its Disorders: The Nature and Treatment of Anxiety and Panic*, 2nd edn. Guilford Press, New York, pp. 380–417.
4. White K.S., Barlow D.H. (2002) Panic disorder and agoraphobia. In Barlow D.H. (ed.) *Anxiety and its Disorders: The Nature and Treatment of Anxiety and Panic*, 2nd edn. Guilford Press, New York, pp. 328–379.
5. Steketee G., Barlow D.H. (2002) Obsessive–compulsive disorder. In: Barlow D.H. (ed.) *Anxiety and its Disorders: The Nature and Treatment of Anxiety and Panic*, 2nd edn. Guilford Press, New York, pp. 516–550.
6. Carter M.M., Tuvorsky J., Barlow D.H. (1994) Interpersonal relationships in panic disorder with agoraphobia: a review of empirical evidence. *Clin. Psychol. Sci. Pract.*, **1**, 25–34.
7. Wittchen H.U., Essau C.A., Von Zerssen D., Krieg J.C., Zaudig M. (1992) Lifetime and six-month prevalence of mental disorders in the Munich follow-up study. *Eur. Arch. Psychiatry Clin. Neurosci.*, **241**, 247–258.
8. Bland R.C., Orn H., Newman S.C. (1988) Lifetime prevalence of psychiatric disorders in Edmonton. *Acta Psychiatr. Scand.*, **77**(suppl. 338), 24–32.
9. Laraia M.T., Stuart G.W., Frye L.H., Lydiard R.B., Ballenger J. C. (1994). Childhood environment of women having panic disorder with agoraphobia. *J. Anxiety Disord.*, **8**, 1–17.
10. Eaton W.W., Kessler R.C., Wittchen H.U., Magee W.J. (1994) Panic and panic disorder in the United States. *Am. J. Psychiatry*, **151**, 413–420.
11. Albano A.M., Chorpita B.F., Barlow D.H. (1996) Childhood anxiety disorders. In: Mash E.J., Barkley F.A. (eds) *Child Psychopathology*. Guilford Press, New York, pp. 196–241.

12. Kearney C.A., Albano A.M., Eisen A.R., Allen W.D., Barlow D.H. (1997) The phenomenology of panic disorder in youngsters: an empirical study of a clinical sample. *J. Anxiety Disord.*, **11**, 49–62.

13. Moreau D.M., Weissman M.M. (1992) Panic disorder in children and adolescents: a review. *Am. J. Psychiatry*, **149**, 1306–1314.

14. Carter M.M., Schultz K.M. (1998) Panic disorder with agoraphobia: its impact on patients and their significant others. In: Carlson J., Sperry L. (eds) *The Disordered Couple*. Brunner/Mazel, Bristol, pp. 29–56.

15. Guarnaccia P.J., Canino G., Rubio-Stipec M., Bravo M. (1993) The prevalence of *ataques de nervios* in the Puerto Rico Disaster Study. *J. Nerv. Ment. Dis.*, **181**, 157–165.

16. Liebowitz M.R., Salman E., Jusino C.M., Garfinkel R., Street L., Cardenas D.L., Silvestre J., Fryer A.J., Carrasco J.L., Davies S., *et al.* (1994) *Ataque de nervios* and panic disorder. *Am. J. Psychiatry*, **151**, 871–875.

17. Hettema J.M., Neale M.C., Kendler K.S. (2001) A review and meta-analysis of the genetic epidemiology of anxiety disorders. *Am. J. Psychiatry*, **158**, 1568–1578.

18. Biederman J., Faraone S.V., Hirshfeld-Becker D.R., Friedman D., Robin J.A., Rosenbaum J.R. (2001) Patterns of psychopathology and dysfunction in high-risk children of parents with panic disorder and major depression. *Am. J. Psychiatry*, **158**, 49–57.

19. Battaglia M., Bertelli S., Politi E., Bernardeschi L., Perna G., Gabriele A., Bellodi L. (1995) Age at onset of panic disorder: influence of familial liability to the disease and of childhood separation anxiety disorder. *Am. J. Psychiatry*, **152**, 1362–1364.

20. Barlow D.H. (2002) Biological aspects of anxiety and panic. In: Barlow D.H. (ed.) *Anxiety and its Disorders: The Nature and Treatment of Anxiety and Panic*, 2nd edn. Guilford Press, New York, pp. 180–218.

21. Emmelkamp P.M.G., Gerlsma C. (1994) Marital functioning and the anxiety disorders. *Behav. Ther.*, **25**, 407–429.

22. Torpy D.M., Measey L.G. (1974) Marital interactions in agoraphobia. *J. Clin. Psychol.*, **30**, 351–354.

23. Webster A.S. (1953) The development of phobias in married women. *Psychol. Monogr.*, **67**, 1–18.

24. Buglass D., Clarke J., Henderson A.S., Kreitman N. (1977) A study of agoraphobic housewives. *Psychol. Med.*, **7**, 73–86.

25. Arrindell W.A., Emmelkamp P.M.G. (1986) Marital adjustment, intimacy and needs in female agoraphobics and their partners: a controlled study. *Br. J. Psychiatry*, **149**, 592–602.

26. McLeod J.D. (1994) Anxiety disorders and marital quality. *J. Abnorm. Psychol.*, **103**, 767–776.

27. Steketee G. (1997) Disability and family burden in obsessive–compulsive disorder. *Can. J. Psychiatry*, **42**, 919–928.

28. Steketee G., Pruyn N. (1998) Family functioning in OCD. In: Swinson R.P., Antony M.M., Rachman S., Richter M.A. (eds) *Obsessive Compulsive Disorder: Theory, Research and Treatment*. Guilford Press, New York, pp. 120–140.

29. Steketee G., Van Noppen B., Lam J., Shapiro L. (1998) Expressed emotion in families and the treatment of obsessive compulsive disorder. *In Session: Psychotherapy in Practice*, **4**, 73–91.

30. Black D.W., Noyes R., Goldstein R.B., Blum N. (1992) A family study of obsessive–compulsive disorder. *Arch. Gen. Psychiatry*, **49**, 362–368.

31. Lenane M.C., Swedo S.E., Leonard H., Pauls D.L., Sceery W., Rapoport J. (1990) Psychiatric disorders in first degree relatives of children and adolescents with obsessive compulsive disorder. *J. Am. Acad. Child Adolesc. Psychiatry*, **29**, 407–412.

32. Pauls D.L., Raymond C.L., Robertson M. (1991) The genetics of obsessive–compulsive disorder: a review. In: Zohar J., Insel T., Rasmussen S (eds) *The Psychobiology of Obsessive–Compulsive Disorder*. Springer-Verlag, New York, pp. 89–100.

33. Swedo S.E., Rapoport J.L., Leonard H., Lenane M., Cheslow D. (1989) Obsessive compulsive disorder in children and adolescents. *Arch. Gen. Psychiatry*, **46**, 335–341.

34. Lensi P., Cassano G.B., Correddu G., Ravagli S., Kunovac J.L., Akiskal H.S. (1996) Obsessive–compulsive disorder: familial-developmental history, symptomatology, comorbidity and course with special reference to gender-related differences. *Br. J. Psychiatry*, **169**, 101–107.

35. Bellodi L., Sciuto G., Diaferia G., Ronci P., Smeraldi E. (1992) Psychiatric disorders in the families of patients with obsessive–compulsive disorders. *Psychiatry Res.*, **42**, 111–120.

36. Amir N., Freshman M., Foa E.B. (2000) Family distress and involvement in relatives of obsessive–compulsive disorder patients. *J. Anxiety Disord.*, **14**, 209–217.

37. Steketee G., Van Noppen B. (2003) Family approaches to treatment for obsessive compulsive disorder. *Braz. J. Psychiatry*, **25**, 43–50.

38. Honjo J., Hirano C., Murase S., Kaneko T., Sugiyama T., Ohtaka K., Aoyama T., Takel Y., Inoko K., Wakabayashi S. (1989) Obsessive compulsive symptoms in childhood and adolescence. *Acta Psychiatr. Scand.*, **80**, 83–91.

39. Riddell M.A., Scahill L., King R., Hardin M.T., Towbin K.E., Ort S.I., Leckman J.E., Cohen D.J. (1990) Obsessive compulsive disorder in children and adolescents: phenomenology and family history. *J. Am. Acad. Child Adolesc. Psychiatry*, **29**, 766–772.

40. Emmelkamp P.M.G., de Haan E., Hoogduin C.A.L. (1990) Marital adjustment and obsessive compulsive disorder. *Br. J. Psychiatry*, **156**, 55–60.

41. Riggs D.S., Hiss H., Foa E.B. (1992) Marital distress and the treatment of obsessive compulsive disorder. *Behav. Ther.*, **23**, 585–597.

42. Livingston-Van Noppen B., Rasmussen S.A., Eisen J., McCartney L. (1990) Family function and treatment in obsessive–compulsive disorder. In: Jenike M., Baer L., Minichiello W.E. (eds) *Obsessive Compulsive Disorder: Theory and Treatment*. Year Book, Chicago, IL, pp. 325–340.

43. Wilborg I.M., Dahl A.A. (1997) The recollection of parental rearing styles in patients with panic disorder. *Acta Psychiatr. Scand.*, **96**, 58–63.

44. Chambless D.L., Bryan A.D., Aiken L.S., Steketee G., Hooley J.M. (2001) Predicting expressed emotion: a study with families of obsessive–compulsive and agoraphobic outpatients. *J. Fam. Psychol.*, **15**, 225–240.

45. Bowlby J. (1988) *A Secure Base*. Basic Books, New York.

46. Goldstein A.J., Chambless D.L. (1978) A reanalysis of agoraphobia. *Behav. Ther.*, **9**, 47–59.

47. Friedman S. (1995) Treating panic disorder with agoraphobia: integrating a family systems and behavioral approach. *In Session: Psychotherapy in Practice*, **1**, 48–68.

48. Leff J., Vaughn C. (1985) *Expressed Emotion in Families: Its Significance for Mental Illness*. Guilford Press, New York.

49. Allsopp M., Verduyn C. (1990) Adolescents with obsessive compulsive disorder: a case note review of consecutive patients referred to a provincial regional adolescent psychiatry unit. *J. Adolesc.*, **13**, 157–169.
50. Cooper M. (1993) A group for families of obsessive–compulsive persons. *Fam. Soc.*, May, 301–307.
51. Calvocoressi L., Lewis B., Harris M., Trufan B.S., Goodman W.K., McDougle C.J., Price L.H. (1995) Family accommodation in obsessive compulsive disorder. *Am. J. Psychiatry*, **152**, 441–443.
52. Calvocoressi L., Mature C., Stanislav K., Skolnick J., Fisk D., Vegso S., Van Noppen B., Price L. (1999) Reliability and validity of the family accommodation scale for obsessive–compulsive disorder. *J. Nerv. Ment. Dis.*, **187**, 636–642.
53. Shafran R., Ralph J., Tallis F. (1995) Obsessive–compulsive symptoms and the family. *Bull. Menninger Clin.*, **59**, 472–479.
54. Hibbs E.D., Hamburger S.D., Lenane M., Rapoport J.L., Kruesi M.J.P., Keysor C.S., Goldstein M.J. (1991) Determinants of expressed emotion in families of disturbed and normal children. *J. Psychol. Psychiatry*, **32**, 757–770.
55. Hibbs E.D., Hamburger S.D., Kruesi M.J.P., Lenane M. (1993) Factors affecting expressed emotion in parents of ill and normal children. *Am. J. Orthopsychiatry*, **63**, 103–112.
56. Stubbe D.E., Zahner G.E.P., Goldstein M.J., Leckman J.F. (1993) Diagnostic specificity of a brief measure of expressed emotion: a community study of children. *J. Child Psychol. Psychiatry*, **4**, 139–154.
57. Hirshfeld D.R., Biederman J., Brody L., Faraone S.V., Rosenbaum J.F. (1997) Associations between expressed emotion and child behavioral inhibition and psychopathology: a pilot study. *J. Am. Acad. Child Adolesc. Psychiatry*, **36**, 205–213.
58. Barlow D.H., O'Brien G.T., Last C.G. (1984) Couples treatment of agoraphobia. *Behav. Ther.*, **15**, 41–58.
59. Cerny J.A., Barlow D.H., Craske M.G., Himadi W.G. (1987) Couples treatment of agoraphobia: a two-year follow-up. *Behav. Ther.*, **18**, 401–415.
60. Arnow B.A., Taylor C.B., Agras W.S., Telch M.J. (1985) Enhancing agoraphobia treatment outcome by changing couple communication patterns. *Behav. Ther.*, **16**, 452–467.
61. Oatley K, Hodgson D (1987) Influence of husbands on the outcome of their agoraphobic wives' therapy. *Br. J. Psychiatry*, **150**, 380–386.
62. Cobb J.P., Matthews A.M., Childs-Clarke A., Blowers C.M. (1984). The spouse as co-therapist in the treatment of agoraphobia. *Br. J. Psychiatry*, **144**, 282–287.
63. Emmelkamp P.M.G., Van Dyck R., Bitter M., Heins R., Onstein E.J., Eisen B. (1992) Spouse-aided therapy with agoraphobics. *Br. J. Psychiatry*, **160**, 51–56.
64. Hafner R.J. (1982) Marital interaction in persisting obsessive–compulsive disorders. *Aust. N. Zeal. J. Psychiatry*, **16**, 171–178.
65. Marks I.M. (1973) New approaches to the treatment of obsessive–compulsive disorders. *J. Nerv. Ment. Dis.*, **156**, 420–426.
66. Chambless D., Steketee G. (1999) Expressed emotion and behavior therapy outcome: a prospective study with obsessive–compulsive and agoraphobic outpatients. *J. Consult. Clin. Psychol.*, **67**, 658–665.
67. Cobb J., McDonald R., Marks I., Stern R. (1980) Marital versus exposure therapy: psychological treatment of co-existing marital and phobic–obsessive problems. *Behav. Anal. Modif.*, **4**, 3–16.
68. Steketee G. (1993) Social support and treatment outcome of obsessive compulsive disorder at 9-month follow-up. *Behav. Psychother.*, **21**, 81–95.

69. Butzlaff R., Hooley J. (1998) Expressed emotion and psychiatric relapse: a meta-analysis. *Arch. Gen. Psychiatry*, **55**, 547–552.
70. Renshaw K.D., Chambless D.L., Rodebaugh T.L., Steketee G. (2000) Living with severe anxiety disorders: relatives' distress and reactions to patient behaviors. *Clin. Psychol. Psychother.*, **7**, 190–200.
71. Peter H., Hand I. (1988) Patterns of patient–spouse interaction in agoraphobics: assessment by Camberwell Family Interview (CFI) and impact on outcome of self-exposure treatment. In: Hand I., Wittchen H.-U. (eds) *Panic and Phobias 2: Treatments and Variables Affecting Course and Outcome*. Springer-Verlag, Berlin, pp. 240–251.
72. Emmelkamp P.M.G., Kloek J., Blaauw E. (1992) Obsessive–compulsive disorders. In: Wilson P.H. (ed.) *Principles and Practice of Relapse Prevention*. Guilford Press, New York, pp. 213–234.
73. Renshaw K.D., Chambless D.L., Steketee G. (2003) Perceived criticism predicts severity of anxiety symptoms after behavioral treatment in patients with obsessive–compulsive disorder and panic disorder with agoraphobia. *J. Clin. Psychol.*, **59**, 411–421.
74. McFarlane W.R. (ed.) (2002) *Multiple Family Groups in the Treatment of Severe Psychiatric Disorders*. Guilford Press, New York.
75. Van Noppen B., Steketee G., McCorkle B.H., Pato M. (1997) Group and multifamily behavioral treatment for obsessive compulsive disorder: a pilot study. *J. Anxiety Disord.*, **11**, 431–446.
76. Gore K.L., Carter M.M. (2001) Family therapy for panic disorder: a cognitive–behavioral interpersonal approach to treatment. In: MacFarlane M.M. (ed.) *Family Therapy and Mental Health: Innovations in Theory and Practice*. Haworth Press, Binghampton, NY, pp. 109–134.
77. Marks I.M., Hodgson R., Rachman S. (1975) Treatment of chronic obsessive–compulsive neurosis with *in vivo* exposure: a 2-year follow-up and issues in treatment. *Br. J. Psychiatry*, **127**, 349–364.
78. Black D.W., Blum N.S. (1992) Obsessive–compulsive disorder support groups: the Iowa model. *Compr. Psychiatry*, **33**, 65–71.
79. Tynes L.L., Salins C., Skiba W., Winstead D.K. (1992) A psycho-educational and support group for obsessive–compulsive disorder patients and their significant others. *Compr. Psychiatry*, **33**, 197–201.
80. Dalton P. (1983) Family treatment of an obsessive–compulsive child: a case report. *Fam. Process*, **22**, 99–108.
81. Fine S. (1973) Family therapy: a behavioral approach to childhood obsessive compulsive neurosis. *Arch. Gen. Psychiatry*, **28**, 695–697.
82. Hafner R.J., Gilchrist P., Bowling J., Kalucy R. (1981) The treatment of obsessional neurosis in a family setting. *Aust. N. Zeal. J. Psychiatry*, **15**, 145–151.
83. Emmelkamp P.M.G., DeLange I. (1983) Spouse involvement in the treatment of obsessive–compulsive patients. *Behav. Res. Ther.*, **21**, 341–346.
84. Mehta M. (1990) A comparative study of family-based and patient-based behavioural management in obsessive–compulsive disorder. *Br. J. Psychiatry*, **157**, 133–135.
85. Hafner R.J. (1992) Anxiety disorders and family therapy. *Aust. N. Zeal. J. Fam. Ther.*, **13**, 99–104.
86. Jenkins J.G., Karno M. (1992) The meaning of expressed emotion: theoretical issues raised by cross-cultural research. *Am. J. Psychiatry*, **149**, 9–21.
87. Thornicroft G., Colson L., Marks I.M. (1991) An inpatient behavioural psychotherapy unit description and audit. *Br. J. Psychiatry*, **158**, 362–367.

88. Grunes M.S., Neziroglu F., McKay D. (2001) Family involvement in the behavioral treatment of obsessive–compulsive disorder: a preliminary investigation. *Behav. Ther.*, **32**, 803–820.
89. Hiss H., Foa E.B., Kozak M.J. (1994) Relapse prevention program for treatment of obsessive–compulsive disorder. *J. Consult. Clin. Psychol.*, **62**, 801–808.
90. Piacentini J., Bergman R.L., Jacobs C., McCracken J.T., Kretchman J. (2002) Open trial of cognitive behavior therapy for childhood obsessive compulsive disorder. *J. Anxiety Disord.*, **16**, 207–219.
91. Waters T.L., Barrett P.M, March J.S. (2001) Cognitive–behavioral family treatment of childhood obsessive–compulsive disorder: preliminary findings. *Am. J. Psychother.*, **55**, 372–387.

6

Families of People with an Eating Disorder

Palmiero Monteleone*, Janet Treasure‡,
Paolo Santonastaso§, Angela Favaro§
and Francesca Brambilla*

*University of Naples SUN, Naples, Italy
‡Thomas Guy House, London, UK
§University of Padua, Padua, Italy

INTRODUCTION

Eating disorders have their onset mostly in late childhood, adolescence and early adulthood. As a consequence, the family of origin is deeply involved in the illness. This applies in particular to anorexia nervosa, where in the majority of cases the onset of the disease is below the age of 16. The emaciation of anorexia nervosa, with all the related physical consequences endangering life, the clearly defined problem of "not eating" and the apparently simple solution "to eat" have a profoundly frustrating and distressing impact on the family. Thus, parents and other relatives are drawn into an intense form of caregiving. Bulimia nervosa has a later age of onset, with the majority of cases occurring over the age of 18, and the symptoms are much more secret. The behaviours are hidden and there is no overt consequence on weight and possibly on general health. Partners or friends may be involved, but the apparent need for care is much less expressed.

The public stigmatization of eating disorders and, in particular, the widespread belief that people with eating disorders are to blame for their illness and that the difficulties they face are self-inflicted [1] may contribute to the difficulties faced by caregivers.

THE IMPACT OF EATING DISORDERS ON THE FAMILY

There are problems in interpreting research in this area, because there have been few studies and most of them have been small. Also, most studies

Families and Mental Disorders. Edited by Norman Sartorius, Julian Leff, Juan José López-Ibor, Mario Maj and Ahmed Okasha. © 2005 John Wiley & Sons Ltd. ISBN 0-470-02382-1

examine cases presenting for treatment at specialized centres or attending events for carers, whose representativeness is doubtful. Research into this area has focused upon the levels of distress and dysfunction in the family, which may be a complex mix of cause and effect. A few studies have examined the caregiving burden and considered models of caregiving within the family.

Anorexia Nervosa

Several features of anorexia nervosa are likely to create frustration and distress within the family. First, every meal becomes a problem, with implications for all aspects of the purchase and preparation of food. This leads to a profound disruption of all social activities, and the family becomes very isolated. Furthermore, it is impossible to disguise the overt signs of the illness, and carers experience high levels of stigma.

An additional burden is related to the associated behaviours, such as excessive activity, compulsions, the need for a rigid timetable, and high standards of cleanliness and tidiness. The parents' anxiety over the patient's physical health is often severe and has a profound impact on their life, disrupting sleep and making them irritable or depressed. The person with an eating disorder is often also angry, hostile and depressed. It is common for parents to be shocked by the changes in their daughter's temper. Moreover, parents are plagued by feelings of inadequacy and self-blame. Individuals with anorexia nervosa strongly defend their behaviours and do not wish to change and to receive help [2]. A recent book by a carer illustrates some of these difficulties [3].

We found high levels of unmet needs and psychological distress in carers of patients with anorexia nervosa [4,5]. Carers also experience a great number of difficulties in their caregiving role [5]. Indeed, the carers of people with anorexia nervosa had higher levels of difficulties and distress than those of people with schizophrenia. Caregivers' distress was related to the levels of unmet needs as well as to the difficulties in the caring role, and there were many negative attributions about the illness [6]. Caregivers conceptualized the illness as arising as part of the patient's personality and believed that they had little control over the illness but that the patient had some control.

Bulimia Nervosa

We consider in this section also eating disorders not otherwise specified that resemble bulimia nervosa.

Several features of bulimia nervosa are likely to create distress within the family. First, the family faces numerous practical difficulties. Large quantities of food are consumed during binges, with the relevant economic burden. The purging behaviour creates problems with bathroom use and function. The patient's preoccupation with weight and shape leads to prolonged grooming/self-care activities and reassurance seeking. Additional behaviours such as stealing, self-harm, alcohol/drug abuse and other forms of impulsivity add to the family's difficulties.

Furthermore, the emotional climate is coloured by anxiety and depression. Carers themselves are also likely to experience a wide range of negative emotions, e.g. anxiety relating to the physical risks associated with the illness, feelings of revulsion and disgust about bingeing and purging behaviours, and feelings of self-reproach and self-blame. Individuals with bulimia nervosa are often ambivalent about their wish to change and to receive help [7].

One study explored the impact of patient factors, carer factors and relationship characteristics on experiences of caregiving and mental health in 112 carers of 68 young subjects with bulimia nervosa/eating disorders not otherwise specified prior to specialist treatment [8]. More than half of the sample reported some mental health problems and a minority (5.4%) were experiencing considerable distress. The profile of General Health Questionnaire scores was very similar to that found in a sample of carers of individuals with anorexia nervosa. The levels of difficulties in most areas of caregiving were comparable to those observed by Treasure et al. [5] in carers of more chronically ill inpatients with anorexia nervosa and higher than those observed in carers of individuals with psychosis. This is surprising, since the sample was young and relatively homogeneous in terms of both short duration of symptomatology and treatment naivety. As in people with anorexia nervosa, dependency and loss were the subscales of the Experience of Care Giving Inventory with the strongest relationship to caregiver mental health problems. A negative experience of caregiving was found to predict carer mental health status. Two relationship factors, expressed emotion (as reported by the patient) and weekly contact hours, were observed to function as predictors of a negative experience of caregiving, jointly accounting for 18% of the variance.

SIBLING, MARITAL AND CHILDREARING ISSUES

Sometimes siblings report feeling left out of the eating disorder and its treatment because parents want to protect them. They generally prefer to be part of the discussions. Their own problems and worries may be neglected. Also, they may be angry and resentful about the effects that the eating disorder has upon the family: for example, their mother may be in tears all the time or the father may shout and be angry. This may lead to some siblings leaving home prematurely.

Although anorexia and bulimia nervosa typically occur in adolescent girls, they often affect adult women. Since these older patients may live with a partner, their disorder may affect the marital relationships and, vice versa, marital relationships may have an impact on the course of the disorder.

The clinical literature, based almost exclusively on descriptive case reports, emphasizes that married patients and their partners often report significant dissatisfaction with their relationship, and consider their marital problems to be the consequence of the patient's eating disorder. It was reported that couples in which one partner had an eating disorder lacked openness, had a low level of marital intimacy, and deficient communication skills [9]. These problems may interfere with the constructive evolution of marriage and may represent an obstacle to recovery from the eating disorder.

Moreover, many of the older women with an eating disorder have children, and the disorder may influence their childrearing practices. Indeed, the mother's preoccupation about shape and weight and her fear of fatness may cause her to underfeed her children and to become critical of her adolescent children's appearance and eating habits. Alternatively, the preoccupation with food, eating and shape may interfere with her sensitivity and responsiveness to children's needs. Studies investigating the childrearing attitudes of mothers with eating disorders have reported that these women are overconcerned about their children's weight and feeding and exhibit a general disruption of parenting. In a controlled study [10], mothers with and without eating disorders and their 1-year-old children were observed at home during both mealtimes and play. As compared to controls, eating disorder mothers were more intrusive with their infants during both mealtimes and play, and expressed more negative emotions during mealtimes but not during play. The children of eating disorder women weighed less than those of control women and their weight was inversely related to the amount of conflict during mealtimes. These changes seem to be specific to mothers with eating disorders: in a study of infants of eating disorder women compared to infants of mothers with postnatal depression and of healthy controls, it was found that the former weighed less than the other two groups [11]. The strongest predictor of infant weight was the extent of the mealtime conflict between the mother's willingness to control the infant's feeding and the infant's need for autonomy during mealtimes. In a subsequent work by the same authors [12], it was evident that the conflict arose not because the mothers intended to be punitive, but because the mother's eating psychopathology disrupted aspects of parental functioning such as the appropriate responsiveness to infant cues preceding the meals and the adequate management of their own concerns around infant self-feeding and food refusal.

UNHELPFUL INTERACTIONS

An eating disorder in the family can lead to a variety of unhelpful reactions and interactions. It is common for parents to have an extreme emotional reaction. They may feel highly anxious and depressed, with thoughts of self-blame, failure and worthlessness. This may be accompanied by perceptions of stigma from other people. Alternatively, some parents become very angry and try to sort out the problem. They then get extremely frustrated when change does not happen. This may lead either to an escalation of the measures of verbal control, e.g. shouting or intimidating, or to withdrawal. A third type of reaction is to avoid facing the difficulty. This involves letting the disorder progress without doing anything, for the fear of upsetting the daughter, or of being blamed or intruded upon if they go and ask for help.

Several parents get into what we call the "compulsive caring" mode, in which they feel they need to do all they can to care for their daughter. They are terrified of saying anything wrong and preoccupied that they have done absolutely everything that is necessary. This often means that the parents take over all responsibility and decision making for their daughter. This can be unhelpful as it encourages the person with anorexia nervosa to regress and become very dependent and ever more demanding. It also gives the implicit message that the world is a threatening place, and that the patient does not have the capacity to deal with it and requires protection. This can prevent the person with anorexia nervosa from changing, maturing and developing new attachments with peers.

Another unhelpful mode of interaction is when a parent tries to logically argue with his/her daughter to make her see the inappropriateness of her behaviour. This may mean that they can spend hours in discussions and arguments. One disadvantage of this pattern of behaving is that it allows the anorexic person to rehearse and articulate her anorexic beliefs. These beliefs are not amenable to any form of logic as they are emotionally rooted. Thus this behaviour tends to perpetuate rather than suppress symptoms. This pattern can easily lead to an escalation of the response, with the parental figure becoming more punitive or angry.

FAMILY BURDEN AND COPING STRATEGIES

It is clear from the above that eating disorders have a profound impact on the patients' families. In spite of this, the family burden in anorexia and bulimia nervosa has rarely been the subject of systematic research.

Santonastaso *et al.* [13] conducted a pilot study exploring burden in families of those with eating disorders and found that the burden of care experienced was comparable to caring for someone with schizophrenia. This study is the only published one including eating disorder participants with a diagnosis other than anorexia nervosa, and the results suggest that carers of individuals with bulimia nervosa may experience fewer difficulties than those caring for individuals with anorexia nervosa.

We assessed the burden in a sample of key relatives of 51 women with bulimia nervosa, purging subtype [14]. We found that the subjective burden was higher than the objective one. Moreover, the relatives' perception of the support received from the social network and professionals, as well as the levels of the positive attitudes toward the patient, were quite high, while the levels of criticism were low. These data suggest that the family of the patients with bulimia nervosa could provide a substantial support in the treatment of this pathology.

Awakening during the night, negative effects on family life and constraints in social activities were the objective burden variables receiving the highest scores among the relatives of bulimic patients. Feelings of loss and depressed mood were the psychological reactions most frequently experienced by those relatives.

No significant correlations were found between the levels of subjective and objective burden, on the one hand, and the relatives' sociodemographic characteristics, the severity of the patients' eating-related psychopathology, the duration of the illness, and the frequency of binge/vomiting episodes, on the other. Moreover, no difference in the levels of burden was observed between the relatives of bulimics with or without comorbid Axis I and/or Axis II psychiatric disorders.

In this sample of key relatives of patients with bulimia nervosa, we also investigated the coping strategies adopted by the relatives. Seeking information about the disorder (88% of the sample), seeking advice about how to behave in critical situations (86%) and seeking spiritual help (84%) were the most frequently adopted strategies. While 50% of the relatives had some form of collusion with the patient, most of them encouraged the patient to maintain her interests and/or to look for some new ones. Interestingly, more than half of the relatives avoided having meals with the patient.

The study of the coping strategies of the families of patients with eating disorders may have significant therapeutic implications, since improving the way in which relatives deal with the burden, especially lowering their levels of criticism and overinvolvement, may have a positive impact on the course and the outcome of the disorder. Furthermore, alleviation of the family's subjective burden may have beneficial effects on the relatives' own mental health.

FAMILY INTERVENTIONS FOR EATING DISORDERS

The role of the family in the treatment of anorexia nervosa was already mentioned in the 19th century as the need to separate the patient from her family (parentectomy) [15], reflecting the implicit belief that parents are faulty with respect to the development and/or the severity of their daughter's illness [16].

The first theories about family interactions and usefulness of family therapy were formulated by Minuchin and colleagues [17] and Selvini Palazzoli [18] in the 1970s. Although the two theories were developed independently, they share some aspects. In both theories, the anorexic family was described as having specific characteristics: the closeness of the relationships within the family, the blurring of boundaries between generations, and a tendency to avoid open disagreement and conflict [19]. Structural family therapy, as developed by Minuchin and co-workers [17], seeks to change dysfunctional transactional patterns within the family system by providing instructions about how to deal with the symptoms, encouraging some types of family interaction and limiting others. Strategic family therapy [18], on the contrary, uses indirect and paradoxical interventions in the attempt to stop the maladaptive circular system adopted by the pathological family.

Subsequent theories and approaches reflect the tendency to develop integrated treatments for patients with eating disorders, combining cognitive, behavioural and family interventions. This integrated approach is the logical consequence of the multifactorial models [e.g. 20] formulated to explain the development of eating disorders. According to Garner's model [20], the family can play a role both in the development of the disorder (as a risk factor) and in the vicious circle that tends to maintain the disorder (maintenance factor). This model suggests that psychoeducational interventions can be useful in the treatment of eating disorders. These interventions, indeed, do not imply that every family with an eating disorder is pathological and needs to be treated. On the contrary, they emphasize the role of parents as educators or co-therapists to help the patient to face the maintenance factors of his/her illness. A psychoeducational intervention can also have the aim of decreasing the negative expressed emotion of the family, that has detrimental effects on the outcome of the disorder [21–23]. Recent models of family therapy usually include psychoeducational and information elements that address the risk and maintenance factors of the disorder and the problem of criticism within the family [19]. Although generally there are few data about the effectiveness of treatments in anorexia nervosa, family therapy represents an exception. Furthermore, in the literature there is an increasing interest in understanding the indications of the different family interventions.

Most of the recent research on family therapy comes from the Maudsley Hospital group [19]. Their model, based on an integration of the structural and the strategic models with psychodynamic elements, represents an empirically based approach shaped by a series of controlled trials [22,24–26]. While one of the limitations of existing studies on the effectiveness of treatments in anorexia nervosa is the lack of differentiation between age-specific groups, the first of the controlled trials of the Maudsley Hospital group indicated that family therapy was specifically more effective than individual supportive therapy in patients with anorexia nervosa with an early onset (less than or equal to 18 years old) and a short history of illness (less than 3 years). The differences regarded weight gain and other more general clinical dimensions [24,27].

The Maudsley model of family therapy limits the use of the typical "strategic" techniques, aiming to help the family to break the usual pattern of conflict avoidance. Since in eating disordered families conflicts are often linked to feelings of guilt and blame [19], in the first phases of therapy these techniques should be used with caution, given the detrimental effects of criticism and hostility on therapy outcome [23] and on treatment engagement [21]. On the contrary, they pay particular attention to familial criticism, analysing both individual and family mechanisms involved in hostility and feelings of guilt. Family interventions in which parents are seen separately from their adolescent daughters seem to be more indicated for families with high levels of criticism and hostility [22]. Moreover, in adolescent anorexia nervosa, therapists usually invite the parents to take control of their daughter's eating [19] as the first step of engaging parents as co-therapists.

The controlled treatment studies assessing the effectiveness of family therapy have shown that, for adolescents with a relatively short history of anorexia nervosa, there is a significant positive response both at the end of treatment and at follow-up [24,25]. The first study compared family therapy with individual supportive therapy performed after an inpatient treatment [24]. A 5-year follow-up confirmed the beneficial effects of family therapy in comparison to individual therapy in patients with adolescent onset and short duration of illness. In patients with adolescent onset and a duration of illness of more than 3 years, there was no difference between family therapy and individual therapy at the end of 5 years. In patients with an age of onset of more than 18 years, individual therapy showed a somewhat better outcome than family therapy, although the difference was not statistically significant [25].

In a study of 90 adolescents with acute anorexia nervosa, traditional inpatient treatment was compared to outpatient individual and family psychotherapy, outpatient group therapy for both patients and their parents treated separately, and no active treatment [28]. The 6-month, 1-year and

2-year follow-ups [28,29] showed that the group that received the out-patient therapy had a significantly better outcome than the no-treatment group.

The study by LeGrange *et al.* [22] randomly assigned 18 adolescent patients with anorexia nervosa to receive either conjoint family therapy (Maudsley model) or a separated family intervention. The difference in weight gain for the two groups was not significant. An extension of this study [26] demonstrated that considerable improvement in nutritional and psychological status occurred in both groups. However, for those patients with high levels of maternal criticism towards the patients, the separated family therapy was superior to the conjoint one. Both groups improved with respect to expressed criticism.

Another controlled trial [30] compared behavioural family system therapy with ego-orientated individual therapy plus family counselling. Both treatments were effective with few differences at the 1-year follow-up. However, the family therapy group showed a significantly greater weight gain and greater change in maternal communication.

Finally, a recent study [31] randomized 25 hospitalized adolescents with restricting anorexia nervosa to receive either family therapy or a family psychoeducational group intervention for 4 months during the inpatient treatment and after discharge. No significant group differences were found on any of the outcome measures, including weight.

Overall, clinical trials including some type of family intervention support the idea that, in adolescent anorexia nervosa, parents should be part of the treatment programme. Evidence also tends to support the idea that family interventions are more useful for cases with onset before the age of 18 and that a separated family counselling or therapy is more indicated in the case of high criticism in the family. More research is needed to explore whether family therapy can be useful in adult patients with anorexia nervosa or in patients with bulimia nervosa. Published studies evaluating the outcome of family treatments in adult patients are less positive than those in adolescents [32,33] with respect to general outcome. The outcome tended to be very similar in patients receiving family therapy and in those receiving individual psychotherapy. So, there are no data to support an additional benefit in the use of some type of family approach in adult patients with anorexia nervosa. Few data are available about which type of treatment tends to be more effective in alleviating the family burden associated with eating disorders [34]. Finally, there are no evidence-based data about the effectiveness of family therapy in normal-weight bulimia nervosa. Since bulimia nervosa usually has an adult onset, treatment research did not consider family therapy as a possible choice. However, family counselling could lead to an improvement of family burden and/or familial criticism, when patients with bulimia nervosa are still living in the family.

In pre-pubertal bulimia nervosa, the involvement of parents is considered essential [35], although no systematic studies are available.

CONCLUSIONS

The relatives of eating disorder patients tend to be overwhelmed by their caring role, which involves being faced with the key symptom at each meal time and often additional night time disturbance. The burden is compounded by the difficulty in understanding the disease. Family members may be confused, angry and desperate because of the disruption to family life and the fear for the patient's mental and physical health. This can lead to vicious circles of unhelpful behaviours and emotions which may worsen the patient's pathology. Thus, family factors can play a role in the maintenance of these disorders and need to be a focus of treatment. Defining and relieving the burden on the patient's relatives is important not only for their well-being, but also for their approach to the disease and their involvement in the cure.

The relationships between family members and patients may have been suboptimal before the onset of the disorder and are further disturbed as a consequence of the disorder. They need to be remodelled in order to provide the patients with an environment that can foster recovery. It is probable that, without this, no therapeutic approach will be successful in the long run.

This does not mean that the relatives of eating disorder patients should always undergo psychological or psychiatric treatments, unless this is dictated by specific psychopathologies. However, including the patient's family within the treatment context with specific programmes aiming to lessen their burden is certainly essential for both their and the patient's well-being.

Family burden may evolve according to two main pathways. The first includes relatives who have clearly understood the significance of the disease and realized the severe mental and physical consequences of the eating disorder, and are anguished because of their apparent incapacity or impossibility to take care of the patient and his/her disorder. They are generally ready to accomplish whatever is requested from them and mostly need support and encouragement to carry on their tasks. The second group includes relatives who, because of sociocultural factors, or pre-existing personal psychopathological impairments, are not able or do not want to understand the core of the problem, or are resistant to the need to change their lifestyle and their intrafamilial relationships. These subjects require a much more complex therapeutic approach.

The family's motivation to be involved in the patient's treatment is the crucial point and needs to be addressed from the time of the initial assessment. There has been a conceptual shift from blaming the family as the cause of the eating disorder to one in which it is the coping response to the illness which may be helpful or not. Thus, family members need to be involved as partners of the treatment team and provided with knowledge and skills to be of help.

At this point, the issue of confidentiality arises. This is a thorny question and often causes problems in that carers are often excluded from getting any information from professionals. There are different rules and expectations about this, which vary with the age of the person with anorexia nervosa. However, independently of age, carers do need to be involved if the risk is high. Basically, there needs to be a balance between issues of confidentiality and those of risk. Concerning medical risk, carers need to know: (a) that a medical and psychological risk assessment is being regularly undertaken; (b) that they will be informed if the threat to health and safety is severe; (c) the danger signs that should alert them to medical risk; and (d) what they should do in the event that they are concerned about health and safety and how they can recruit help when necessary.

Concerning the illness in general, they need to know: (a) what are the general causes of an eating disorder; (b) what one can expect in terms of outcome and prognosis; (c) the evidence base for treatment and management; (d) the general maintaining factors of an eating disorder; and (e) the best strategies to help someone with an eating disorder.

In conclusion, the family of the patient with an eating disorder has a central role in both the evolution of the disorder and its management. At the moment, there is enough evidence favouring the parents' involvement in the treatment of children and adolescents with anorexia nervosa, but the effectiveness of the family participation in the treatment of adults with eating disorders is not yet adequately supported. In addition, few data are available about which type of treatment tends to be more effective in alleviating the family burden associated with eating disorders. These areas should be more deeply investigated in the future.

REFERENCES

1. Crisp A.H., Gelder M.G., Rix S., Meltzer H.I., Rowlands O.J. (2000) Stigmatisation of people with mental illnesses. *Br. J. Psychiatry*, **177**, 4–7.
2. Blake W., Turnbull S., Treasure J.L. (1997) Stages and processes of change in eating disorders. Implications for therapy. *Clin. Psychol. Psychother.*, **4**, 186–191.
3. Smith G. (2004) *Anorexia and Bulimia in the Family*. John Wiley & Sons, Chichester.
4. Haigh R., Treasure J.L. (2003) Investigating the needs of carers in the area of eating disorders: development of the Carers' Needs Assessment Measure (CaNAM). *Eur. Eat. Disord. Rev.*, **11**, 125–141.

5. Treasure J., Murphy T., Szmukler G., Todd G., Gavan K., Joyce J. (2001) The experience of caregiving for severe mental illness: a comparison between anorexia nervosa and psychosis. *Soc. Psychiatry Psychiatr. Epidemiol.*, **36**, 343–347.

6. Haigh R., Whitney J., Weinman J., Treasure J. (2002) Caring for someone with an eating disorder: an exploration of carers' illness perceptions, distress, experience of caregiving, and unmet needs. Unpublished manuscript.

7. Treasure J.L., Katzman M., Schmidt U., Troop N., Todd G., de Silva P. (1999) Engagement and outcome in the treatment of bulimia nervosa: first phase of a sequential design comparing motivation enhancement therapy and cognitive behavioural therapy. *Behav. Res. Ther.*, **37**, 405–418.

8. Winn S., Perkins S., Walwyn R., Schmidt U., Eisler I., Treasure J., Berelowitz M., Dofge L., Frost S., Jenkins M., *et al.* (2003) Predictors of mental health problems and negative caregiving experiences in carers of individuals with bulimia nervosa. Unpublished manuscript.

9. Van Den Broucke S., Vandereycken W., Vertommen H. (1995) Mental communication in eating disorder patients: a controlled observational study. *Int. J. Eat. Disord.*, **17**, 1–22.

10. Stein A., Wolley H., Cooper S.D., Fairburn C.G. (1994) An observational study of mothers with eating disorders and their infants. *J. Child Psychol. Psychiatry*, **35**, 733–748.

11. Stein A., Murray L., Cooper P., Fairburn C.G. (1996) Infant growth in the context of maternal eating disorders and maternal depression: a comparative study. *Psychol. Med.*, **26**, 569–574.

12. Stein A., Woolley H., McPerson K. (1999) Conflict between mothers with eating disorders and their infants during mealtimes. *Br. J. Psychiatry*, **175**, 455–461.

13. Santonastaso P., Saccon D., Favaro A. (1997) Burden and psychiatric symptoms on key relatives of patients with eating disorders: a preliminary study. *Eat. Weight Disord.*, **2**, 44–48.

14. Monteleone P., Santonastaso P., Magliano L., Favaro A., Fiorillo A., Maj M. (2003) Assessment of family burden and coping strategies among the relatives of patients with bulimia nervosa. Unpublished manuscript.

15. Harper G. (1983) Varieties of parenting failure in anorexia nervosa: protection and parentectomy revisited. *J. Am. Acad. Child Psychiatry*, **22**, 134–139.

16. Vandereycken W., Kog E., Vanderlinden J. (1988) *The Family Approach to Eating Disorders*. Publishers Marketing Association, New York.

17. Minuchin S., Rosman B.I., Baker I. (1978) *Psychosomatic Families: Anorexia Nervosa in Context*. Harvard University Press, Cambridge, MA.

18. Selvini Palazzoli M. (1974) *Self-Starvation: From the Intrapsychic to the Transpersonal Approach to Anorexia Nervosa*. Chaucer, London.

19. Dare C., Eisler I. (1997) Family therapy for anorexia nervosa. In: Garner D.M., Garfinkel P.E. (eds) *Handbook of Treatment for Eating Disorders*. Guilford Press, New York, pp. 307–324.

20. Garner D.M. (1993) Pathogenesis of anorexia nervosa. *Lancet*, **341**, 1631–1635.

21. Szmukler G.I., Eisler I., Russell G.F.M., Dare C. (1985) Anorexia nervosa: parental "expressed emotion" and dropping-out of treatment. *Br. J. Psychiatry*, **47**, 265–271.

22. LeGrange D., Eisler I., Dare C., Russell G.F.M. (1992) Evaluation of family therapy in anorexia nervosa: a pilot study. *Int. J. Eat. Disord.*, **12**, 347–357.

23. Van Furth E.F., Van Strien D.C., Martina L.M.L., Van Son M.J.M., Hendrickx J.J.P., Van England H. (1996) Expressed emotion and the prediction of outcome in adolescent eating disorders. *Int. J. Eat. Disord.*, **20**, 19–31.
24. Russell G.F.M., Szmukler G.I., Dare C., Eisler I. (1987) An evaluation of family therapy in anorexia nervosa and bulimia nervosa. *Arch. Gen. Psychiatry*, **44**, 1047–1056.
25. Eisler I., Dare C., Russell G.F.M., Szmukler G.I., LeGrange D., Dodge E. (1997) Family and individual therapy in anorexia nervosa. A 5-year follow-up. *Arch. Gen. Psychiatry*, **54**, 1025–1030.
26. Eisler I., Dare C., Hodes M., Russell G., Dodge E., LeGrange D. (2000) Family therapy for adolescent anorexia nervosa: the results of a controlled comparison of two family interventions. *J. Child Psychol. Psychiatry*, **41**, 727–736.
27. Morgan H.G., Russell G.F.M. (1975) Value of family background and clinical features as predictors of long-term outcome in anorexia nervosa: four-year follow-up study of 41 patients. *Psychol. Med.*, **5**, 355–371.
28. Crisp A.H., Norton K., Gowers S., Halek C., Bowyer C., Yeldham D., Levett G., Bhat A. (1991) A controlled study of the effect of therapies aimed at adolescent and family psychopathology in anorexia nervosa. *Br. J. Psychiatry*, **159**, 325–333.
29. Gowers S., Norton K., Halek C., Crisp A.H. (1994) Outcome of outpatient psychotherapy in a random allocation treatment study of anorexia nervosa. *Int. J. Eat. Disord.*, **15**, 165–177.
30. Robin A.L., Siegel P.T., Koepke T., Moye A.W., Tice S. (1994) Family therapy versus individual therapy for adolescent females with anorexia nervosa. *J. Develop. Behav. Pediatr.*, **15**, 11–116.
31. Geist R., Heinmaa M., Stephens D., Davis R., Katzman D.K. (2000) Comparison of family therapy and family group psychoeducation in adolescents with anorexia nervosa. *Can. J. Psychiatry*, **45**, 173–178.
32. Hall A., Crisp A.H. (1987) Brief psychotherapy in the treatment of anorexia nervosa: outcome at one year. *Br. J. Psychiatry*, **151**, 185–191.
33. Dare C., Eisler I., Russell G., Treasure J., Dodge E. (2001) Psychological therapies for adults with anorexia nervosa. Randomised controlled trial of out-patient treatments. *Br. J. Psychiatry*, **178**, 216–221.
34. Favaro A. (2002) What about family burden in eating disorders? In: Maj M., Halmi H., López-Ibor J.J., Sartorius N. (eds) *Eating Disorders*. John Wiley & Sons, Chichester, pp. 420–422.
35. Lask B., Bryant-Waugh R. (1997) Prepubertal eating disorders. In: Garner D.M., Garfinkel P.E. (eds) *Handbook of Treatment for Eating Disorders*. Guilford Press, New York, pp. 476–483.

7

Families of Children with a Mental Disorder

Simon G. Gowers and Claudine Bryan

University of Liverpool, Liverpool, UK

INTRODUCTION

Classification is an aid to communication and research. An effective classi-fication system of children's mental health problems should provide useful pointers to aetiology, choice of treatment and prognosis and also to the likelihood of associated difficulties, of which the impact on the family is but one.

Some aspects of child psychopathology, such as behavioural disturbance, seem to reflect extremes on a continuum that extends into the normal range, with many or all children exhibiting lesser degrees of the same features. Sometimes the demarcation between normal and abnormal is an arbitrary issue of degree, but sometimes the cut-off is justified, because the symptom or behaviour is bimodal in distribution or because those children at the extremes for a dimension may differ qualitatively in other important res-pects from those in the normal range.

Classification in Child Psychiatry

The current versions of the International Classification of Diseases of the World Health Organization (ICD-10) [1] and the *Diagnostic and Statistical Manual* of Mental Disorders of the American Psychiatric Association (DSM-IV) [2] have converged into very similar classifications compared to the many differences between earlier versions of the two systems. Indeed, the research version of the ICD-10 details criteria that are almost identical to the DSM-IV criteria. There has been a move away from diagnostic labels

Families and Mental Disorders. Edited by Norman Sartorius, Julian Leff, Juan José López-Ibor, Mario Maj and Ahmed Okasha. © 2005 John Wiley & Sons Ltd. ISBN 0-470-02382-1

TABLE 7.1 The major categories of child and adolescent mental disorders with ICD-10 codes

Developmental disorders	Emotional disorders	Disruptive behavioural disorders
Mental retardation (F70–79)	Anxiety disorders (F93, F46)	Conduct disorder (F91)
Specific developmental disorders of speech and language (F80)	Fears and phobia (F93.1, F40)	Oppositional defiant disorder (F91.3)
Specific developmental disorders of scholastic skills (F81)	Obsessive–compulsive disorder (F42)	Hyperkinetic disorder (F90)
Pervasive developmental disorders (F84)	Depressive disorder (F32)	
	Stress and adjustment disorders (F43)	
	Somatization disorder (F45.0)	

based on aetiology and pathogenesis in favour of those that describe clinical features without assumptions of aetiology.

The main categories of child psychiatric disorder can be grouped into developmental disorders, emotional (internalizing) disorders and disruptive behavioural (externalizing) disorders (see Table 7.1).

The ICD-10 includes a section F90 to F98—behavioural and emotional disorders with onset usually occurring in childhood and adolescence. The emotional disorders which present in childhood, in particular, may be either specific to that stage of development—such as separation anxiety disorder of childhood—or have features which are not age-specific, such as obsessive–compulsive disorder, which is therefore classified in the main section of ICD-10. Increasingly, children are recognized as suffering adult-type disorders, and the main section of the classification system should be used unless there is a definite developmental component.

The developmental disorders comprise a heterogeneous group of delays or abnormalities in development which are related to biological maturation. They are not strictly psychiatric disorders but are generally considered in mental health classification systems because they render children at high risk of associated psychosocial problems. So, for example, a family with a child with mental retardation may require help with the management of associated behavioural or emotional disorders as well as special education, rather than treatment of the generalized developmental disorder.

There are a number of disorders which do not fit neatly into the above classification, such as the eating disorders (anorexia nervosa and bulimia nervosa) and psychoses (both rare before completion of puberty), as well as tic disorders (F95), best considered as developmental disorders.

Comorbidity is extremely common in child mental health [3], with many children meeting criteria for more than one disorder. For example, those with hyperactivity commonly meet criteria for oppositional defiant disorder or conduct disorder.

Multiaxial Classification

Diagnostic labels are often too restricting when it comes to describing a child with learning difficulties or physical problems as well as a mental disorder. ICD-10 provides a multiaxial version to enable difficulties in different areas to be coded on different axes without assigning precedence to any one, as follows: Axis 1—Psychiatric disorder; Axis 2—Specific delays in development (e.g. specific reading disorder); Axis 3—Intellectual level; Axis 4—Medical condition; Axis 5—Psychosocial adversity.

Epidemiology

The overall prevalence of child psychiatric disorder depends on the threshold applied. The Isle of Wight study [4], which was the first large epidemiological study of child psychiatric disorder, suggested that approximately 7% of children in middle childhood suffered a psychiatric disorder, with conduct and mixed disorders being approximately twice as common as emotional disorders. Subsequent studies have suggested that this is an underestimate, with many reporting prevalence rates of at least twice this level. However, a number of these studies have merely recorded whether children are showing a particular set of symptoms or behaviours regardless of whether they have a significant impact in terms of social impairment, distress or disruption. Prevalence rates from subsequent epidemiological surveys give the following figures: 17.6% in 11-year olds in Dunedin, New Zealand [5]; 18.1% in 4–16-year-olds in Ontario, Canada [6]; 17.95% in 4–16-year-olds in Puerto Rico [7]; and 9.5% in 5–16-year-olds in England and Wales [8].

All epidemiological studies have demonstrated that the prevalence of disorder increases with age. To some extent, this finding is an inevitable consequence of age being a definitional feature of several disorders. Enuresis cannot be diagnosed, for example, before the age of 5, while some features of conduct disorder require the child to have a degree of independence from parental supervision. Verhulst and Koot [9] reviewed 49 surveys and computed an average prevalence rate of 12.9% for child psychiatric disorders. This later review suggested that emotional disturbances and disorders of disruptive behaviour were equally common, with rates of 6–8%. Community samples have shown that only a small proportion (typically between 10% and 30%) of children with mental disorders have had contact with specialist mental health services. In the British National Survey of 10 000 5- to 15-year-olds [8], for example, only 27% of children with a psychiatric disorder had been in contact with specialist child mental health services, while 30% had not had contact with any professional. This study found that disorders involving disruptive behaviour and those of longer duration were more likely to be referred.

FAMILY BURDEN AND STRESS

Caring for a child with a psychiatric disorder may have a significant impact on the family. There is a large body of research evidence to suggest that parents of a child with a psychiatric disorder are likely to experience increased burden and parenting stress, when compared to parents of healthily developing children [10–12]. The impact, however, is likely to vary with the nature of the child's disorder and also a number of family variables. Episodic disorders with an acute onset will have a different effect on family life compared with chronic disorders. In addition, the same disorder can present different challenges to the family at different ages. For example, aggressive behaviour will become more challenging as the child gets bigger, while difficulties in social communication in autism may present new problems as the child enters adolescence.

Family structure and economic stability are also important determinants of family burden. Two parents in a supportive relationship are likely to be more able to face the child's needs than an unsupported single parent. Socio-economic disadvantage will add to the burden of a child's mental disorder. Given that externalizing disorders are more prevalent in economically disadvantaged families, the double burden of financial and emotional stress is very common. In turn, the stresses on the family will impact on the child's mental health problem, to the extent that a circular relationship of cause and effect between family adversities and the child's mental disorder may be seen to operate.

The term "caregiver burden" is often used to describe the wide range of physical, psychological, emotional, social and financial problems that family caregivers may experience [10]. Day-to-day family life is likely to be seriously affected by the child's disorder and in many cases family relationships will be adversely affected. Raising a child with attention-deficit/hyperactivity disorder (ADHD) has been found to cause substantial burden to all family members, including problems with interactions between parent and child, sibling and child, and increased levels of marital discord [11]. Furthermore, research has found that mothers of autistic children report less parental competence and marital satisfaction and more family stress and adjustment problems when compared to mothers of Down syndrome children, or those of developmentally normal children [12,13]. The level of parental stress and marital dissatisfaction experienced appears to be directly associated with the reported severity of the child's behavioural disturbance [14], and this will depend on the nature of the child's disorder, with externalizing disorders causing considerably more stress than internalizing disorders. Much of the research conducted in recent years has focused on externalizing disorders, because of the wide range of challenging behavioural and social problems these children display. They are also responsible for high levels of burden, and consequently these disorders are far more common in referrals to child and adolescent mental health services (CAMHS) than are internalizing disorders [15]. The following section will therefore focus mostly on the externalizing disorders of childhood and developmental disorders.

Mental Health Problems in Other Family Members

Families of children with psychiatric disorders are more likely to suffer mental health problems themselves, and these in turn will impact on their parenting and caring abilities. There are a number of possible explanations. First, a parental mental health problem may have an aetiological role in the child's difficulties; for example, a depressive illness in a parent may contribute to separation anxiety in a child. Second, the child's disorder may adversely affect a parent and, consequently, his/her parenting ability; for example, a hyperactive child may contribute to a parent's depressed mood. Finally, the same factors may contribute to the development of disorder in both the parent and child. The factor may be genetic, a psychosocial adversity, or major catastrophe such as a war. For example, it is suggested that up to 25% of children with ADHD will have a parent with ADHD [16]. Siblings are also likely to be at increased risk of displaying symptoms, as it is reported that first-degree relatives of those with ADHD are 68% more likely to present with ADHD themselves than are controls [17]. Genetic studies suggest that the siblings of children with ADHD have higher incidences of behaviour, mood and anxiety disorders [18] and are more likely to suffer from a "subclinical" level of ADHD [19] than siblings of unaffected children.

Clearly, parents will often be faced with the difficulty of not only caring for the index child, but also for siblings with a higher rate of other, or sub-threshold disorders.

It is likely that adults with ADHD will experience specific parenting difficulties and that their symptoms of inattention, impulsivity and over-activity will lead to an inconsistent parenting style [20]. They may also have difficulties in organizing daily family life. These symptoms are likely to make it difficult for parents to deal with the burden that comes with caring for a child with ADHD and also may compromise their ability to engage effectively in treatment for their child's condition.

Lainhart [21] has reviewed the occurrence of psychiatric problems in the parents and siblings of children with autism, and suggested that these families may be at increased risk of developing mental health problems both because of the stress and burden of caring for the autistic child, and because of predisposing biological factors. Depression in particular has been found to be increased in the first-degree relatives of autistic individuals, and it is suggested that this is not completely due to the burden of care, particularly because in many cases the maternal depression was present before the birth of the affected child [22,23]. Siblings of autistic children may also be more likely to display social or language development difficulties themselves [24]. A review of genetic studies [25] reveals that there is likely to be a strong genetic link in the development of autism. Siblings of autistic individuals have been found to have a 3% rate of autism themselves, a 6% rate of another pervasive developmental disorder, and a wide range of cognitive and social deficits, likely to represent a broader phenotype of autism [26]. Caring for more than one child with a psychiatric disorder is likely to significantly increase the burden and stress experienced by parents.

Parenting Competence

It is perhaps not surprising that mothers of children affected by a psychiatric disorder might report less parental competence than those raising a developmentally normal child [13], because many of these parents feel ill-equipped to deal with their child's needs and challenging behaviours. A study of families of children with autism found that parents reported significantly lower efficacy scores than the parents of normally developing children of similar ages, and that perceived stress levels correlated negatively with the measure of efficacy [27]. This aspect of burden is likely to vary according to the place of the child in the family. For example, if parents have already raised two healthy children, and their third child is affected by a mental disorder, they are likely to have more confidence in their abilities as parents than if it were their first child who was affected. They will also be able to use some of the parenting skills they have learnt in dealing with the healthy children and apply these to the more difficult child. The perceived burden caused by a child has been found to vary according to the parent's gender, with fathers of autistic children reporting lower perceived parenting competence than mothers do [27]. Although there is much evidence to suggest that parenting stress will be greater in families with an affected child, it may be the developmental delay as much as the behavioural deviance which is responsible. A comparison between families with an autistic child, families with a child matched on gender and chronological age, and families with a child matched on gender and developmental level suggested that some aspects of the stress reported by caregivers of the autistic children were more similar to those reported by the parents of the normally developing children of matched developmental age, than those of normally developing children of matched chronological age [28], so it may be important to consider which children ought to be used as a comparison group when assessing parental stress factors.

Impact on Siblings

Siblings are also likely to be affected when there is a child with a psychiatric disorder in the family. Studies looking at the family relationships of children with ADHD, autism and learning disabilities have found that siblings report less warmth, closeness and satisfaction in the relationship than typical siblings do [29,30]. Furthermore, siblings of affected children have been found to experience difficulties themselves, including higher levels of anxiety, increased worries about the future [31], lower self-esteem [32] and feelings of rejection from their parents [33]. They may also be more likely to exhibit problem behaviours themselves [34], perhaps because of the anxiety and rejection they feel, or because they are copying the behaviours exhibited by their sibling [35]. Although it seems extremely likely that problem behaviours exhibited by siblings are in part due to the influence of the family environment, as we have discussed, in some cases they may have inherited a partial syndrome of the disorder affecting their sibling. Consequently, an interaction of these genetic and environmental factors is likely to make them vulnerable to social, academic and emotional difficulties [36].

These effects have been found to differ depending on the sex and birth order of the sibling, with younger siblings and girls older than the disabled child experiencing increased anxiety, while boys older than the affected sibling have been found to show increased acceptance [37]. It has been further suggested that siblings may experience difficulties in peer relationships, and these may be increased when there are no other normally developing siblings in the family for them to identify with. Siblings may experience feelings of embarrassment or shame, and these can result in them trying to hide their brother's or sister's difficulty from their friends to avoid teasing or bullying at school. However, it is noteworthy that many siblings of children with a mental disorder also report positive aspects of their relationship [29], and some studies have found that, overall, parents tend to hold a less positive perception of their children's relationships with each other than the siblings themselves do [29,30].

Family Life

As well as having a significant impact on relationships between family members, caring for a child with a psychiatric disorder is also likely to disrupt other areas of family life. For example, it has been found that parents of children with a range of emotional and behavioural disorders, including depression, reactive attachment disorder and ADHD, are likely to make employment adjustments to accommodate caring for the child. These include choosing a job that requires less concentration and in which they can work fewer hours, so as to be available to care for the child themselves rather than use day care or an after-school centre [38]. Parents in this study also often reported that the job they were in was very different from the career they had originally planned to pursue. Perhaps in spite of such adjustments, it appears that parents of affected children are likely to be less productive at work in that they are more likely to suffer concentration difficulties, and their work is more likely to be interrupted by phone calls about their child or absences to deal with a difficult situation that has arisen [38,39]. Interestingly, it appears that maternal employment may be indirectly associated with *reduced* conduct problems in ADHD children [40]. Through employment, the stress of caring for the ADHD child was reduced, which led to greater parenting well-being (measured in terms of stress, self-efficacy and satisfaction), and in turn to a decreased frequency of child conduct problems [40].

Practical issues, such as organizing holidays or family days out, are likely to require greater consideration and planning. For example, mothers of autistic children have reported that their children frequently disrupt the planning of family activities, restrict family travel and cause more last-minute changes of plan compared with mothers of developmentally normal children [13]. Many parents will find it difficult to take time away for themselves, because they may feel unable to leave the child in the care of somebody else, and this in turn can increase the strain on the parents' relationship and lead to further marital dissatisfaction and discord. Although extended family and grandparents can provide a source of great support for some parents coping with a child's psychiatric disorder, others have reported receiving frequent criticism of their parenting style from their own parents or in-laws [41,42]. These negative comments are likely to decrease parents' feelings of competence and self-esteem, and their isolation will be increased if they feel unable to rely on close family members for support.

In some cases, either parent's loss of confidence in their parenting ability or the need to devote special attention to the sick child may lead them to curtail the decision to have further children.

Financial Burden

When parents adjust their occupations and choose to work fewer hours so they can be available for the child, there is likely to be some financial impact on the family in terms of loss of earnings. However, this is not the only financial implication of having a child with a mental health problem. In fact, research suggests that there is a substantial financial burden to the family across the child's lifetime. Scott *et al.* [43] conducted a follow-up study of 142 ten-year-old children, who had been diagnosed with conduct disorder or who had no problems, to assess the overall cost of conduct disorder. "Cost" was measured in terms of a range of factors, which included crime, extra educational provision, foster or residential care, state benefits and health costs. They found that, by age 28, the children who had been diagnosed with conduct disorder had incurred costs that were 10 times higher than those with no problems. In terms of family burden, the pilot study they conducted prior to this, looking at children aged between 4 and 8 with conduct disorder, found that the mean extra cost for these children was £15 282 a year, as compared to children with no problems, and that 31% of this cost was covered by the families. This is equal to a mean additional cost of £4737 per year for each family. Other child psychiatric disorders are likely to be equally costly to the family. Jarbrink and Knapp [44] studied the cost of autism in Britain and suggested that, for the family of a child with autism and an additional learning disability, the lifetime cost of the disorder in terms of family expenses alone was likely to be somewhere in the region of £30 800. This is again a great financial burden for a family to manage. Parents of children with intellectual, physical or learning disabilities may also manage significant additional financial burdens, which include the cost of private teachers, specific learning courses, consultations, private doctors and other therapies [45].

Psychological Burden

In some cases, the burden of caring for an affected child has also been seen to have a significant impact on the parents' psychological well-being, and this is reflected in the increased rates of mental health problems among these parents. As discussed earlier, parents may be more likely to suffer mental health problems because of a genetic susceptibility or biological link with their child's disorder, but research also suggests that the burden and stress of caring for the child everyday can lead to increased psychiatric problems among parents. Many studies have found increased levels of parental depression [e.g. 46] and it has been suggested that in at least some parents it is most likely that the stress of caring for the child has caused the depression to develop [47]. Evidence also suggests that parents are at greater risk of alcohol-related problems [11,48,49], especially if there is a family history of increased alcohol consumption. Pelham *et al.* [50] studied parents of children with externalizing disorders such as ADHD, conduct disorder or oppositional defiant disorder following interactions with boys trained to act either like normal children or like children with one of the externalizing disorders, and found that the parents who had a family history of alcohol problems showed increased drinking following their interaction with deviant boys, as compared to parents with a similar history who interacted with normal boys.

An aspect of psychological impact that is often overlooked is the grief reaction many parents will experience on learning their child has a mental illness [51]. Alongside this, parents may experience feelings of guilt, wondering if they have done something wrong to cause their child to become ill, or whether, genetically, they may have played a part in their child developing the disorder. These feelings may be further increased by the perceived stigma that still surrounds psychiatric disorders. A study of the attitudes of 51 mothers [42] found that those whose children had ADHD expected that mothers of children who did not have ADHD would hold harsh views of the disorder, even though generally this was not the case. Families of affected children often worry about how other parents will react to their child's problem behaviour in public or in school, and how this might reflect on the perception of their parenting ability. Feeling stigmatized by their child's disorder in this way is likely to lead to an increase in the feelings of depression and social isolation that these parents already experience.

Positive Aspects

Although the research and evidence reviewed so far suggests that having a child with a psychiatric disorder can cause substantial family burden, there is also evidence to suggest that the impact is not necessarily all negative. This is particularly true in the area of sibling relationships. Kendall [33] performed a qualitative study with siblings of children with ADHD and found that some siblings reported positive feelings and pride about assisting with caring for their affected sibling. Other research has suggested that siblings show greater maturity and responsibility than peers of their age, and become more altruistic and tolerant in nature, through living with an autistic sibling [52,53]. There is also evidence to suggest that siblings of a child who is disabled in some way are more likely to go into caring professions when they are older [54], because of the experience they had within their own family. One study of siblings of ADHD children showed that they displayed *greater* peer competence and psychosocial adjustment in school when their ADHD siblings were rated as displaying more severe behavioural symptoms leading to conflict at home [19]. It is suggested that one possible explanation is that interacting with and caring for the ADHD child has taught the sibling better social skills than they would otherwise have acquired.

Families affected by child psychiatric disorders may develop wider and stronger social support networks than other families would have done, and evidence suggests that for children identified by screening as being at high risk for ADHD, these stronger support systems lowered the chances of treatment for ADHD being accessed during the 12 months before and after the assessment screening [55]. Although caring for a child with a psychiatric disorder has often been found to produce increased marital strain and dissatisfaction, in some cases it may have a positive effect on the relationship. For example, parents of children with disabilities have reported that their own relationship was strengthened by coping with their child, and that they experienced feelings of great satisfaction and strength [45]. This finding is supported by Akerley [56], who found that the divorce rate was significantly lower than average among parents with an autistic child.

COPING

The extent to which a family adjusts to coping with a child with a psychiatric disorder will vary. Eiser [57] suggests that, for the family of a child with a chronic disease, certain resistance and risk factors will play a part in determining the extent to which the disease impacts on family life. Resistance factors include intrapersonal factors, such as temperament, competence, motivation and problem-solving ability, and also social–ecological factors such as family environment, social support, family members' adaptation and utilitarian resources. Risk factors include the severity of the disease, care demand and related psychosocial stressors. Factors such as these are also likely to apply to the coping ability of a family of a child with a psychiatric disorder, where the same resistance and risk factors are likely to impact on the adjustment and burden experienced by each family.

Coping Styles and Strategies

Parents' methods of coping with their child's diagnosis are likely to change over time. Many parents report negative feelings, including despair, grief, self-blame and sorrow [45], when their child is first diagnosed. As time passes, the support they receive from professionals, family and friends will assist them in developing adaptive and positive coping strategies. Gray [58] found that parents' experiences do seem to improve over time, and it may be that the initial burden caused to the family becomes easier to cope with. In a 10-year longitudinal study of families of children with autism, he found that many parents reported improvements in their psychological health and in their relationships with wider family members. They also found that stigmatizing reactions appeared to have declined, and that over the 10 years they had developed more effective coping strategies for the stressful situations that arose [58].

Heiman [45] studied the concept of resilience, "the ability to withstand and rebound from crisis and distress", in parents whose children had intellectual, physical or learning disabilities. They identified three factors that enabled parents to function "in a resilient way": open discussions with family, friends and professionals, a positive relationship between parents, and continuous support for the family. Parents reported that an intensive programme that included education, therapy and psychological support enhanced their coping ability. This has important implications for treatment.

Social Support

Social support is suggested to be an important factor in a family's coping ability. Research has shown that social support can reduce reported stress in mothers of children with autism and that lower levels of social support can be predictive of maternal depression and anxiety [59,60]. Informal support may be perceived to be more effective than formal support [59] and in some cases use of community resources has been reported to be associated with increased maternal distress. It is suggested that this could be because mothers are more likely to seek out community help at the point when they are most distressed about their child's behaviour, in which case the support offered could have become associated with distress. Alternatively, the community support may have been perceived to be insufficient or ineffective, hence increasing the mothers' distress [61].

Lam et al. [62] found that carers of children with learning disabilities with high expressed emotion rated a significantly higher number of behaviours as "definite problems" and rated social support as significantly less helpful than the carers with low expressed emotion, even though there was no actual difference between the social support available or the numbers of problem behaviours between the two groups. This suggests that the level of expressed emotion may predict a carer's perceived stress and burden, and can affect the perceived efficacy of social support, which will again have an effect on stress levels.

The Voluntary Sector: Help with Coping

Many families struggling to cope with a child's psychiatric disorder have found that vital information and support is available to them through the voluntary sector. There are a vast number of charities set up to deal with child mental health, and these offer a wide range of services, including telephone helplines, often staffed by parents who have coped with a child's mental health problem themselves. They generally issue leaflets and publications which offer further information, organize training courses and conferences to educate parents and professionals, and provide information on local support groups that parents can get involved with, as well as assistance in finding out what services and support are available, and what rights and responsibilities parents have in caring for their child. The Internet is also a valuable resource for parents and there are many websites dedicated to child mental health problems. One such website for child ADHD is www.adders.org, which provides background information about the disorder, lists of articles or books that parents might be interested in reading, information about support groups in countries across the world and up-to-date news and research about the disorder. It also provides chat forums so that parents can share experiences and views of their child's disorder. Some of the websites dedicated to child psychiatric disorders are set up by parents who have experienced the burden of caring for a child with such a disorder themselves. The website www.conductdisorders.com was originally set up by a parent as a message board, so that parents of children with conduct disorder could contact each other. It now has many members and provides support and information about conduct disorders, ADHD, autism, bipolar disorder and other disorders. These are just two examples of many such websites available for ADHD and conduct disorder, but similar ones are also available for other childhood disorders, including autism (e.g. www.mugsy.org) and learning disabilities (e.g. www.bild.org.uk, www.learningdisabilities.org.uk).

Many parents receive valuable practical support in coping with their child from charitable organizations. The UK-based charity Mencap works with people with learning disabilities and their families or carers (www.mencap.org.uk) and has community support teams based across the country to provide support on issues such as education, housing, employment and leisure activities for people with learning disabilities and their families. It is also running a campaign for local authorities to provide more support for parents and carers, including respite.

There are also many charities set up to deal with general mental health issues rather than a specific disorder, such as the Mental Health Foundation, MIND and Young Minds.

Many of these charities carry out extensive research and treatment programmes. The National Autistic Society (NAS), founded in 1962, encompasses a wide range of services for people with autism and their families. It provides support for parents whose pre-school child has just been diagnosed with autism and has set up an early intervention programme known as the NAS EarlyBird Programme. The aim of this programme is to assist parents in understanding what the diagnosis of autism means for them and their child, help them to structure interactions with their child so as to develop communication and build strategies to pre-empt and manage difficult behaviours. The programme is currently being offered in a number of countries and offers weekly group parent training over a 3-month period. A recent efficacy study [63,64] showed that the programme significantly reduced parental stress, altered parents' communication style and resulted in parents perceiving their children more positively. These results were all maintained at 6-month follow-up. Satisfaction data also showed that a significant majority of parents felt the programme had increased their confidence in managing their child's disorder.

FAMILY INTERVENTIONS

Research into interventions and treatments available for child psychiatric disorders has recognized the importance of considering and addressing family factors that may impact on the disorder, and of including parents in the interventions, as benefits are likely to be sustained longer after treatment if parents are actively involved [65]. When considering young children, particularly those of pre-school age, it seems reasonable to assume that, as parents are likely to be heavily involved in all areas of their child's life at this time, treatment will need to include them in order to be optimally effective.

For certain disorders, such as oppositional defiant disorder and conduct disorder, researchers have suggested that parents are sometimes lacking in necessary parenting skills [e.g. 66], which provides another rationale for including, or even focusing specifically, on parents when treating the child's problem behaviours. A range of psychological approaches involving parents are used in child and adolescent mental health, including psycho-education, individual behavioural work, parental counselling, family therapy, parent training and humanistic parenting programmes [67].

The following section reviews the evidence for the effectiveness of the more common family interventions in the various disorders.

Family Therapy

Conjoint family therapy developed from the notion that problems in the family system might manifest themselves in the symptomatic behaviour of the identified child. Family systems theory suggests that the traditional idea that a child's behaviour can be explained in terms of linear causality has limitations. Family members are seen as being interdependent, a change in one affecting other members in different ways [68]. Hence, a circular model of causality lies at the heart of the theory. Over the past 50 years, family therapy approaches have undergone a succession of transformations, based on the rapidly evolving theory, but generally empirical research has lagged behind the theory, with very few randomized controlled trials demonstrating their effectiveness. Furthermore, it is often unclear which elements of the family therapeutic process constitute the essential agents of change [69]. Structural family therapy developed by Minuchin in the 1960s focuses on the "here and now", with little reference to the child's history. Change is brought about through action rather than insight. It is based on a model of a healthy or normative family with clear boundaries in relationships [68]. The therapist is active and directive. In strategic family therapy [70], the therapist uses a range of strategies to bring about change in presenting symptoms, rather than imposing a normative structure on the family.

The narrative approach is a more recent development focusing on the stories people have about themselves, which guide their lives [71], and has been developed in association with attachment theory [72].

Parent Training

By far the most widely researched psychological intervention in child psychiatry to date is parent training, and this has been applied most in the externalizing disorders. Parent training began in the USA in the 1960s and drew heavily on principles from behavioural learning theory [73]. Since its initial focus on child behaviour problems at home, parent training has expanded considerably so that, alongside these, it can now address multiple child features, including behaviour or academic difficulties at school, peer relationships, problem-solving and communication skills, as well as parent factors such as confidence in parenting, stress and depression [67]. The programmes work by forming a collaborative relationship between the family and programme facilitators, with the aim of engaging families. In this method, rather than being told what they should be doing with their children by "experts", parents' own experience and knowledge of their children is recognized and they are seen to be the experts on their own child's behaviour. In this way parents and professionals bring their own expertise to the programme and work together to achieve their aims.

Programmes may be run either individually with one or both parents to address in detail their specific difficulties, or in a group format, where parents help each other by offering solutions or suggestions. Materials are often used as a basis for discussion, commonly videotapes, which show parents interacting with children in situations likely to occur in a family. These are shown to the group, and the group leader then instigates a group discussion about ways of handling the situation. Role-playing is also often a feature of group parent training, through which parents are taught skills such as problem solving, interactive play and reinforcement skills. Programmes typically follow a structured curriculum over a number of weekly sessions (average 10–12) in which parents are taught the behavioural principles of managing their child's problem behaviours. Research comparing different ways of delivering a distance-learning version of the parent training suggests that an individually self-administered videotape modelling treatment is more effective in reducing children's deviance if therapist consultation is available, than if there is no therapist involvement in the treatment [74]. Furthermore, comparison of an individually administered videotape modelling treatment, a group discussion videotape modelling treatment, a group discussion treatment and a waiting-list control group suggested that, although there were relatively few differences between the outcomes of the three treatment conditions, the group discussion videotape modelling treatment was consistently favoured in terms of any differences found [75] and only parents from this group showed stable improvements at a 3-year follow-up [74].

Conduct Disorder

Parent training is the best-evaluated intervention available for treating conduct problems in children. Although many studies have focused on groups of children aged 7 or older [76], research has suggested that, as children get older, their behaviour problems are likely to become entrenched and so early intervention in the pre-school years is now considered critical [77].

Webster-Stratton [78] described the treatment of 34 families of children with conduct disorder, aged between 3 and 8 years, attending 9 weekly 2-hour sessions of parent training. One-month post-treatment, mothers' reports and independent observations in the home suggested that behaviour problems had significantly decreased, and these gains appeared to be maintained at a 1-year follow-up. A replication of this study [79], using a larger sample of 101 families, followed a similar design except that treatment length was 10 weeks. Again, behaviour problems were significantly reduced 1 month post-treatment, as reported by both parents and teachers, when compared to an untreated waiting list control group, and at 1-year follow-up according to parent reports. The control group was no longer available for comparison at the 1-year follow-up time because they had been treated.

Although there is much evidence for the efficacy of parent training, results have not always been maintained at follow-up. Many studies have failed to use a long-term follow-up and, for those that did, it is reported that 25% to 46% of parents reported continuing child behaviour problems that fell into the clinical range. Additionally, 26% of teachers reported that children from treated families still had significant behavioural difficulties [74].

One of parent training's main limitations in effectiveness may be that, by focusing exclusively on parenting skills, individual child risk factors are not being addressed. The Incredible Years training series [80] is a comprehensive set of programmes aimed at parents, teachers and children. This builds on the idea that parent training may not be enough, and other factors need to be targeted in preventing or treating early-onset conduct problems. The main objectives of the series are to reduce conduct problems in children, to promote social, emotional and academic competence in children, to promote parental competence and strengthen families, and to promote teacher competence and strengthen school–home connections [80]. The series includes parent training programmes such as BASIC, using group discussion of video vignettes, ADVANCE, which addresses other family risk factors such as depression and lack of social support, and SCHOOL, which teaches parents how to support their child's education. There is also a teacher training programme aimed at enhancing classroom management skills, and a child training programme known as Dina Dinosaur Social Skills and Problem-Solving Curriculum, which addresses issues such as peer relationships, problem solving and controlling anger using videotape modelling and fantasy play with puppets. The programmes have been evaluated in a number of randomized studies by Webster-Stratton and colleagues, reporting results for the BASIC programme in reducing child conduct problems and improving parent–child interactions [74,81–83] and for ADVANCE in improving parents' communication, problem solving and collaboration [84].

With regards to the addition of a training programme for the children themselves, Kazdin et al. [85] found that combining child and parent training produced more successful outcomes, in terms of reported aggressive behaviour, than child training alone or parent training alone did.

Webster-Stratton and Hammond [86] studied this further using a sample of 97 children aged 4–7 years who met DSM-III-R criteria for a diagnosis of either conduct disorder or oppositional defiant disorder. Participants were randomly allocated to one of four conditions—child training (following the Dinosaur School curriculum), parent training (BASIC+ADVANCE), a combination of both the child and parent training programmes or a waiting-list control group. Assessment methods included parent reports and independent observations in the home and at the clinic. Initial results, 2 months post-treatment, indicated that the combined treatment produced more significant improvements across a broader range of variables. In terms of clinical significance, an overall reduction of at least 30% in deviant behaviours during mother–child interaction was reported by 73.7% of the child training group, 60% of the parent training group and 95% of the combined group at 1-year follow-up. This study provides some evidence of the potential usefulness of including child skills training elements in a treatment programme. Webster-Stratton and Hammond [86] suggest that further child training programmes should be developed, ideally to be used alongside parent training or as a useful alternative when parents are unable or unwilling to attend training themselves.

The Fast Track Prevention Trial is a large-scale early-intervention study looking at the prevention of conduct problems, being run by the Conduct Problems Prevention Research Group in the United States [87]. The intervention is based on a developmental model of antisocial behaviour, with the understanding that there are multiple determinants and risk factors, including those of the child and the parents, which need to be addressed by any intervention. The study identified 891 high-risk children, who were allocated to intervention or control conditions and will be followed up from Grade 1 through to Grade 10. The multi-component intervention condition includes an adapted version of the PATHS Curriculum (Promoting Alternative Strategies, 88) delivered by Grade 1 teachers throughout the year, parent training and skills groups, child social skills training groups, academic tutoring and "peer-pairing" sessions.

Outcome data have so far been reported from assessments at the end of Grades 1 and 3 [87,89]. Some positive findings have emerged: for example, at the end of Grade 1, children in the intervention group had progressed significantly more than control children in their acquisition of skills, which according to the developmental model ought to act as critical protective factors. Parenting behaviours and peer relationships showed improvements. At the end of Grade 3, teachers' reports indicated significantly lower rates of aggressive, disruptive and disobedient behaviours for intervention children than they had at Grade 1, and parental reports suggested positive changes in problem behaviours for intervention children over the previous 12 months. The positive effect on parenting behaviours reported at the end of Grade 1 was maintained, while that on peer relationships was not. Overall, most effect sizes were modest, especially considering what might have been expected for such an intensive intervention. However, the authors highlight the fact that the sample was drawn from the extreme end of high risk. They also point out that the real test of the effectiveness of the intervention will come when the children enter adolescence.

Hyperactivity

Although psychostimulants are the current treatment of choice for ADHD, parents and professionals are sometimes uncomfortable with the use of medications in young children, and may prefer to consider psychological approaches as a first line of treatment. Furthermore, figures suggest that up to 25% of children do not respond positively to medication [90], in which case behavioural and family interventions would be indicated. Although such approaches are highly unlikely to remove all ADHD symptoms, they can help parents learn how to have greater control over their child's behaviour and how to prevent unacceptable behaviours [91].

Parent behavioural training is also generally welcomed, and randomized controlled trials have suggested it can play an important role in the treatment of ADHD [e.g. 92]. Parental counselling and support is another popular approach [93], offering parents the chance to reflect on the parenting process and to explore their feelings about the child. A randomized trial that compared these two approaches against a waiting list control group [94] found that although both treatment groups differed significantly from controls on measures of ADHD symptoms, maternal well-being and paternal sense of competence at the end of treatment, the parent training group had significant reductions in ADHD symptoms, and a significant increase in maternal adjustment, when compared to the other treatment group and the control group.

Where psychostimulants are used, it has been suggested that psychological approaches should be used alongside medication to improve long-term behavioural outcome [95]. The National Institute of Mental Health (NIMH)'s Multimodal Treatment of Children with ADHD (MTA) Cooperative Group [96] conducted a 14-month multimodal treatment study in order to compare the effectiveness of medication management alone, intensive behavioural treatment alone, and a combination of the two against standard community care. The study recruited 579 children aged between 7 and 9.9 years and meeting the DSM-IV criteria for ADHD combined type, and randomly allocated them to one of the above four treatment groups. Medication management consisted of titration of dosage against behaviour followed by monthly visits; behavioural treatment included parent training, child-focused training and a school-based intervention. Combined treatment involved both of these, and standard community care was that which would usually be available to the child. Results suggested that combined treatment and medication management alone were significantly more effective than behavioural treatment alone or standard community care. For the core ADHD symptoms, the combined treatment appeared to offer little benefit over medication alone, and for other areas of functioning few differences were found among any of the treatments. However, significantly lower doses of medication were used in the combined treatment arm, suggesting that this might be a more acceptable form of treatment for those parents who are concerned about the side effects of larger doses of medication. Results of the consumer satisfaction measures from the MTA study did reveal that the combined treatment was judged more favourably by parents than treatment with medication alone. It is possible that longer-term application of the behavioural treatments alongside medication could reveal further benefits of this approach over medication alone.

Autistic Spectrum Disorders

In recent years there has been a shift in approaches to autistic spectrum disorders from provider-based recommendations to collaborations between families and professionals and from child-centred approaches to family-centred approaches [97]. Intensive behavioural interventions have been popular approaches, often based on the applied behavioural analysis (ABA) principles of Lovaas [98]. This programme involves 40 hours per week of structured and intense 1:1 input in the home setting over a period lasting for two or more years. A fully trained programme team of at least three people is involved with each family. Lovaas's work with institutionalized children during the 1960s and 1970s highlighted the importance of parent involvement in the intervention, showing that gains in verbal communication were lost when treatment ended, unless the child moved back with their parents, who could work to maintain the skills learnt. Lovaas [98] compared a treatment group who received the intensive 40-hour-per week programme with a group who received only 10 hours of the same treatment per week and a no-treatment control group. He found that 47% of children in the intensive treatment group had "recovered" and achieved "normal functioning" by age 7 when they entered mainstream education. Although these results were questioned (e.g. [99]), particularly in terms of how "recovery" should be defined or measured, a follow-up study of Lovaas's sample by McEachin et al. [100], when the children had reached a mean age of 13 years, suggested that the majority of those who received the intensive treatment had maintained the gains made in terms of intelligence and adaptive behaviour.

Since these initial seemingly impressive results, the implementation of intensive home-based behavioural interventions has increased dramatically, so that, by mid-1999, approximately 250 Lovaas-style programmes have been established in the UK [101]. However, a number of other early-intervention programmes using behavioural methods and involving parent and child training have also developed, some of which are based on Lovaas's principles. Dawson and Osterling [102] compared eight such programmes: Douglass, Health Sciences Centre, LEAP, May Institute, Princeton, TEACCH, Walden Preschool and the Lovaas Approach. They found that around half the children in all of these programmes appeared to respond positively and all or most children made significant gains. It should be added that, apart from the Lovaas Approach, no comparisons were made with control groups. In commenting on these results, Connor [103] states that ideally a randomized controlled trial, with thorough outcome assessment to compare the benefits of various programmes, is needed.

Depressive Disorders

One of the most popular and best-researched interventions for depression in child and adolescent populations is cognitive–behaviour therapy (CBT). Although the majority of research has focused on adolescent depression, there is a small literature on childhood depressive disorders. Brent *et al.* [104] state that family involvement in the child's treatment is critical, and describe a number of reasons why this is likely to be beneficial: among them, the possible reduction of drop-out and the fact that involving parents offers a chance both to reduce parental distress and to address issues such as lack of support and cohesion in the family, both of which can interfere with the treatment's potential effectiveness [105].

CBT approaches aim to improve depressed mood by modifying both depressive cognitions and behaviour patterns [106]. Although parents will usually be involved in the treatment of younger children, the main focus is on the child, and the aim is for a collaborative relationship to be formed between therapist and child, so that they can work towards solving the problem together. The CBT may be delivered individually or in a group-based setting. Research in an adolescent population (14–18 years) has indicated that there is little long-term benefit of a combined treatment of group-based CBT and parent training and psychoeducation over the CBT alone [107], although it could be that the parent component would prove more useful in a younger patient population. In cases where individual or group CBT has been tried with little success, and there are wider family issues that may need addressing, family therapy might be a more appropriate treatment approach, so that family members can become more involved in the treatment and therapeutic work can be done focusing on specific relationships in the family.

Family therapy has been investigated as an approach to the grief reaction of children following the death of a parent. Black and Urbanowicz [108] randomly assigned children to a 6-session family therapy programme conducted in the home by a bereavement counsellor, or to a non-treatment control group. The family therapy treatment appeared to be effective in both the short and long term, with results indicating that, on average, a treated child fared better than 69% of control cases 1 and 2 years later and, in terms of parent health problems, the surviving parent fared better than 73% of controls at 1 year and 92% of controls 2 years after treatment.

Anxiety Disorders

CBT has been the treatment of choice for childhood anxiety disorders, and many trials focused solely on the child and obtained significant improvements as compared to controls [e.g. 109,110]. However, as with depressive disorders, it has been suggested that the family can play a vital role in treatment efficacy. For example, Klein and Pine [111] make the point that it would be difficult to effectively treat a child suffering from severe separation anxiety without involving the parents.

A number of research studies have investigated the addition of family or parent treatment components for children's anxiety disorders. For example, Graziano and Mooney [112] found that self-instructional training for children with a night fear, combined with a concurrently run parent training component, teaching parents to modify the child's fears using reinforcement techniques, resulted in clinically significant improvements in the child's behaviour at bedtime, as compared to an untreated control group. Mendlowitz et al. [113] studied children with a variety of anxiety disorders and compared three treatments: child only, parent only and treatment of the parent and child together. Although the results did suggest that there were greater improvements in the children who had been treated together with their parents, there were no independent assessments of outcome. Rather, parental report alone was used, and it is difficult to judge the external validity of this outcome.

In the first randomized controlled trial of CBT plus family anxiety management training [114] in the treatment of children with severe anxiety disorders, an individual CBT approach based on Kendall et al.'s [115] treatment manual and using an adapted version of the *Coping Cat Workbook*

[116] was compared with a second treatment group who received the same individual programme, and an additional family anxiety management treatment module [117], in which parents and children were seen together. Immediately following treatment, 88% of cases who received the combined individual and family treatment showed clinically significant recovery, compared with 61% who had received only the individual treatment. These results were maintained at 1-year follow-up, suggesting that the addition of the family anxiety management programme resulted in a highly effective treatment for the child's anxiety disorder. Interestingly, when a longer-term follow-up was conducted (5–7 years later), the two treatments appeared to be equally effective, with 87% of the individual and 86% of the combined treatment group being diagnosis free. The effectiveness of the combined treatment appeared to depend on the child's age, so that, for younger children (7–10 years), the addition of the family anxiety management training resulted in significantly more children being diagnosis free, whereas for older children (11–14 years), individual CBT seemed to be sufficient. A further study [118] comparing group CBT alone against the same treatment with an added family management component also yielded positive results. At 1-year follow-up, 85% of the children in the combined condition were diagnosis free, compared with 65% of the group CBT alone condition. These results suggest that the CBT can be effectively delivered in a group setting, and that the addition of the family management component did have added benefits for treatment outcome.

However, two recent studies [119,120] have shown no significant benefit of an additional parent training component at follow-up, suggesting that for some children a more cost-effective individual or group CBT approach may be sufficient. As suggested by the results from Barrett *et al.*'s [114] study, certain child characteristics such as age may be important in determining who will benefit from an additional family component to treatment. There is also evidence that, for anxious parents, a family component addressing parents' anxiety can improve treatment outcome for the child [121]. It may be important to take factors such as these into account at assessment, so that a treatment approach appropriate to each family's needs can be chosen.

Selective serotonin reuptake inhibitors (SSRIs) have been extensively researched in populations of adults suffering from a variety of anxiety disorders and have been shown to be effective. A placebo-controlled study of SSRIs in children [122] suggested significant effects of the medication for children with mixed anxiety disorders, compared to controls. There are, however, significant recent concerns about adverse effects of these drugs in children, with uncertainties over whether they will be licensed for use. As discussed previously with ADHD, there may be benefits of adding a family-based treatment alongside the medication, especially in conditions such as separation anxiety. However, as yet, there have been no reported findings of the efficacy of such combined treatments [111].

Obsessive–Compulsive Disorder

Treatment for childhood obsessive–compulsive disorder (OCD) often begins with educating the family about the disorder [123], so that parents have some knowledge about how to deal with their children's behaviours and rituals. Drug therapy has been widely used in paediatric populations, generally clomipramine or SSRIs. However, behaviour therapy is also used, the most common form of which is exposure and response prevention (ERP). This approach was originally developed for adults and involves exposure to cues that usually induce obsessive thoughts and rituals, with maintenance of this exposure for at least an hour with no ritualizing or until discomfort is reduced [123]. Shafran [124] suggests that one consideration of the use of ERP in children is whether they are able to understand the treatment, and this is an area where the involvement of family members can help. In a review of the literature, March [125] suggested that there is some evidence for the beneficial effect of parent-assisted ERP in assisting the child to confront the ritual-inducing cues without engaging in the behaviours that they would usually associate with these.

As discussed with other child psychiatric disorders, a combined programme of drug treatment and behavioural therapy may be a useful approach to OCD. March et al. [126] studied the effectiveness of a combined drug treatment and CBT treatment for children and adolescents with OCD. The CBT treatment included a psychoeducational component for children and parents, child training in mapping, anxiety management training, exposure with response prevention and parent training in how to support their children and reinforce the skills they were learning. At the end of treatment and at an 18-month follow-up, 80% of the children were found to show substantial clinical improvement. Unfortunately, there was no control group included for comparison in this study.

Family Factors that May Affect Treatment Outcome

When parents are an integral part of their child's treatment, it is important to take into account family factors that can have an impact on the effectiveness of the approach. Research has suggested that family background factors such as social class and marital status, maternal factors such as depression and family history of alcoholism, and child factors such as comorbidity or severity of the disorder, are likely to predict the outcome of parent training in particular [e.g. 79]. It appears likely that increased treatment acceptability will lead to increased adherence and therefore greater effectiveness [90] and it is important that the views of parents are considered when choosing an appropriate treatment. This is particularly relevant with the use of medications, as discussed earlier, where some parents may wish to use lower doses or avoid their use altogether if possible.

With regard to the impact of maternal mental health on the outcome of parent training for child ADHD, Sonuga-Barke *et al.* [127] assessed mothers' level of ADHD symptoms and categorized them as high, medium or low. All mothers received parent training and the children's problem behaviours were then reassessed. Results showed that children whose mothers had displayed a high level of ADHD symptoms themselves showed little or no change in behaviour following the parent training, whereas children whose mothers had only displayed a low level of ADHD symptoms showed a marked reduction in their ADHD symptoms. There was also a strong association between the level of maternal ADHD symptoms and measures such as perceived parental competence, parenting satisfaction and depression. It is suggested that up to 25% of children with ADHD will have a parent who also has the diagnosis [16], and parent training programmes may need to be adjusted for these families, for example, using shorter sessions or reducing the requirement for higher-level organizational functions.

Webster-Stratton *et al.* [128] studied the families of 99 children with conduct problems who were randomly assigned to receive a child training programme based on the Dinosaur School curriculum, or to a waiting-list control group. Children who received the training programme showed significant improvement in aggressive and non-compliant behaviour as compared to controls. The results of those who did and did not make progress with the treatment were compared on factors of comorbidity with ADHD, parenting discipline factors and family risk factors such as low income, marital distress and maternal depression. Results indicated that negative parenting practices, such as use of harsh discipline and critical remarks, were related to unsuccessful child training, but other family risk factors were not.

A recent study [129] demonstrated that although maternal mental health difficulties such as depression, history of abuse and substance abuse led to poorer parenting, as measured by parent reports and independent observations, these risk factors did not have an effect on the engagement in or outcome of parent training programmes. In some cases, the mothers with mental health risk factors were more engaged in the programme than those without the risk factors. Every effort was made in this study to make the parent training programme accessible to all: for example, child care, meals and transportation were provided, and these may have been important factors in increasing attendance and engagement, and therefore the effectiveness of the programme.

CONCLUSIONS

Children generally live within a family setting of some sort and, in early and middle childhood, family relationships are the most significant in the child's life. Even where organic and constitutional factors operate, these relationships will often have a significant effect on the presentation of child mental health problems, and parents' and siblings' lives will themselves be affected by the more severe disorders, emotionally, practically and sometimes financially. The past two decades have seen a tremendous growth in family-based interventions with proven benefits in good quality treatment trials. The Internet has also opened up a range of supports for families to supplement those provided by the voluntary sector. The burden on the family of a child with mental health problems is often lessened by the provision of information and support, while the formal therapies generally focus on marshalling family resources and promote coping through a greater sense of empowerment.

REFERENCES

1. World Health Organization (1992) *The ICD-10 Classification of Mental and Behavioural Disorders. Clinical Descriptions and Diagnostic Guidelines.* World Health Organization, Geneva.
2. American Psychiatric Association (1994) *Diagnostic and Statistical Manual of Mental Disorders*, 4th edn. American Psychiatric Association, Washington, DC.
3. Caron C., Rutter M. (1991) Comorbidity in child psychopathology: concepts, issues and research strategies. *J. Child Psychol. Psychiatry*, **32**, 1063–1080.
4. Rutter M., Tizard J., Whitmore K. (eds) (1970) *Education, Health and Behaviour.* Longman, London.
5. Anderson J.C., Franz C.P., Williams S., McGee R., Silva P.A. (1987) DSM-III disorders in pre-adolescent children. *Arch. Gen. Psychiatry*, **44**, 69–76.
6. Offord D.R., Boyle M.H., Szatmari P., Rae-Grant N.I., Links P.S., Cadman D.T., Byles J.A., Crawford J.W., Blum H.M., Byrne C. (1987) Ontario Child Health Study II. Six-month prevalence of disorder and rates of service utilization. *Arch. Gen. Psychiatry*, **44**, 832–836.
7. Bird H.R., Canino G., Rubio-Stipec M., Gould M.S., Ribera J., Sesman M., Woodbury M., Huertas-Goldman S., Pagan A., Sanchez-Lacay A. (1988) Estimates of the prevalence of child maladjustment in a community survey in Puerto-Rico. *Arch. Gen. Psychiatry*, **45**, 1120–1126.
8. Meltzer H., Gatward R., Goodman R., Ford T. (2000) *The Mental Health of Children and Adolescents in Great Britain.* The Stationery Office, London.

9. Verhulst F., Koot H. (1995) *The Epidemiology of Child and Adolescent Psychopathology*. Oxford University Press, Oxford.
10. Dowdell E.B. (1995) Caregiver burden: grandmothers raising their high risk grandchildren. *J. Psychosoc. Nurs. Ment. Health Serv.*, **33**, 27–30.
11. Hankin C.S. (2001) ADHD and its impact on the family. *Drug Benefits Trends*, **13**(Suppl. C), 15–16.
12. Sanders J.L., Morgan S.M. (1997) Family stress and adjustment as perceived by parents of children with autism or Down Syndrome: implications for intervention. *Child. Fam. Behav. Ther.*, **19**, 15–32.
13. Rodrigue J.R., Morgan S.B., Geffken G. (1990) Families of autistic children: psychological functioning of mothers. *J. Clin. Child Psychol.*, **19**, 371–379.
14. Morris M.M. (2001) Parental stress and marital satisfaction in families of children with attention deficit/hyperactivity disorder. *Dissertation Abstracts International*, **61**, 7–A.
15. Kazdin A.E., Weisz J.R. (2003) Context and background of evidence-based psychotherapies for children and adolescents. In: Kazdin A.E., Weisz J.R. (eds) *Evidence-Based Psychotherapies for Children and Adolescents*. Guilford Press, London, pp. 3–21.
16. Faraone S.V., Biederman J. (1997) Do attention deficit hyperactivity disorder and major depression share familial risk factors? *J. Nerv. Ment. Dis.*, **185**, 533–541.
17. Rutter M., Silberg J., O'Connor T., Simonoff E. (1999) Genetics and child psychiatry I: Advances in quantitative and molecular genetics. *J. Child Psychol. Psychiatry*, **40**, 3–18.
18. Faraone S.V., Biederman J., Lechman B.K., Spencer T., Norman D., Seidman L.J., Kraus I., Perrin J., Chen W.J., Tsuang M. (1993) Intellectual performance and school failure in children with attention deficit hyperactivity disorder and in their siblings. *J. Abnorm. Psychol.*, **102**, 616–623.
19. Smith A.J., Brown R.T., Bunke V., Blount R.L., Christophersen E. (2002) Psychosocial adjustment and peer competence of siblings of children with attention deficit/hyperactivity disorder. *J. Attention Disord.*, **5**, 165–177.
20. Weiss M., Hechtman L., Weis G. (2000) ADHD in parents. *J. Am. Acad. Child Adolesc. Psychiatry*, **39**, 1059–1061.
21. Lainhart J.E. (1999) Psychiatric problems in individuals with autism, their parents and siblings. *Int. Rev. Psychiatry*, **11**, 278–298.
22. Biderman J., Faraone S.V., Keenan K., Benjamin J., Krifcher B., Moore C., Sprich S., Ugaglia K., Jellinek M.S., Steingard R., *et al.* (1992) Further evidence for family-genetic risk factors in attention deficit hyperactivity disorder (ADHD): patterns of comorbidity in probands and relatives in psychiatrically and pediatrically referred samples. *Arch. Gen. Psychiatry*, **49**, 728–738.
23. Piven J., Chase G.A., Landa R., Wzorek M., Gayle J., Cloud D., Folstein S.E. (1991) Psychiatric disorders in the parents of autistic individuals. *J. Am. Acad. Child Adolesc. Psychiatry*, **30**, 471–478.
24. Piven J., Palmer P. (1999) Psychiatric disorder and the broader autism phenotype: evidence from a family study of multiple-incidence autism families. *Am. J. Psychiatry*, **156**, 557–563.
25. Rutter M. (2000) Genetic studies of autism: from the 1970s into the millennium. *J. Abnorm. Child Psychol.*, **28**, 3–14.
26. Bolton P., Macdonald H., Pickles A., Rios P., Goode S., Crowson M., Bailey A., Rutter M. (1994) A case–control family history study of autism. *J. Child Psychol. Psychiatry*, **35**, 877–900.

27. Belchic J.K. (1996) Stress, social support, and sense of parenting competence: a comparison of mothers and fathers of children with autism, Down syndrome and normal development across the family life cycle. *Dissertation Abstracts International*, **57**, 2–A.

28. Mann C. (1996) Stress, coping and adaptation in families with young autistic children. *Dissertation Abstracts International*, **56**, 11.

29. Robertson K. (2002) Relationships between boys with autism and their siblings. *Dissertation Abstracts International*, **63**, 3–A.

30. Stone K.L. (2000) An investigation of sibling relationships of children with ADHD and their older siblings. *Dissertation Abstracts International*, **60**, 8–B.

31. Bagenholm A., Gillberg C. (1991) Psychosocial effects on siblings of children with autism and mental retardation: a population-based study. *J. Ment. Defic. Res.*, **35**, 291–307.

32. Prystalski S.M. (1998) The effects of autism on sibling relationships. *Dissertation Abstracts International*, **58**, 8–B.

33. Kendall J. (1999) Sibling accounts of ADHD. *Fam. Process*, **38**, 117–136.

34. Hastings R.P. (2003) Behavioural adjustment of siblings of children with autism. *J. Autism Develop. Disord.*, **33**, 99–104.

35. Hames A. (1998) Do the younger siblings of learning-disabled children see them as similar or different? *Child Care Health Develop.*, **24**, 157–168.

36. Bauminger N., Yirmiya N. (2001) The functioning and well-being of siblings of children with autism: behavioural–genetic and familial contributions. In: Burack J.A., Charman T. (eds) *The Development of Autism: Perspectives from Theory and Research*. Lawrence Erlbaum Associates, Mahwah, NJ, pp. 61–80.

37. Coleby M. (1995) The school-aged siblings of children with disabilities. *Develop. Med. Child Neurol.*, **37**, 415–426.

38. Rosenzweig J.M., Brennan E.M., Ogilvie A.M. (2002) Work–family fit: voices of parents of children with emotional and behavioural disorders. *Social Work*, **47**, 415–424.

39. Hankin C.S., Wright A., Gephart H. (2001) The burden of attention-deficit/hyperactivity disorder. *Drug Benefit Trends*, **13**, 7–13.

40. Harvey E. (1998) Parental employment and conduct problems among children with attention-deficit/hyperactivity disorder: an examination of child care workload and parenting well-being as mediating variables. *J. Soc. Clin. Psychol.*, **17**, 476–490.

41. Gray D.E. (1998) *Autism and the Family*. Thomas, Springfield, IL.

42. Norvilitis J.M., Scime M., Lee J.S. (2002) Courtesy stigma in mothers of children with attention deficit/hyperactivity disorder: a preliminary investigation. *J. Attention Disord.*, **6**, 61–68.

43. Scott S., Knapp M., Henderson J., Maughan B. (2001) Financial cost of social exclusion: follow up study of antisocial children into adulthood. *Br. Med. J.*, **323**, 191–194.

44. Jarbrink K., Knapp M. (2001) The economic impact of autism in Britain. *Autism*, **5**, 7–22.

45. Heiman T. (2002) Parents of children with disabilities: resilience, coping and future expectations. *J. Develop. Phys. Disabil.*, **14**, 159–171.

46. Anastopoulos A.D., Guevremont D.C., Shelton T.L., DuPaul G.J. (1992) Parenting stress among families of children with attention deficit hyperactivity disorder. *J. Abnorm. Child Psychol.*, **20**, 503–520.

47. Faraone S.V., Biederman J., Chen W.J., Milberger S., Warburton R., Tsuang M.T. (1995) Genetic heterogeneity in attention-deficit hyperactivity disorder

(ADHD): gender, psychiatric comorbidity and maternal ADHD. *J. Abnorm. Psychol.*, **104**, 334–345.

48. Pelham W.E., Lang A.R., Atkeson B., Murphy D.A., Gnagy E.M., Greiner A.R., Vodde-Hamilton M., Greenslade K.E. (1997) Effects of deviant child behaviour on parental distress and alcohol consumption in laboratory interactions. *J. Abnorm. Child Psychol.*, **25**, 413–424.

49. Pelham W.E., Lang A.R. (1999) Can your children drive you to drink?: Stress and parenting in adults interacting with children with ADHD. *Alcohol Health Res. World*, **23**, 292–298.

50. Pelham W.E., Lang A.R., Atkeson B., Murphy D.A., Gnagy E.M., Greiner A.R., Vodde-Hamilton M., Greenslade K.E. (1998) Effects of deviant child behaviour on parental alcohol consumption: stress-induced drinking in parents of ADHD children. *Am. J. Addict.*, **7**, 103–114.

51. Mohr W.K., Regan-Kubinski M.J. (2001) Living in the fallout: parents' experiences when their child becomes mentally ill. *Arch. Psychiatr. Nurs.*, **15**, 69–77.

52. Howlin P. (1988) Living with impairment: the effects on children of having an autistic sibling. *Child Care Health Develop.*, **14**, 395–408.

53. McHale S., Sloan J., Simeonsson R. (1986) Relationships of children with autistic, mentally retarded and non-handicapped brothers and sisters. *J. Autism Develop. Disord.*, **16**, 399–415.

54. Cantwell D., Baker L. (1984) Research concerning families of children with autism. In: Schopler E., Mesibov G. (eds) *The Effects of Autism on the Family*. Plenum Press, New York, pp. 41–63.

55. Bussing R., Zima B.T., Gary F.A., Mason D.M., Leon C.E., Sinha K., Garvan C.W. (2003) Social networks, caregiver strain, and utilization of mental health services among elementary school students at high risk for ADHD. *J. Am. Acad. Child Adolesc. Psychiatry*, **42**, 842–850.

56. Akerley M.S. (1984) Developmental change in families with autistic children. In: Schopler E., Mesibov G.B. (eds) *The Effects of Autism on the Family*. Plenum Press, New York, pp. 85–98.

57. Eiser C. (1990) *Chronic Childhood Disease: An Introduction to Psychological Theory and Research*. Cambridge University Press, Cambridge.

58. Gray D.E. (2002) Ten years on: a longitudinal study of families of children with autism. *J. Intellect. Develop. Disabil.*, **27**, 215–222.

59. Boyd B.A. (2002) Examining the relationship between stress and lack of social support in mothers of children with autism. *Focus Autism Other Develop. Disab.*, **17**, 208–215.

60. Weiss M.J. (2002) Hardiness and social support as predictors of stress in mothers of typical children, children with autism, and children with mental retardation. *Autism*, **6**, 115–130.

61. Podolski C.L., Nigg J.T. (2001) Parental stress and coping in relation to child ADHD severity and associated child disruptive behaviour problems. *J. Clin. Child Psychol.*, **30**, 503–513.

62. Lam D., Giles A., Lavander A. (2003) Carers' expressed emotion, appraisal of behavioural problems and stress in children attending schools for learning disabilities. *J. Intellect. Disabil. Res.*, **47**, 456–463.

63. Shields J. (2000) The NAS EarlyBird Programme: autism-specific early intervention for parents. *Prof. Care Mother Child*, **10**, 53–54.

64. Shields J. (2001) The NAS EarlyBird Programme: partnership with parents in early intervention. *Autism*, **5**, 49–56.

65. Grizenko N. (1997) Outcome of a multimodal day treatment for children with severe behaviour problems: a five-year follow-up. *J. Am. Acad. Child Adolesc. Psychiatry*, **36**, 989–997.

66. Patterson G.R. (1982) *Coercive Family Process*. Eugene, Castalia.

67. Scott S. (2002) Parent training programmes. In: Rutter M., Taylor E. (eds) *Child and Adolescent Psychiatry*, 4th edn. Blackwell, Oxford, pp. 949–967.

68. Minuchin S. (1974) *Families and Family Therapy*. Harvard University Press, Cambridge, MA.

69. Jacobs B.W., Pearse J. (2002) Family therapy. In: Rutter M., Taylor E. (eds) *Child and Adolescent Psychiatry*, 4th edn. Blackwell, Oxford, pp. 968–982.

70. Haley J. (1976) *Problem Solving Therapy*. Jossey-Bass, San Francisco, CA.

71. White M. (1995) *Re-Authoring Lives: Interviews and Essays*. Dulwich Centre, Adelaide, South Australia.

72. Byng-Hall J. (1995) *Rewriting Family Scripts*. Guilford Press, London.

73. Skinner B.F. (1953) *Science and Human Behaviour*. Macmillan, New York.

74. Webster-Stratton C. (1990) Long-term follow-up of families with young conduct problem children: from pre-school to grade school. *J. Clin. Child Psychol.*, **19**, 144–149.

75. Webster-Stratton C., Kolpacoff M., Hollinsworth T. (1988) Self-administered videotape therapy for families with conduct-problem children: comparison with two cost-effective treatments and a control group. *J. Consult. Clin. Psychol.*, **56**, 558–566.

76. Nixon R.D.V. (2002) Treatment of behaviour problems in preschoolers: a review of parent training programs. *Clin. Psychol. Rev.*, **22**, 525–546.

77. McMahon R.J. (1994) Diagnosis, assessment, and treatment of externalising problems in children: the role of longitudinal data. *J. Consult. Clin. Psychol.*, **62**, 901–917.

78. Webster-Stratton C. (1985) Mother perceptions and mother–child interactions: comparison of a clinic-referred and a non-clinic group. *J. Clin. Child Psychol.*, **14**, 334–339.

79. Webster-Stratton C., Hammond M. (1990) Predictors of treatment outcome in parent training for families with conduct problem children. *Behav. Ther.*, **21**, 319–337.

80. Webster-Stratton C. (2001) The incredible years: parents, teachers and children training series. *Residential Treat. Children Youth*, **18**, 31–45.

81. Webster-Stratton C. (1984) Randomised trial of two parent-training programs for families with conduct-disordered children. *J. Consult. Clin. Psychol.*, **52**, 666–678.

82. Webster-Stratton C. (1989) Systematic comparison of consumer satisfaction of three cost-effective parent training programs for conduct problem children. *Behav. Ther.*, **20**, 103–115.

83. Webster-Stratton C., Hollinsworth T., Kolpacoff M. (1989) The long-term effectiveness and clinical significance of three cost-effective training programs for families with conduct-problem children. *J. Consult. Clin. Psychol.*, **57**, 550–553.

84. Webster-Stratton C. (1994) Advancing videotape parent training: a comparison study. *J. Consult. Clin. Psychol.*, **62**, 583–593.

85. Kazdin A.E., Esveldt-Dawson K., French N.H., Unis A.S. (1987) Effects of parent management training and problem-solving skills training combined in the treatment of antisocial child behaviour. *J. Am. Acad. Child Adolesc. Psychiatry*, **24**, 416–424.

86. Webster-Stratton C., Hammond M. (1997) Treating children with early-onset conduct problems: a comparison of child and parenting training interventions. *J. Consult. Clin. Psychol.*, **65**, 93–100.

87. Bierman K.L., Coie J.D., Dodge K.A., Greenberg M.T., Lochman J.E., McMahon R.J., Pinderhughes E.E. (2002) Evaluation of the first 3 years of the fast track prevention trial with children at high risk for adolescent conduct problems. *J. Abnorm. Child Psychol.*, **30**, 19–35.

88. Kusche C.A., Greenberg M.T. (1994) *The PATHS Curriculum*. Developmental Research and Programs, Seattle, WA.

89. Bierman K.L., Coie J.D., Dodge K.A., Greenberg M.T., Lochman J.E., McMahon R.J., Pinderhughes E.E. (1999) Initial impact of the fast track prevention trial for conduct problems: I. The high-risk sample. *J. Consult. Clin. Psychol.*, **67**, 631–647.

90. Gage J.D., Wilson L.J.. (2000) Acceptability of attention-deficit/hyperactivity disorder interventions: a comparison of parents. *J. Attention Disord.*, **4**, 174–182.

91. Anastopoulos A.D., Farley S.E. (2003) A cognitive–behavioural training program for parents of children with attention-deficit/hyperactivity disorder. In: Kazdin A.E., Weisz J.R. (eds) *Evidence-Based Psychotherapies for Children and Adolescents*. Guilford Press, London, pp. 187–203.

92. Anastopoulos A.D., Shelton T.L., DuPaul G.J., Guevremont D.C. (1993) Parent training for attention-deficit hyperactivity disorder: its impact on parent functioning. *J. Abnorm. Child Psychol.*, **21**, 581–596.

93. Davis H., Spurr P. (1998) Parent counselling: an evaluation of a community child mental health service. *J. Clin. Child Psychol.*, **19**, 98–110.

94. Sonuga-Barke E.J.S., Daley D., Thompson M., Laver-Bradbury C., Weeks A. (2001) Parent-based therapies for pre-school attention-deficit/hyperactivity disorder: a randomised, controlled trial with a community sample. *J. Am. Acad. Child Adolesc. Psychiatry*, **40**, 402–408.

95. Ialongo N.S., Horn W.F., Pascoe J.M. (1993) The effects of a multimodal intervention with attention-deficit hyperactivity disorder children: a nine month follow up. *J. Am. Acad. Child Adolesc. Psychiatry*, **32**, 182–189.

96. The MTA Cooperative Group (1999) A 14-month randomised clinical trial of treatment strategies for attention-deficit/hyperactivity disorder. *Arch. Gen. Psychiatry*, **56**, 1073–1086.

97. Becker-Cottrill B., McFarland J., Anderson V. (2003) A model of positive behavioural support for individuals with autism and their families: the family focus process. *Focus Autism Other Develop. Disab.*, **18**, 113–123.

98. Lovaas O.I. (1987) Behavioural treatment and normal educational and intellectual functioning in young autistic children. *J. Consult. Clin. Psychol.*, **55**, 3–9.

99. Schopler E., Short A., Mesibov G. (1989) Relation of behavioural treatment to normal functioning. *J. Consult. Clin. Psychol.*, **57**, 162–164.

100. McEachin J.J., Smith T., Lovaas O.I. (1993) Long-term outcome for children with autism who received early intensive behavioural treatment. *Am. J. Ment. Retard.*, **97**, 359–372.

101. Johnson E., Hastings R.P. (2001) Facilitating factors and barriers to the implementation of intensive home-based behavioural intervention for young children with autism. *Child. Care Health Develop.*, **28**, 123–129.

102. Dawson G., Osterling J. (1997) Early intervention in autism. In: Guralnick M. (ed.) *The Effectiveness of Early Intervention*. Brookes, Baltimore, MD, pp. 307–326.

103. Connor M. (1998) A review of behavioural early intervention programmes for children with autism. *Educ. Psychol. Pract.*, **14**, 109–117.

104. Brent D.A., Gaynor S.T., Weersing V.R. (2002) Cognitive–behavioural approaches to the treatment of depression and anxiety. In: Rutter M., Taylor E. (eds) *Child and Adolescent Psychiatry*, 4th edn. Blackwell, Oxford, pp. 921–937.

105. Brent D.A., Kolko D., Birmaher B. (1998) Predictors of treatment efficacy in a clinical trial of three psychosocial treatments for adolescent depression. *J. Am. Acad. Child Adolesc. Psychiatry*, **37**, 906–914.

106. Moore M., Carr A. (2000) Depression and grief. In: Carr A. (ed) *What Works with Children and Adolescents? A Critical Review of Psychological Interventions with Children, Adolescents and their Families.* Taylor & Francis/Routledge, London, pp. 203–232.

107. Lewinsohn P., Clarke G., Hops H., Andrews J. (1990) Cognitive behavioural treatment for depressed adolescents. *Behav. Ther.*, **21**, 385–401.

108. Black D., Urbanowicz M. (1987) Family intervention with bereaved children. *J. Child. Psychol. Psychiatry*, **28**, 467–476.

109. Kendall P.C. (1994) Treating anxiety disorders in children: results of a randomised clinical trial. *J. Consult. Clin. Psychol.*, **62**, 100–110.

110. Kendall P.C., Flannery-Schroeder E., Panichelli-Mindel M. (1997) Therapy for youths with anxiety disorders: a second randomised clinical trial. *J. Consult. Clin. Psychol.*, **65**, 366–380.

111. Klein R.G., Pine D.S. (2002) Anxiety disorders. In: Rutter M., Taylor E. (eds) *Child and Adolescent Psychiatry*, 4th edn. Blackwell, Oxford, pp. 486–509.

112. Graziano A., Mooney K. (1980) Family self-control instruction and children's night time fear reduction. *J. Consult. Clin. Psychol.*, **48**, 206–213.

113. Mendlowitz S.L., Manassis K., Bradley S. (1999) Cognitive–behavioural group treatment in childhood anxiety disorders: the role of parent involvement. *J. Am. Acad. Child Adolesc. Psychiatry*, **38**, 1223–1229.

114. Barrett P., Dadds M., Rappee R. (1996) Family treatment of childhood anxiety: a controlled trial. *J. Consult. Clin. Psychol.*, **64**, 333–342.

115. Kendall P., Kane M., Howard B., Siqueland L. (1990) *Cognitive–Behavioral Therapy for Anxious Children. Treatment Manual.* Workbook Publishing, Admore, PA.

116. Kendall P. (1992) *Coping Cat Workbook.* Workbook Publishing, Admore, PA.

117. Sanders M., Dadds M. (1993) *Behavioural Family Intervention.* Pergamon Press, New York.

118. Barrett P.M. (1998) Evaluation of cognitive–behavioural group treatments for childhood anxiety disorders. *J. Clin. Child Psychol.*, **27**, 459–468.

119. Spence S.H., Donovan C., Brechman-Toussaint M. (2000) The treatment of childhood social phobia: the effectiveness of a social skills training-based, cognitive–behavioural intervention, with and without parental involvement. *J. Child Psychol. Psychiatry All. Discipl.*, **41**, 713–726.

120. Heyne D., King N.J., Tonge B.J., Rollings S., Young D., Pritchard M., Ollendick T.H. (2002) Evaluation of child therapy and caregiver training in the treatment of school refusal. *J. Am. Acad. Child Adolesc. Psychiatry*, **41**, 687–695.

121. Cobham V.E., Dadds R., Spence S.H. (1998) The role of parental anxiety in the treatment of childhood anxiety. *J. Consult. Clin. Psychol.*, **66**, 893–905.

122. RUUP Anxiety Study Group (The Research Units on Pediatric Psychopharmacology) (2001) Fluvoxamine treatment of anxiety disorders in children and adolescents. *N. Engl. J. Med.*, **344**, 1279–1285.

123. Rapoport J.L., Swedo S. (2002) Obsessive–compulsive disorder. In: Rutter M., Taylor E. (eds) *Child and Adolescent Psychiatry*, 4th edn. Blackwell, Oxford, pp. 571–592.

124. Shafran R. (1998) Childhood obsessive–compulsive disorder. In: Graham P. (ed.) *Cognitive Behaviour Therapy for Children and Families*. Cambridge University Press, Cambridge, pp. 45–73.

125. March J. (1995) Cognitive behavioural psychotherapy for children and adolescents with OCD: a review and recommendations for treatment. *J. Am. Acad. Child Adolesc. Psychiatry*, **34**, 7–18.

126. March J., Mulle K., Herbel B. (1994) Behavioural psychotherapy for children and adolescents with OCD: an open trial of a new protocol-driven treatment package. *J. Am. Acad. Child Adolesc. Psychiatry*, **33**, 333–341.

127. Sonuga-Barke E.J.S., Daley D., Thompson M. (2002) Does maternal ADHD reduce the effectiveness of parent training for pre-school children's ADHD? *J. Am. Acad. Child Adolesc. Psychiatry*, **41**, 696–702.

128. Webster-Stratton C., Reid J., Hammond M. (2001) Social skills and problem-solving training for children with early-onset conduct problems: who benefits? *J. Child Psychol. Psychiatry*, **42**, 943–952.

129. Baydar N., Reid J.M., Webster-Stratton C. (2003) The role of mental health factors and program engagement in the effectiveness of a preventive parenting program for Head Start mothers. *Child Develop.*, **74**, 1433–1453.

8

Families of People with Drug Abuse

A. Hamid Ghodse and Susanna Galea

St George's Hospital Medical School, University of London, UK

INTRODUCTION

The families of individuals with drug abuse carry a significant burden when dealing with their drug abusing relatives. Reactions to the problem may vary from an assumption of responsibility resulting in an enmeshed and paternalistic approach, to an absolute disownership of and disengagement from the problem. Whatever grade of responsibility is employed by family members, the influence on family dynamics is profound. The family, as a unit, strives to regain stability and homeostasis, developing complex coping strategies and interactions which may contribute to the chronic course of the individual's drug abusing career. The awareness of such family processes and interactions is of utmost importance in understanding the nature and progression of the problem of drug abuse by the family member.

Drug abuse within a family context may be understood from a different perspective. A family member's drug abuse may be the symptom of dysfunctional family dynamics and interactions, serving to displace the focus of conflict. Drug abuse may be the coping behaviour, driven by the motivation to achieve stability and equilibrium within the family, with the drug use behaviour itself contributing to ongoing dysfunctional dynamics within the family. In such a situation, the evaluation of the interactions between the drug abuser and family members provides an understanding of the contribution of the dysfunctional family dynamics to the aetiology, as well as the nature and progression of drug use.

Family-based interventions, within the field of drug abuse, aim to unravel the complex relationship between drug abuse and family dynamics. Drug abuse is understood from theoretical frameworks such as the 'family systems' theory [1,2] and the 'stress–coping–health' theory

Families and Mental Disorders. Edited by Norman Sartorius, Julian Leff, Juan José López-Ibor, Mario Maj and Ahmed Okasha. © 2005 John Wiley & Sons Ltd. ISBN 0-470-02382-1

[3,4], and an attempt is made to disentangle family processes which contribute to the ongoing problematic behaviour. Effective family-based interventions recognize specific needs of the family as a unit as well as specific needs of the different family members. The focus is not the drug abuser, but how family interactions and family processes may contribute to the behaviour of the different family members. Family approaches are designed to empower family members to alter their functioning within the family system, with the goal of altering the nature and progression of drug abuse, making the problem more bearable for each family member or completely alleviating the problem within the family.

This chapter looks at drug abuse within a family context and provides a review of the burden faced by the families of subjects with drug abuse and of the available interventions empowering the families to alleviate the problem. Throughout effort has been made to focus and refer to the use of drugs, as opposed to the use of alcohol. However, alcohol has been mentioned when literature on drugs falls short and when a distinction between the two is arbitrary or has not been made in the literature.

UNDERSTANDING THE FAMILY BURDEN

Drug abuse is a multidimensional behaviour, with multiple biological, psychological and social components involved in the genesis, nature and progression of the condition. The extent of the burden carried by the family of a subject with drug abuse is determined by such biological, psychological and social components of the addictive behaviour. Similarly, the nature of the drug abuse is determined, to a significant extent, by the adaptation of the family to the abuse.

Literature on families of subjects abusing substances mostly refers to individuals abusing alcohol and heroin. There is very little written about families of abusers of other substances. The family burdens, systems and structures of alcohol and heroin abusing subjects were described as being very similar, leading to the assumption that families of subjects with drug abuse behave in similar ways, independent of what substance is being abused. Another observation reinforcing such similarities is that most substance users use more than one substance, so that a description of family behaviour according to substance may be arbitrary. However, these assumptions should be interpreted with some caution—empirical evidence suggests that the family processes of subjects abusing benzodiazepines and/or cannabis are very different and less dysfunctional than those of subjects abusing opiates and/or alcohol. Such differences may not necessarily only be due to substance-specific effects, but also due to socio-cultural aspects in relation to the substance. For example, families of subjects abusing alcohol in Western countries may behave very differently from those in developing countries. There is a socio-cultural acceptance of alcohol use in the Western world, whereas in developing countries use of alcohol is less acceptable and may even go against held religious beliefs. Similarly, the family processes of an individual abusing heroin may be very different to those where the individual abuses cannabis, because the socio-cultural backgrounds of these families may be very different.

In this section, the burden carried by family members is described in terms of the biological, psychological and social components of drug abuse. Concepts underlying the processes and interactions of families with increased risk of transgenerational drug abuse are described. An analysis of frequently recognized needs of the family as a unit, as well as the various family members, is presented.

The Extent of the Problem: Epidemiological Data

The past decade has witnessed an increase in globalization of the drug market [5]. Problematic drug use is now reported by several countries, including those within the developing world, particularly those countries close to or involved in the main trafficking routes. In the 1990s, 134 countries and territories reported that they faced a drug abuse problem. This spread is less dramatic than that occurring in the 1980s, and in fact some of the countries have reported stabilization and others a decline. However, overall, the number of countries and territories reporting an increase in problematic drug use for all major drug types remains higher than those reporting a decline or stabilization. For example, in 1998, 41% of countries reported an increase, 27% a reduction and 32% stabilization.

There are an estimated 180 million drug users all over the world—an equivalent of 3% of the global population or 4.2% of the population aged 15 and above [5] (see Table 8.1). Globally, the most widely used substance is cannabis, followed by amphetamine-type stimulants, cocaine-type substances and opiates. However, consumption rates vary depending on geographical location, reflecting availability and cultural trends. For example, the problematic use of opiates is most common within Europe and Asia (reported by 100% of countries), accounting for around 75% of all treatment demand in both regions, whereas they account for around 25% in North America. On the other hand, the abuse of cocaine-type substances is most prevalent in the Americas (reported by 85% of countries) and accounts for 61% of the overall treatment demand.

Drug-related morbidity and mortality parallel the increase in globalization. Within the European Union, an estimated 7000–9000 acute drug-related deaths occur each year, with most of the victims being in their 20s and 30s

TABLE 8.1 Estimated world annual prevalence of drug abusers in the late 1990s (adapted from 5)

	Illicit drugs	Cannabis	Amphetamine-type stimulants	Cocaine	Opiates
Global number of people (in millions)	180.0	144.1	28.7	14.0	13.5
Percentage of global population	3.0	2.4	0.5	0.2	0.2
Percentage of global population aged 15 and above	4.2	3.4	0.7	0.3	0.3

[6]. In the UK, the National Programme on Substance-Misuse Deaths reported coroner notifications on 1498 drug-related deaths in 2001, with only 65% of these having a history of drug abuse/dependence [7].

A high proportion of adolescents and young adults use drugs and account for most of the globally reported drug use. In the European Union, reported prevalence rates of drug use among young adults, aged from 15 to 34, are approximately two times those among adults as a whole [6]. Sutherland and Shepherd [8], in a study of 4516 subjects aged 11–16, found that the prevalence for regular use of illicit drugs ranged from 1.2% in 11-year-olds to 31.8% in 16-year-olds. UK data also demonstrate a gradual increase in notified addicts under 21 years of age: for example, there is a steady increase from 1989 to 1995, with a sharp increase of 35% between 1995 and 1996 [9].

Over the past decade, there has been an ongoing increase in the use of substances among the female population. The UK Home Office Index of Addicts shows a gradual increase in new female addicts, with the number almost tripling from 1988 to 1996. However, the proportion of females in the total number of addicts gradually declined [9].

The increase in drug availability and the spread of drug abuse across countries, ethnic groups, age groups, genders and roles result in an increased impact of drug abuse on family life. It is difficult to estimate precisely the extent of the impact on families and family members; however, Velleman and Templeton [10] suggest that a subject with drug abuse is likely to have a negative impact on at least two family members. Using the data from the World Drug Report of 180 million illicit drug users, this translates to around 360 million family members affected by a relative's drug use. Findings from a survey carried out in the UK in 1996 indicate that 35% of young men and 27% of young women aged 16–19 had used some form of drug in the previous year [11]. Conservatively extrapolating these data to the impact on families in the UK, one can expect that around one in every three families in the UK is affected by drug use by a family member. These figures do not take into consideration individuals with an alcohol problem. Although both estimates are very crude, they indicate that the impact/burden on families is significantly large. However, such interpretations should be made with caution, as the figures are potentially influenced by several confounding factors, such as family size, frequency of family contact, and what 'family' means to that particular drug abuser. Of note is the fact that a significant proportion of drug abusers presenting to services would have burnt their bridges with their nuclear family years previously, and their 'mother' might be replaced by a significant close friend. In such cases, the 'family' consists of immediate significant others. Thus, the impact of drug abuse can have a 'ripple effect', influencing a large number of people in society, which in turn has an impact on the drug abuser.

The family plays an important role in the treatment of the family member with drug abuse. Often it is the family that brings the drug abuser to treatment. Brisby *et al.* [12] showed how partners, families and friends contribute to around 40% of calls to alcohol advice centres. Also, drug users perceive the family as the most helpful support in their recovery. In countries where the family is the central nucleus within society, such as Greece, Malta and African countries, the family plays a significant role in referral to treatment, exerting pressure on the drug abuser to seek treatment. The coping behaviour adopted by the family also contributes to the treatment pathway chosen by the drug abuser.

Epidemiological data from several countries support the concept that the family burden of drug abuse within varied societies is profound. The globalization of drug markets and increased availability of drugs make the differences between different cultures less prominent. However, the initiation of drug use at younger ages, and the increase of drug use across all ages, make the impact on the family more significant.

Biological Vulnerability: The Genetic Milieu

Use of substances often runs in families and across generations. Children of substance using parents have a higher risk of developing drug abuse than children of parents who do not use substances. It is unclear whether this familial pattern is due to genetic factors or to shared family environments. The extent of the contribution of genetic and environmental factors in the development, nature and progression of drug abuse varies from one individual to another, and from one family to the next. In either case, a comprehensive family history on assessment is crucial in understanding the risk and protective factors involved in the drug using behaviour. A family history of substance abuse is one of the most valid predictors of risk for the genesis and progression of substance use [13]. The case of Ms X, described in the Appendix of this chapter, provides a prototype family, where combined genetic and environmental determinants contribute to a significant family burden.

Most of the evidence supporting a genetic contribution to drug abuse within a family context derives from twin and adoption studies. Pickens *et al.* [14], in a study involving monozygotic and dizygotic male and female twin pairs, reported a moderate level of heritability in males, but not in females, for substance abuse or dependency. The monozygotic male concordance rate was 63% (22% for females), as compared to 44% (15% for females) in dizygotic twins. Similarly, Enoch and Goldman [15] reported heritability for stimulant and opioid use ranging from 0.11 to 0.45. Tsuang *et al.* [16], in a study involving a large number of twin pairs, found that 0.34% of the variance between twins was attributed to genetics, 0.28% to their shared environment, and 0.38% to their non-shared environment. Several findings from twin studies indicate increased genetic links in males, as opposed to females, where the environmental components may have more of a contribution.

In a study involving adoptees, Meller *et al.* [17] reported that a history of abuse of drugs in the biological family was associated with drug abuse in the adoptee, supporting contributions of shared genetic factors.

Such genetic components are believed to work through various mechanisms. One mechanism may be a genetically inherited vulnerability altering the endogenous reward pathways, from which drugs obtain their reinforcing properties [18,19]. Another mechanism described is that of sharing a genetic vulnerability to a behavioural trait, such as sensation-seeking behaviour, which links consequent disorders such as antisocial personality disorder and substance use disorder [18,20–22]. Whatever the mechanism, substance abuse is not believed to be regulated through a single gene—it is a multigenetic disorder, with several genes contributing to an increased vulnerability to expression of substance-seeking behaviour [23]. Similarly, individuals may inherit genes that decrease the vulnerability for substance use—for example, the gene responsible for D1 receptors, which has been shown to be responsible for a reduction in cocaine use in animals [19].

Despite evidence of genetic factors involved in the preponderance of drug abuse in families, genetic loading alone is unlikely to result in use of substances. It is the specific interaction between genetic factors and environmental factors which results in the development of drug abuse.

The Family Environment: Processes, Systems and Structures

The family environment plays an important role in the clustering of drug abuse in families. Behaviour within the family provides the ingredients for the expression of intrinsic vulnerability to substance use. The family processes, structure and systems also play a role in the nature and progression of substance use by another family member.

Drug abuse does not always run in families. The significant environment contributing to the genesis of the disorder may be the environment outside the family. Peer pressure [8,9] and increased drug availability [5,9] may be two factors increasing the risk for the development of substance use. The contribution and interaction of genetic factors, family environment and the external environment to the development and maintenance of drug use by a family member is complex and difficult to determine in individual cases, highlighting the importance of making as comprehensive an assessment as possible.

Whatever mechanisms are at play, the effects of drug abuse on family dynamics are marked. Dysfunctional family dynamics may have guided the family member to a pathway to use drugs, and to continue using drugs. The effects of drug abuse within this family context may produce functional changes shifting the family towards stability. On the other hand, dysfunctional family dynamics may develop in an attempt to cope with drug abuse by the relative. The use of drugs by Ms X (see Appendix) had profound effects on family dynamics, and use of drugs by the family influenced Ms X's behaviour. As Ms X's life cycle and drug use progressed, it was the family dynamics that contributed to her deterioration. However, despite the underlying dysfunction, the family still played an important role in bringing Ms X into treatment and in keeping her engaged in treatment.

Addiction, like other human dysfunctional behaviours, can be perceived as existing between or among people, with the whole family considered as ill. The dysfunction lies within the interaction patterns of the various family members [4,24]. The family interaction, as viewed from a systemic framework [1,2], is forever shifting in order to maintain homeostasis. The use of drugs by the family member is the behaviour that develops in order to achieve the required equilibrium and stability within the family function. The reaction of the family to drug abuse, whether dysfunctional or not, is also an attempt at achieving such equilibrium for survival.

Several commonalities and typologies of dysfunctional families of subjects with drug abuse have been described in the literature. Kaufman [25] explored family interactions of heroin addicts and classified them according to dysfunctions described by Minuchin [26]:

- *Enmeshed interaction*: the family interacts through overinvolvement and ineffective closeness, at the expense of the autonomy of the different members. The family system deals with stress by intense emotional reactions.

- *Disengaged interaction*: the interaction is distant and lacks emotion. Closeness and a sense of belonging between family members are lacking, allowing each family member to be a single unit.

Studies identified that most of the family relatives of heroin addicts interacted dysfunctionally. Of the mother–child relationships, 88% were enmeshed and 3% were disengaged. On the other hand, 41% of father–child relationships were enmeshed and 42% disengaged [25].

The enmeshed relationships between mother and child are described as symbiotic [27]. Mothers take on their child's drug abuse problem as their own. They behave in similar dysfunctional ways, such as taking tranquillizers, which they may share with their child for psychosomatic complaints. Such behaviours can be explained using the 'stress–coping–health' framework [3,4], explaining substance abuse problems as constituting a family stress, giving rise to signs of strain in the relatives, many times in the form of physical or psychological ailments. The enmeshed relationship is also evident when the mother gets overinvolved in the illegal activities of the child, for example, becoming an accomplice when trying to cover the child's behaviour, or herself carrying out illegal activities, such as shoplifting, thus sharing the child's problem.

Enmeshment can also be seen in sibling interaction, where the enmeshed sibling may assist the drug abuser in drug taking. Examples would include offering financial support, providing the substance for the abuser or injecting the abuser.

Interactions are also determined by cultural differences. In his study of narcotic addicts, Kaufman [25] observed that enmeshment was more frequent in Jewish, Greek and Italian families, whereas disengagement was more common in Puerto Rican families.

Stanton [27] explored the dysfunctional patterns of families with a subject with drug abuse and described the patterns which distinguished such families from other dysfunctional families:

- *Increased frequency of multigenerational substance use problems*, together with increased frequency of other addictive behaviours, such as gambling. This phenomenon, as described earlier in the chapter, is likely to be the result of shared genetic and family environments.
- *Frequent primitive expressions of conflict through ineffective overinvolvement.* For example, no direct expression of anger, but inappropriate emotive outbursts.
- *Overt alliances and triangulations in the family system*, for example, coalitions between the mother and the drug abuser, effectively splitting the family and reducing the other family relationships to disengaged interaction. This was more frequently observed in opiate and amphetamine

addicts, as opposed to cocaine and barbiturate addicts [28], although users of one substance only are not so prevalent.

- *Frequent themes of premature/unexpected death or traumatic losses within the family*, with the suggestion that drug abuse was a result of the inability of the family to effectively resolve grief [29,30]. This phenomenon is understood through the 'family systems' theory. The overwhelming feeling of loss experienced by the family serves as a threat for the family system, with the potential for the family to break up. Drug abuse provides the abuser with a mechanism for dealing with stress, making the addict helpless and dependent on the family, i.e. adopting the sick role. Through this incapacity there is family unification, making the addict a saviour. The concept can also be explained through the stress–coping–health framework. The family stress resulting from traumatic losses is reduced through drug abuse, either by shifting the distress from the loss to the drug abuse and/or by the abuser enacting destructive behaviour, with mock separations, for example, by overdoses, in order to unify the family and aid the family to work through unresolved grief. Unresolved family grief is also seen as responsible for the cohesion and ongoing contact between family members. Some studies [31,32] have shown that the majority of addicts maintained regular contact with their families. Such frequency of contact was also observed across cultures, e.g. among heroin addicts in Italy and Thailand. Families of drug abusers are unable to separate/lose contact due to their ongoing need to reduce the family stress resulting from unresolved grief. Specific traumatic losses that were studied in families of substance users include loss of a family member [32] and emigration [33].
- *Pseudo-individuation*. Families of drug abusers have an intense fear of separation [32]. The drug abuser is highly dependent on the family and resists taking on responsibility. The use of drugs serves two functions. The first function is to reinforce the dependence of the drug abuser on the family and reinforce the need for the family to care for the abuser, so that all parties feel close. The second function is to give the abuser a sense of autonomy when using the drug. The subculture of drug abuse is not shared with the family and the pharmacological effects of the drug provide a sense of power and omnipotence which is only experienced by the drug abuser. This gives a false sense of individuation and autonomy. These brief mock separations by the drug abuser also continue to enhance family closeness.
- *Difficulties in adjusting to cultural changes*. This stems from the observation that the offspring of immigrant families have increased risk of developing substance abuse. This has been explained by the instability of the parents, being unable to respond to the needs of their children, and at times also looking for support from their children. The use of drugs

allows the user to reverse the parental need and to deal with unresolved loss issues.

- *Poor communication.* Several studies refer to the difficulties in communication within the family environment. Feelings are not expressed freely, with gestures of love and affection frequently lacking. Interpersonal conflicts are dealt with counterproductively. Family interaction can also be cold and lifeless, becoming alive when dealing with the problem of substance use [34]. Such reports of poor communication tie in with the frequency of enmeshed and disengaged family interactions described earlier in this section. In such cases drug abuse serves as a tool for communication. The shift in focus on the drug abuser provides a sense of closeness which bridges the gap left due to the poor communication. Poor communication between family members can also result in inconsistent limit setting. 'Good' behaviour may be ignored, easily forgotten and not praised, whereas 'bad' or deviant behaviour may be at times punished and at times rewarded. In this context, drug abuse is perceived as resulting from conflicting messages given by the family to the abusing relative. The mechanisms underlying this behaviour could be understood by applying the 'social disorganization and strain' theoretical framework, which states that a social system, for example, the family, with no internal consensus on norms and values, breeds deviant behaviour [35].

As indicated earlier in the chapter, most studies exploring family function involve families of heroin and alcohol users, with the assumption that families of substance users, whatever the substance of abuse, function in similar ways. However, some differences, possibly a result of both substance-specific effects and the socio-cultural aura of the substance, have been reported in the literature [28]. For example, the families of opiate addicts were described as characteristically having one enmeshed, 'weak and ineffectual' parent and a disengaged or 'overpowering tyrant' other. This prototype was also described by Stanton [27,36] in studies involving American families of opiate addicts, which also reported that the over-involved parent was more likely to be the opposite sex parent. In contrast, cocaine abusers typically had positive and functional family backgrounds, with a warm mother and encouraging father. In cocaine families, it is believed that it is the family drive for success which drives the subject to cocaine use. Families of amphetamine addicts, on the other hand, characteristically had domineering and manipulative mothers and disengaged and ineffectual fathers. Barbiturate users typically described disengaged fathers and enmeshed, symbiotic mothers. It is important to note that such studies describe these differences as substance-specific differences, without giving much consideration to the possibility that such differences in family function may be a result of socio-cultural differences in family dynamics.

Another finding which contributes to drug abuse clustering in families and across generations is that a significant proportion of drug abusers marry other substance abusers [36,37]. The marriage is perceived as an attempt at seeking an interaction similar to that of the family of origin, as well as an attempt at ensuring that the drug abuser does not separate from the family of origin. As described earlier on, strong dysfunctional interactions are at play among family members, making the drug abuser and family members stick together. Marriage to another drug abuser ensures that such cohesion in the family of origin will be maintained. Ineffective closeness is seen between the drug abuser and the drug abusing spouse, with frequent marital disagreements, permitting both drug abusers to reinstate the cohesion with their family of origin. Similarly, if the drug abuser has been away from the family home for a while, a crisis tends to occur in the family of origin, bringing the abuser back home.

The extent and effects of dysfunction in families of drug abusers are constantly changing. Although dynamics and processes may be continuously dysfunctional, the stress and strain faced by the family may not be continuously difficult to cope with. Similarly, the drug abusing behaviour may go through phases of comparative stability. These fluctuations parallel the different developmental stages that the family experiences. For example, when Ms X was pregnant (see Appendix), both the mother and stepfather went through a stable phase in their drug using career, with the stepfather also managing to abstain completely. Matching stability was also seen in Ms X herself. In contrast, the sister went through a chaotic phase with markedly increased self-destructive behaviour. This may be interpreted as fear of being separated from the family of origin, given that the family was focused on Ms X's pregnancy. The sister maintained homoeostasis for the family, ensuring the family remained unified.

Hence, the family goes through various stages in its life cycle, with some stages being recognized as stress or crisis stages; for example, birth of the first child, children leaving home, death of a parent. Families with dysfunctional interaction have difficulty adjusting to such stages within their life cycle and tend to remain 'stuck' in trying to cope with the stress [38]. These crisis stages can also be considered as traumatic losses, which have been described as contributing to drug use within the family context.

The description of the family environment given above shows the complexity of the burden imposed on the family of a subject with drug abuse. Theoretical frameworks have been applied to clarify the burden. However, several mechanisms may be contributing to the behaviour within the family. Also, many studies describe family dysfunction from a cross-sectional analysis, giving little consideration to the fluctuations in stress and strain that the family may go through. On the other hand, most families exhibit a need for cohesion, irrespective of the substance being used, the dysfunction at play and the culture from which they come, indicating the important role the family has in the progress and engagement of the drug abuser in treatment.

What Is the Effect? The Needs of Families of Subjects with Drug Abuse

Vulnerability of the family of a subject with drug abuse is not only quantified by genetic predisposition and dysfunctional family processes and interaction. It is also determined by other effects these predispositions may have. For example, besides having to deal with the problem of drug abuse, Ms X's family (see Appendix) also had to deal with the stigma experienced by the sister when she moved to a different neighbourhood. This perceived positive 'fresh start' was changed to a stressful life event, which increased the family burden. This subsection will describe some of the effects on families of drug abusers which increase family vulnerability.

Physical Effects

Families of subjects with drug abuse experience a range of physical problems, considered to be the expression of the stress imposed on them. Such families frequently consult primary health care services with repetitive or chronic physical ailments, which highlight the importance of primary care workers addressing the contextual aspect of the physical issues [39]. A study by Velleman et al. [40] distinguished between short-term and long-term physical effects. Short-term effects included excessive tiredness and lack of energy, while long-term effects included ulcers, raised blood pressure and shingles.

A survey and a qualitative study carried out in Scotland [41] reported a significant prevalence of colds and flu, heart problems and stomach problems.

The drug abusers themselves also have an increased risk of developing physical problems. There is a higher incidence of hepatitis C and human immunodeficiency virus (HIV) infections in the drug abuse population, when compared to the general population [9,42]. The complications of these conditions can be increasingly traumatic, shifting the family focus onto physical priorities. The family has the increased burden of dealing with specific health issues. This is illustrated in the Appendix, when the sister develops physical health problems due to self-harm.

The high prevalence of physical problems increases the vulnerability of the family. This is likely to mobilize them into dealing with physical conditions, shifting the spotlight away from the drug abuse. The homoeostasis is once again established and the family stays together. Physical problems are also perceived by society as 'unfortunate situations' which, although likely to be instigated by drug abuse, are not brought on by choice. This serves to reduce the stigma faced by the family.

Psychological Effects

Earlier on in the chapter it was shown how enmeshment within the family may contribute to a relative (e.g. mother) sharing the drug taking behaviour by requiring tranquillizers for psychological problems. Families of drug abusers have been described as experiencing increasing stress, anxiety, loneliness, depressive episodes, guilt and suicide ideation. Longer-term effects such as chronic depression and anorexia are also common [40]. Relatives also report an increase in addictive behaviours such as smoking, alcohol use and excessive eating.

Children within the family also have a high risk of exhibiting behavioural disorders, poor school performance and delinquent behaviour [43,44]. Child abuse and neglect is more prevalent in families with substance use. The presence of dysfunction in the family with unclear roles and boundaries requires a family member to take on 'parental responsibility'. Often this role is taken on by the child.

Bekir et al. [45] described two possible responses by the child to such situations: (a) rebellious response, with behavioural problems, anger and withdrawal, and (b) rescuing response (making decisions, taking on parental tasks and experiencing humiliation at the situation).

The drug abusing subject is also at increased risk of developing comorbid mental disorders. The UK National Outcome Treatment Study reported that 10% of patients with a substance misuse problem had a psychiatric admission within a 2-year period prior to their point of contact with drug and alcohol services [46]. The US Epidemiological Catchment Area general population study [47] reported a lifetime prevalence for mental disorder of 53% among individuals with a drug problem. This figure did not include individuals with an alcohol problem and the most common mental problems were anxiety and mood disorders. The risk of suicide is also markedly increased in patients with a substance misuse problem, especially when comorbid mental disorder is also evident [48]. This can have significant effects on the family dynamics, either serving to increase the family vulnerability and stress, or to strengthen the family closeness through the 'mock' separations.

Families of drug abusers are also more prone to domestic violence. The inability of the family to resolve interpersonal conflicts and to share ineffective overinvolvement gives rise to outbursts of anger and aggression, which may result in domestic violence. Domestic violence is associated with increased psychological/psychiatric morbidity, in its own right, contributing further to the impact of drug abuse on the family.

Psychological problems can have profound effects on the vulnerability of the family. Once again the family dynamics shift towards the survival route, with consequent deterioration or stability of the drug abuser. Psychological effects, for family members, may be an unconscious 'blessing' or 'curse'.

Social Effects

Social effects experienced by the family reflect the social consequences of drug abuse. One effect may be financial hardship. The family may have had money stolen by the drug abuser, or they may be paying money for the drug abuser's treatment or paying for his/her drugs. Some family members may also be unemployed, which is likely to add to the financial strain. Unemployment is reported to be markedly higher in families of substance users [41].

The effect of the criminal activity associated with drug abuse can be devastating on the family. The discussion of this extends beyond the scope of this chapter. However, of note is the fact that the family's fear of separation [27] may have become a reality through criminal activity, i.e. criminal activity separating the abuser from the family through sanctions, such as custody. The family may thus experience another loss and may have to find another mode of functioning. On the other hand, this could be the last straw for family survival.

Social effects are associated with increased social isolation and increased stigma for the family. Such spiralling effects make it more difficult for the family to seek appropriate measures to resolve the family problem.

The effects and needs of families of drug abusers are not static and are determined by the nature of drug abuse and the extent of the dysfunction within the family. Although the family has been discussed as a single unit, the effects may be different for different family members. Velleman *et al.* [40] found that partners of drug abusers, when compared to the parents of drug abusers, experienced more mood changes, domestic violence and financial difficulties. Siblings are more at risk of becoming drug users themselves, than other family members [41]. The subjective experience of stress is more pronounced in the parents, especially the mother, increasing the risk of physical and psychological effects.

The demands on the family are also once again partly determined by the type of substance used, linking substance-specific effects with socio-cultural effects. The use of illegal substances is associated with a higher prevalence of negative social effects, when compared with use of legal substances, such as benzodiazepines. Relatives feel less constrained financially by users of prescribed drugs, and the more tolerant attitude of society results in decreased social isolation. Similarly, the enmeshed relationship between mother and abuser is less likely to result in the mother taking on illegal activities, if the substance abused is one that society tolerates more readily.

A comprehensive assessment of a drug abuser should aim to identify the effects of drug abuse on family life. The demands made on family members and their increased vulnerability make drug abuse in the family more difficult to cope with.

COPING WITH THE BURDEN

The effect of the burden of drug abuse on the family depends on the coping style adopted by the family to deal with the problem. Coping styles are, to some extent, determined by the interaction and communication within the family. For example, enmeshed and overinvolved family systems are more likely to adopt the coping style of engagement. Coping styles may also vary with different family members within each family, as well as with the stage of change that both the family and the drug abuser may be in.

The term 'coping', as used in this chapter, does not signify effectiveness or success. Coping can be both adaptive and maladaptive. A coping style may be appropriate and effective in dealing with drug abuse within the family, at a particular stage in the family's life cycle, but may be highly inappropriate and maladaptive at other times and may 'enable' the drug using behaviour. The coping styles described in this section provide frameworks which can be applied to facilitate the understanding of family reaction.

When attempting to match treatment/intervention with the needs of the drug abuser and/or family, it is important to consider what coping mechanisms are at play. If the family coping style is one of withdrawal, the family is unlikely to engage in treatment. In such cases, application of motivational enhancement techniques may be the most appropriate intervention. Similarly, in 'co-dependence', such as when relatives conceal the problem from others by making excuses for the drug abuser, counselling may be the most appropriate technique, aiming at trying to reduce the frequency of such behaviour.

Typologies of coping styles adopted by families of substance users have been described in the literature [3,49–52]. The working typology that appears to have gained most popularity is that described by Orford *et al.* [51]. They identified eight common coping styles: controlling, emotional, avoidance/withdrawal from user, inaction, tolerance, support for the user, confrontation/assertion and independence. The styles found to be most effective were 'confrontation' and 'support for the user'. However, such findings were interpreted with caution and the authors highlighted that typologies oversimplify the family's reaction, and their usefulness was only in providing some structure to a complex behaviour. They also noted that mechanisms of coping may combine two or more coping styles at different times: for example, combining the 'controlling' and 'support for the user' styles when bringing a patient to treatment.

In a later study, Orford *et al.* [53] reclassified the typologies into three categories: engagement, toleration and withdrawal. They found that there was only weak support for the eight typologies, and that the family shifted from being engaged, tolerant and withdrawing according to the nature and progression of substance use. The typologies identified in the previous research were considered to be different facets of the engaged, tolerant and withdrawing styles. For example, some forms of engagement may be emotional and controlling and others more assertive.

Family members adopting the engaged style are actively engaged in trying to resolve the problem. They confront the drug abuser and offer their support to bring about change. The family has the subjective experience of control over the problem.

The tolerant style involves accepting the situation, but overall remaining inactive; that is, the family does not try to resolve it. This is observed in the Appendix, where the mother lends money to the sister knowing that it will be spent on drugs. This coping style rarely brings on change; its benefit is the achievement of stability in the family function. It usually makes the family feel powerless and anxious, associated with feelings of guilt.

The withdrawal style involves the family avoiding interaction with the user. They step back, shifting all responsibility of the problem onto the drug user. There is an underlying drive for independence, which potentially mobilizes the drug user to bring on change. The family feels more in control of the situation and members are able to continue living their lives.

Orford *et al.* [53] explored and compared these coping styles in two different cultures. They suggested that coping typologies were universal and could be applied to varying cultures; however, some cultures were more likely to apply one coping style than another. For instance, in their study, relatives in the South West of England were more likely to adopt the withdrawal coping style than the relatives in Mexico City. This coping style was also found to be associated with more health problems than the other styles [53].

Another approach to understanding the complexity of family coping is to establish adopted coping styles in the context of family adjustment to drug abuse. For example, the family may initially adopt the tolerant style, later adopting engagement, and eventually withdrawal, until they go back through the cycle through the tolerant style [53,54]. Hence, just as the substance user goes through stages of change in his/her drug abusing career, the family can be seen as going through similar stages [55,56]. The cycle of change described by Prochaska and DiClemente [55] specifically refers to stages that a drug abuser goes through. The application of the same stages to family behaviour is ideal, and allows comparison of family adjustment and drug abuser adjustment; however, the stages do not always match the behaviour exhibited by the family. In other words, the cycle is not an exact fit when it describes family adjustment.

The comparison of family adjustment with drug abuser adjustment is useful in understanding the behaviour within the family. The stage of change of the drug abuser may not always parallel that of the family, triggering a phase of deterioration for either the drug abuser or the family or both. Engagement in treatment is also affected by the stages of change of the drug abuser and the family and whether they are parallel.

The Stage of Pre-Contemplation

When the family is first confronted by the problem of drug abuse by one of its relatives, their initial reaction may be one of denial. They are unwilling to acknowledge the problem, despite evidence to the contrary. Episodes clearly related to drug abuse are minimized and considered to be one-off events, and rationalized as happening due to stress or some other ailment. The family may try to avoid getting emotionally involved, actively intellectualizing the problem. When other people bring up the issue of drug abuse, family members may react with anger and irritability and may try to change the topic of discussion.

The coping position within this stage of change is typically the tolerant style. This implies that it is unlikely to effect change, but it maintains family stability and equilibrium. Denial or pre-contemplation avoids family conflict and only has short-term effectiveness in adjustment.

In comparison with siblings, parents are more likely to behave in a pre-contemplative way, because they are usually more shocked by the drug abuse than siblings, who may already be aware of the ongoing problem [40].

The Stage of Contemplation

As time passes and the drug use continues, negative effects become increasingly more common. The family starts accepting that a problem exists and that maintaining equilibrium in family dynamics is no longer of benefit to the family. Stress in the family intensifies and children within the family may exhibit behavioural problems and poor academic performance. Family members become increasingly unhappy with the situation and with their relationship with the drug abuser.

As the family experiences one crisis after another with disorganization of family dynamics, family members become more determined that something must change. Hence, the family gradually shifts from tolerance to engagement. This stage of change lies somewhere in between two styles, demonstrating that more than one coping style may be adopted at the same time. The experience of powerlessness associated with a tolerant style gradually changes to a recognition of an ability to do something about the drug abuse problem, which is characteristic of the engaged method.

Siblings are often described as being in the contemplative stage when the parents are in the pre-contemplative stage. They feel resentful and angry with the drug abuser, understanding that the negative consequences for the family were the result of drug abuse. They try to protect their parents from the impact of drug abuse, enabling them to stay in the pre-contemplative stage [40].

The Stage of Preparation

This stage of change is facilitated by the engaged style of coping. The family has definite intentions to effect change. They verbalize their concerns about the problem, openly acknowledging the impact of drug abuse on the family. They widen their knowledge about the issue by, for instance, obtaining leaflets and searching the Internet. They explore ways of seeking help and establishing contact with relevant services.

Family members experience a desire to resolve the problem and frequently confront the drug abuser about the matter. They put increasing pressure on the drug abuser to change his/her behaviour to reduce/abstain from using drugs, or to establish contact with treatment services. Their approach is usually a mixture of support, encouragement and anger. It is not difficult to understand how dysfunctional family dynamics with poor communication, giving praise and punishment inappropriately, can enable the drug abuser to stay in this stage of change. If the family are inconsistent in their boundaries, norms and values, they will be inconsistent in their attitudes and feelings—at times rewarding and at other times punishing the same behaviour.

The engaged coping style characteristic of this stage can effect change through consistency and perseveration.

The Stage of Action

The family is now mobilized into doing something about the problem. Family members start taking more family responsibilities, such as increasing their work commitments to overcome their financial burden. Children may assume parental roles and older siblings might leave the family environment to pursue their goals in life. The underlying agenda of such behaviour is to restore stability in the family system and to induce change in the drug abuser.

At this stage, family members may serve as the vehicles driving the drug abuser to treatment. They may also seek treatment for themselves, which to some extent depends on service availability.

The action stage is associated with hope and a feeling of achievement by family members. The coping style characteristic of this change is again engagement.

The Stages of Maintenance and Relapse

Although action brings on change, the chronic nature of drug abuse requires perseverance and ongoing encouragement from the family, in order for that change to be maintained. The reorganization of the family system may be difficult for the family to accept and maintain, and unless they receive suitable support, they may relapse back to their previous methods of functioning.

On the other hand, once change has occurred, family members may wish to disengage from their relationship with the substance abuser, to focus on other issues in life, thus adopting the withdrawal style of coping. Thus, this stage may be characterized by efforts to separate or divorce, which are unlikely to maintain the change.

Unless appropriate support is in place, family dynamics will revert back to familiar ways of functioning and the whole family once again feels reassured, despite the reinforcement of dysfunctional behaviour. Any separations or divorce are reconciled and the family is once again unified in 'relapse'.

Thus, the exploration of a family's coping style is incomplete unless understood in the context of the family's readiness to change. However, the cycle of change was designed to describe the behaviour of substance users, and its application to family behaviour may have some limitations. For instance, families do not always react by denial to the discovery of drug abuse, but may leap instantly into the action stage by rushing the experimental cannabis abuser to specialist services. Another example is the family that enters the cycle at the contemplation stage, interpreting adolescent behaviour as due to drug use, even if this was not the case. The pre-contemplative stage is not synonymous with denial. Pre-contemplation within a substance user refers to not having an intention to change, perceiving the use of substances as having more benefits than harm. Denial, on the other hand, is a reaction that blocks recognition of substance use, due to an underlying awareness that the issue is associated with more harm than benefit. Thus, describing the family in denial as being in the pre-contemplative stage is slightly inaccurate. Nevertheless, the cycle offers a useful framework for exploring coping behaviours of families of subjects with drug abuse. The understanding of family adjustment is crucial to the application of effective family-based interventions.

EMPOWERMENT: ALL IS NOT DOOM

Understanding the burden carried by a family of a subject with drug abuse, as well as exploring the family's unique way of functioning, interacting and coping, provides the basis for the development of strategies aimed at guiding the family to alleviating or eliminating the problem. The 'ripple effect' of drug abuse highlights the importance of addressing the family burden. Failing to address the burden may have negative consequences on society and the drug abuser within the family, which further contributes to the family burden.

Interventions targeted at the drug abuser have beneficial effects for both the family and society. The health care costs of families of substance users are comparatively high in the years prior to the drug abuser's engagement with services, but tend to drop sharply thereafter [57]. Beneficial effects for society can also be substantial, and in fact a UK study [58] reported that £1 spent on treatment of a drug abuser saves £3 expenditure for the criminal justice system.

Family-based interventions empower the families to bring on change in family function, blocking the 'ripple effect' of drug abuse and facilitating harm-reduction or abstinence of the drug abuser. The chronicity and repetition of family dynamics in Ms X's family (see Appendix) is a clear indication of the need for a more integrative approach to treatment.

The Aims of Family-Based Interventions

The purpose of family-based interventions is to work with relatives in order to reduce the impact of drug abuse on the family and to increase the chances of success in the treatment of the drug abuser. There are a variety of approaches with the family as the focus of the intervention. Although such approaches are varied in intensity and structure, and have developed from varied theoretical perspectives, they all share one common concept: that families play a role in the course of drug abuse and that drug abuse equally has an important role in family well-being.

The aims of family-based interventions, as described by Copello and Orford [59], are: (a) to bring drug abusers into treatment and to maintain their engagement in treatment; (b) to increase the benefits of treatment of the drug abuse and family functioning; and (c) to reduce the impact and reduce harm for family members and significant others.

Such aims indicate that the family-based interventions have broader outcomes than those related to drug abuse, namely, improved physical, psychological and social health of the family. When measured through such indicators, family-based interventions are more than an adjunctive treatment modality for drug abuse [57].

There are no specific indications for the implementation of family-based interventions. Their usefulness can be universal. However, specific interventions may be more effective for specific family systems, coping styles and stages of readiness to change in either the family or the drug abuser. Also, some families and their drug abusing relatives may be more at risk than others and may have an increased need for family-based approaches, than other families. Such high-risk families are those with the greatest effects/needs mentioned earlier on in the chapter.

Types of Family-Based Interventions

A variety of family-based interventions are outlined in Table 8.2. Interventions have been classified according to a tier model suggested by the Health Advisory Service [60]. The advantages of using a tier classification are that it allows a comprehensive inclusion of family-based interventions, provides a schematic way of analysing whether all family needs are being met, provides a framework against which to measure service provision and permits analysis of the ease of access of such interventions by the family.

Effectiveness of Family-Based Interventions

Over the years family-based interventions have been given insufficient credit. Research on the effectiveness of such approaches focused on outcome indicators specific to the drug abuser, for example, reduction in injecting behaviour, reduction in criminal activity and retention in

TABLE 8.2   A tier classification of family-based interventions

Tier	Intervention	Structure/indication/usefulness
Tier 1 Easy access services offering an initial point of contact, advice, information and referral on to other services	Telephone helplines	Counselling skills approach to provide support and advice Particularly useful for the family in the preparation stage of change Also of benefit to the drug abuser
	Education and information (e.g. leaflets/Internet sites)	Useful at any stage of change
	Family-oriented prevention sessions	Increase drug awareness Useful to shift the family from a stage of pre-contemplation to contemplation and preparation
	Brief interventions (e.g. general practitioner, social services)	Provision of information specific to the need of the particular family Gateway system channelling families to appropriate services Address physical, psychological and social needs associated with drug abuse by a family member Useful at any stage of change
	Personal coping skills training (e.g. stress management, anger management)	Aimed at improving the coping abilities of family members, reducing the impact of drug abuse Usually not specific to drug abusing families/stresses related to drug abuse Useful at any stage of change
	Diversionary activities (e.g. sports, drama)	Provide the opportunity for family members to distract their attention to activities not related to drug abuse. Permit a temporary escape from the problem, with the aim of reducing family stress Not specific to drug abusing families Useful at any stage of change, but may facilitate denial or withdrawal if used in the pre-contemplative stage
	Advocacy	Advice, support and confidence to decrease the effects of vulnerability and stigma, empowering family members to make informed decisions and to recognize their rights

continued

TABLE 8.2 (*continued*)

Tier	Intervention	Structure/indication/usefulness
Tier 1 (*continued*)	Advocacy (*continued*)	Useful at any stage of change, but may facilitate denial by shifting "blame" onto rights not fulfilled, as opposed to "resistance to change"
	Respite	Provides opportunity for family members to take time away from problem Not usually specific for families of drug abusers Useful at any stage of change
Tier 2 More structured interventions, addressing situations where drug use is, or is likely to be, a significant issue	Support groups (self-help, facilitator-led)	Provide a safe nonjudgmental environment to verbalize issues of concern, to learn more about drug abuse and its effects on the family, to increase awareness of ways of coping and to reduce the impact of stigma and isolation Effective in reducing family stress and improving family health Useful at any stage of change
	Befriending	Offers one-to-one support to those family members finding it difficult to attend support groups Useful at any stage of change, but particularly when the family is ambivalent about openly acknowledging the problem
	Parental skills training	Address family dysfunction through the provision of guidelines on parental roles and skills Does not explore specific dysfunction of particular families, but provides general guidelines Useful at any stage of change. Particularly useful at maintenance stage, in delaying/preventing relapse
	Structured counselling (individual, couples, group)	Addresses impact of drug abuse on family interaction and health Provides opportunity for family members to verbalize concerns Less intense than psychotherapy Useful at any stage of change

continued

TABLE 8.2 (*continued*)

Tier	Intervention	Structure/indication/usefulness
Tier 3 More specialized interventions aimed at working with multiple and complex drug-related problems	Unilateral family therapy	Sessions with partner/significant other, addressing impact of drug abuse, coping strategies and interaction Aims to (a) improve health and well-being of the family; (b) increase the likelihood of the drug abuser to seek treatment; (c) slow down the progression of drug abuse Useful when drug abuser is resisting help (pre-contemplation/contemplation) and when the partner/significant other is in action stage. Prolongs maintenance stage
	Community reinforcement training	Structured approach with significant others: (a) reassurance that responsibility for using drugs lies with drug abuser, despite family dysfunction; (b) recognition of dysfunctional behaviour in the family; (c) instillation of hope by providing structure; (d) encouragement of significant others to find brief escape routes away from the problem Useful when drug abuser is resisting help (pre-contemplation/contemplation) and when the significant others are in action stage. Prolongs maintenance stage
	Behavioural couples therapy	With couples—exploring the impact of the dysfunction on drug abuse and vice versa Improves retention to treatment Useful when couples are in action stage. Prolongs maintenance stage
	Family therapy (e.g. brief strategic family therapy, multidimensional family therapy)	Focus on the family as a unit in the establishment and progression of drug abuse In-depth and intensive approach, to preserve family and reduce drug abuse Useful when family is in action stage. Prolongs maintenance stage

continued

TABLE 8.2 (*continued*)

Tier	Intervention	Structure/indication/usefulness
Tier 3 (*continued*)	Social behaviour and network therapy	Variant of family therapy, starting with the drug abuser and extending to significant others in the treatment process Useful when drug abuser is in action stage and significant others are in contemplation/preparation. Engagement shifts significant others to action stage
Tier 4 Interventions aimed at the most complex cases, involving interagency working	Therapeutic communities for families	Provides opportunity for the family to spend time within a therapeutic environment Useful for well-motivated families (action/maintenance) with severe dysfunction

treatment. Family-based interventions have wider implications and outcome indicators, including improved family health. Research demonstrating such wide implications is sparse, and so effectiveness studies on family-based interventions report conservative outcomes.

One of the first studies demonstrating a positive outcome was that reported by Stanton *et al.* [61]. They demonstrated that two thirds of heroin addicts showed a dramatic decrease in their drug taking behaviour following 10 sessions of family therapy.

More recently, a meta-analysis [62] compared family or couples therapy with other therapies. Patients receiving family or couples therapy showed a bigger reduction in drug use and an improvement in treatment retention, when compared with those receiving individual counselling, peer group therapy, and family psychoeducation. However, there was no difference between those receiving family therapy and those having relatives' groups.

A randomized controlled trial [63] examined whether intensive family-focused interventions were effective in reducing parental drug use and preventing initiation of drug use in their children. The interventions consisted of family skills training, as well as "home-based case management" assisting the family in the application of such skills to the family life. The intervention package was structured with well-defined sessions. Families included in the study were those with the parent(s) on methadone maintenance. Twelve-month follow-up revealed an improvement in parental ability to abstain from using drugs in crisis situations and to apply family rules and boundaries. They showed a reduction in frequency of drug use and a reduction in family conflict. However, the study failed to demonstrate significant beneficial effects on child behaviour, although 12 months may not be a long enough period to demonstrate such findings.

Brief strategic family therapy was evaluated against group counselling of adolescents with cannabis use as well as conduct disorder [64]. Brief strategic family therapy was associated with significantly greater reductions in use of cannabis, based on self-reports. Family function was also significantly improved in the 'brief strategic family therapy' group, whereas there was no improvement in the 'group counselling' group.

There are several other studies in the literature reporting positive outcomes when family-based interventions are applied. The involvement of significant others in treatment, for instance through community reinforcement training [65] or social behaviour and network therapy [66], has been shown to improve outcomes. Interventions aimed at addressing the effects of drug abuse on the physical and psychological health of family members, through primary care interventions, have also been shown to provide positive outcomes [39]. Despite such strong evidence, the implementation of family-based interventions is far from satisfactory. A survey in the USA found that couples-based programmes were only provided by 27% of services surveyed [67].

The reasons for the scarcity of family-based interventions are unclear. However, empirical evidence suggests that the cost–benefits of such interventions are only just starting to be appreciated and that they have been perceived as being 'too intensive' [67]. Another reason is that, although several studies have reported positive outcomes, methodological rigour is not the stronghold of some of the research.

CONCLUSIONS

Drug abuse by a family member has biological, psychological and social implications for the family. The genetic predispositions within the family, as well as the family interaction, constitute a family environment that contributes to the initiation, nature and progression of the drug abusing behaviour. The complex dynamics of the interplay of such processes has been described in this chapter. The coping behaviour adopted by families and its relationship to the stage of readiness to change within the family have also been discussed. The provision of family-based interventions to empower such families is sparse and the literature supporting their effectiveness is limited. However, the range of interventions described highlights their role alongside the various tiers of service provision, demonstrating the importance of addressing drug abuse within a family context, as a family problem.

APPENDIX: CASE HISTORY

Ms X, a 20-year-old, injecting, multiple substance user, referred herself to the Community Drug and Alcohol Team, claiming she wanted to be 'clean'. She reported using around 1.5 g of heroin intravenously, around 1 g of cocaine, mostly snorted, but some taken intravenously, mixed with heroin, and 60 mg of diazepam tablets taken orally, on a daily basis. She also used 2–4 ecstasy tablets once a week. Ms X had been using such amounts for about 3 months prior to the referral, but had a longer history of drug abuse dating back about 5 years.

Ms X's family structure consisted of mother, stepfather and sister (2 years older). Her biological father had left the family home when Ms X was 4 years of age, but maintained contact with the family. The stepfather had come onto the scene in the past 5 years.

The chronology of events in Table 8.3 demonstrates the burden carried by the family and the impact of the family on drug abuse and related behaviour by Ms X.

TABLE 8.3   Chronology of events

Chronology/ age of Ms X	Events/behaviour within the family environment	Events/behaviour related to Ms X
Birth	Mother and biological father abusing cannabis, alcohol and cocaine Drug dealing providing finances. Both parents unemployed Poor parental skills Sister physically abused by father Sister with temper tantrums	Perceived as a "sweet" and "affectionate" child Mother describes better bonding with Ms X than with sister
4 years old	Biological father leaves family home Financial crisis Sister with behavioural problems, both at school and at home	Ms X talks in "baby-language" and finds it difficult to be weaned off her dummy
4½ years old	Mother employs consistent approach in the family; boundaries clear Mother stops using alcohol and cocaine Income support Sister's behaviour markedly improved	Warmth and affection between mother and Ms X

continued

Table 8.3 (*continued*)

Chronology/ age of Ms X	Events/behaviour within the family environment	Events/behaviour related to Ms X
5 years old	Sister caught smoking cannabis (from mother) Mother reacts by increasing warmth towards sister; also increases own use of cannabis and restarts smoking cocaine	Mother unable to cope. Ms X sent to grandmother
5½ years old	Mother re-establishes contact with biological father Worsening of sister's behavioural problems	Ms X is back with family Ms X reported as being difficult to manage at school
6–14 years old	Repetitive separations and reconciliations with biological father, associated with worsening and improvements in sister's behavioural problems, drug use in the family and financial situation Sister started self-cutting at the age of 11 and got into trouble with the police at the age of 12, for shoplifting	Ms X's care shared between mother and grandmother Worsening of behavioural problems, both at school and at home, including smoking cannabis (from parents)
15 years old	Mother starts relationship with stepfather, who is a non-drug/ alcohol user Mother abstinent from all substances Sister admitted to a psychiatric secure unit, due to repetitive self-harm, antisocial behaviour and use of cannabis, heroin, cocaine, benzodiazepines and alcohol	Ms X starts using heroin. Starts as intravenous use, on a twice a week basis
15–17 years old	Increased disharmony between mother and daughters. No expression of affection/warmth from mother to daughters. Several outbursts of anger Mother and stepfather maintain abstinence Sister has a child and is housed by authorities; stability in both drug and mental health issues	Escalation of drug use by Ms X
18 years old	Sister and child isolated and not accepted by neighbourhood. Accused of introducing drugs to the area. Sister claims otherwise. Results in rapid worsening of drug use and incidents of self-harm by sister	Ms X leaves family home and settles at grandmother's place Reduces use of drugs from daily to twice weekly

continued

Table 8.3 *(continued)*

Chronology/ age of Ms X	Events/behaviour within the family environment	Events/behaviour related to Ms X
18 years old *(continued)*	Mother starts using cocaine and cannabis and introduces substances to stepfather Stepfather starts using alcohol daily Mother lends money to sister due to financial crisis	
19 years old	Mother, stepfather and sister using alcohol and drugs daily Child under the care of Social Services; placed in a foster home	Ms X's drug use worsens Returns to family home
20 years old	Mother reduces amount of daily drug use Mother facilitates Ms X's move to seek treatment	Ms X refers herself to drug and alcohol services
21 years old	No change in use of drugs and alcohol Sister continues to self-harm	Ms X stable on medication and well engaged with services
22 years old	Mother stops cocaine use and reduces cannabis use to alternate days Stepfather becomes abstinent Mother and stepfather focus their attention on Ms X's pregnancy. Increased care associated with love gestures Sister's condition continues to deteriorate	Ms X becomes pregnant Maintains stability in drug use

The chronology of events describes the fluctuations in family dynamics. The family works its way through repetitive losses and crises, which strengthen the family relationships and reinforce the family dysfunction. Drug use is an integral part of family function and shifts from one member to the other, depending on who takes on the role of saviour.

REFERENCES

1. Bateson G. (1971) The cybernetics of "self": a theory of alcoholism. *Psychiatry*, **34**, 1–18.
2. Bowen M. (1974) Alcoholism as viewed through family systems theory and family psychotherapy. *Ann. N. Y. Acad. Sci.*, **233**, 115–122.
3. Moos R.H., Cronkite R., Finney J.W. (1990) *Alcohol Treatment: Context, Process and Outcome*. Oxford University Press, New York.

4. Orford J. (1998) The coping perspective. In: Velleman R., Copello A., Maslin J. (eds) *Living with Drink: Women who Live with Problem Drinkers*. Longman, London, pp. 128–149.

5. United Nations Office for Drug Control and Crime Prevention (2000) *World Drug Report 2000*. Oxford University Press, Oxford.

6. European Monitoring Centre for Drugs and Drug Addiction (2003) *The State of the Drugs Problem in the European Union and Norway: Annual Report 2003*. Office for Official Publications of the European Communities, Luxembourg.

7. Ghodse H., Oyefeso A., Webb L., Schifano F., Pollard M., Jambert-Gray R., Corkery J. (2002) *Drug-Related Deaths as Reported by Coroners in England & Wales: Annual Review 2001 & np-SAD Surveillance Report No. 9, Including Drug-related Deaths in Scotland in 2001*. National Programme on Substance-Misuse Deaths, European Centre for Addiction Studies, St George's Hospital Medical School, London.

8. Sutherland I., Shepherd J.P. (2001) Social dimensions of adolescent substance use. *Addiction*, **96**, 445–458.

9. Ghodse H. (2002) *Drugs and Addictive Behaviour: A Guide to Treatment*, 3rd edn. Cambridge University Press, Cambridge.

10. Velleman R., Templeton L. (2002) Family interventions in substance misuse. In: Petersen T., McBride A. (eds) *Working with Substance Misusers: A Guide to Theory and Practice*. Routledge, London, pp. 145–152.

11. Office for National Statistics and Equal Opportunities Commission (1998) *Social Focus on Women and Men*. The Stationery Office, London.

12. Brisby T., Baker S., Hedderwick T. (1997) *Under the Influence: Coping with Parents who Drink Too Much—A Report on the Needs of the Children of Problem Drinking Parents*. Alcohol Concern, London.

13. Merikangas K.R., Avenevoli S. (2000) Implications of genetic epidemiology for the prevention of substance use disorders. *Addict. Behav.*, **25**, 807–820.

14. Pickens R.W., Svikis D.S., McGue M., Lykken D.T., Heston L.L., Clayton P.J. (1991) Heterogeneity in the inheritance of alcoholism: a study of male and female twins. *Arch. Gen. Psychiatry*, **48**, 19–28.

15. Enoch M.A., Goldman D. (1999) Genetics of alcoholism and substance abuse. *Psychiatr. Clin. North Am.*, **22**, 289–299.

16. Tsuang M.T., Lyons M.J., Eisen S.A., Goldberg J., True W., Lin N., Meyer J.M., Toomey R., Faraone S.V., Eaves L. (1996) Genetic influences on DSM-III-R drug abuse and dependence: a study of 3372 twin pairs. *Am. J. Med. Genet.*, **67**, 473–477.

17. Meller E., Enz A., Goldstein M. (1988) Absence of receptor reserve at striatal dopamine receptors regulating cholinergic neuronal activity. *Eur. J. Pharmacol.*, **155**, 151–154.

18. Zuckerman M. (1999) *Vulnerability to Psychopathology: A Biosocial Model*. American Psychiatric Association, Washington, DC.

19. Vanyukov M.M., Tarter R.E. (2000) Genetic studies of substance abuse. *Drug Alcohol Depend.*, **59**, 101–123.

20. Zuckerman M., Neeb M. (1979) Sensation seeking and psychopathology. *Psychiatry Res.*, **1**, 255–264.

21. Zuckerman M. (1986) Sensation seeking and the endogenous deficit theory of drug abuse. *NIDA Research Monograph*, **74**, 59–70.

22. Koopmans J.R., Boomsma D.I., Heath A.C., Van Doornen L.J. (1995) A multivariate genetic analysis of sensation seeking. *Behav. Genet.*, **25**, 349–356.

23. Hardie T.L. (2002) The genetics of substance abuse. *AACN Clinical Issues*, **13**, 511–522.
24. Orford J. (1990) Alcohol and the family: an international review of the literature with implications for research and practise. In: Kozlowski L.T., Anis H.M., Cappell H.D., Glaser F.B. (eds) *Research Advances in Alcohol and Drug Problems*. Plenum Press, New York, pp. 81–155.
25. Kaufman E. (1981) Family structures of narcotic addicts. *Int. J. Addict.*, **16**, 273–282.
26. Minuchin S. (1975) *Families and Family Therapy*. Harvard University Press, Cambridge, MA.
27. Stanton M.D. (1980) A family theory of drug abuse. In: Lettieri D.J., Sayers M., Wallenstein Pearson H. (eds) *Theories on Drug Abuse: Selected Contemporary Perspectives*. National Institute of Drug Abuse Research, Washington, DC, pp. 147–156.
28. Spotts J.V., Shonts F.C. (1980) A life-theme theory of chronic drug abuse. In: Lettieri D.J., Sayers M., Wallenstein Pearson H. (eds) *Theories on Drug Abuse: Selected Contemporary Perspectives*. National Institute of Drug Abuse Research, Washington, DC, pp. 59–70.
29. Stanton M.D. (1977) The addict as saviour: heroin, death and the family. *Fam. Process*, **16**, 191–197.
30. Coleman S.B. (1980) Incomplete mourning and addict/family transactions: a theory for understanding heroin abuse. In: Lettieri D.J., Sayers M., Wallenstein Pearson H. (eds) *Theories on Drug Abuse: Selected Contemporary Perspectives*. National Institute of Drug Abuse Research, Washington, DC, pp. 83–89.
31. Vaillant G. (1966) A 12-year follow-up of New York narcotic addicts: some social and psychiatric characteristics. *Arch. Gen. Psychiatry*, **15**, 599–609.
32. Stanton M.D., Todd T.C., Heard D.B., Kirschner S., Kleiman J.I., Mowatt D.T., Riley P., Scott S.M., Van Deusen J.M. (1978) Heroin addiction as a family phenomenon: a new conceptual model. *Am. J. Drug Alcohol Abuse*, **5**, 125–150.
33. Vaillant G. (1973) A 20-year follow-up of New York narcotic addicts. *Arch. Gen. Psychiatry*, **29**, 237–241.
34. Hanson K.J., Estes N.J. (1977) Dynamics of alcohol families. In: Estes N.J., Heineman E. (eds) *Alcohol: Development, Consequences and Interventions*. C.V. Mosby, St Louis, MO, pp. 67–75.
35. Merton R.K. (1968) Anomie, anomia and social interaction: contexts of deviant behaviour. In: Clinard M. (ed.) *Anomie and Deviant Behaviour*. Free Press, New York, pp. 213–242.
36. Stanton M.D. (1979) Drugs and the family. *Marriage Fam. Rev.*, **2**, 1–10.
37. Bloch S., Hafner J., Harari E., Szmukler G.I. (1994) *The Family in Clinical Psychiatry*. Oxford University Press, Oxford, pp. 173–194.
38. Haley J. (1973) *Uncommon Therapy*. Norton, New York.
39. Mental Health Foundation (1999) *Working with the Families of People with Alcohol and Drug Problems: The Development and Evaluation of a Package for Use in Primary Care*. Mental Health Foundation, London.
40. Velleman R., Bennett G., Miller T., Orford J. (1993) The families of problem drug users: a study of 50 close relatives. *Addiction*, **88**, 1281–1289.
41. Effective Interventions Unit (2002) *Supporting Families and Carers of Drug Users: A Review*. Scottish Executive, Edinburgh.
42. European Monitoring Centre for Drugs and Drug Addiction (2003) Hepatitis C: a hidden epidemic. In: *Drugs in Focus: Bimonthly Briefing of the European*

Monitoring Centre for Drugs and Drug Addiction, November–December 2003. Office for Official Publications of the European Communities, Luxembourg.

43. Markowitz R. (1993) Dynamics and treatment issues with children of drug and alcohol abusers. In: Shulamith L., Ashenberg S. (eds) *Clinical Work with Substance Abusing Clients.* Guilford Press, New York, pp. 214–229.

44. Dore M.M., Kaufman E., Nelson-Zlupko L., Granfort E. (1996) Psychosocial functioning and treatment needs of latency age children from drug-involved families. *Fam. Soc.,* **77**, 595–603.

45. Bekir P., McLellan T., Childress A.R., Gariti P. (1993) Role reversals in families of substance misusers: a transgenerational phenomenon. *Int. J. Addict.,* **28**, 613–630.

46. Gossop M., Marsden J., Stewart D. (1998) *NTORS at One Year: The National Treatment Outcome Research Study.* Department of Health, London.

47. Regier D.A., Farmer M.E., Rae D.S., Locke B.Z., Keith S.J., Judd L.L., Goodwin F.K. (1990) Comorbidity of mental disorders with alcohol and other drug abuse: results from the Epidemiological Catchment Area (ECA) study. *JAMA,* **264**, 2511–2518.

48. Oyefeso A., Ghodse H., Clancy C., Corkey J. (1999) Suicide among drug addicts in the UK. *Br. J. Psychiatry,* **175**, 277–282.

49. Endler N.S., Parker J.D. (1990) Multidimensional assessment of coping: a critical evaluation. *J. Personal Soc. Psychol.,* **58**, 844–854.

50. Mattlin J.A., Wethington E., Kellser R.C. (1990) Situational determinants of coping and coping effectiveness. *J. Health Soc. Behav.,* **31**, 103–122.

51. Orford J., Rigby K., Miller T., Tod A., Bennett G., Velleman R. (1992) Ways of coping with excessive drug use in the family: a provisional typology based on the accounts of 50 close relatives. *J. Commun. Appl. Psychol.,* **2**, 163–183.

52. Orford J., Natera G., Davies J., Nava A., Mora J., Rigby K., Bradbury C., Bowie N., Copello A., Velleman R. (1998) Tolerate, engage or withdraw: a study of the structure of families coping with alcohol and drug problems in South West England and Mexico City. *Addiction,* **93**, 1799–1813.

53. Orford J., Natera G., Velleman R., Copello A., Bowie N., Bradbury C., Davies J., Mora J., Nava A., Rigby K., *et al.* (2001) Ways of coping and the health of relatives facing drug and alcohol problems in Mexico and England. *Addiction,* **96**, 761–774.

54. Steinglass P., Bennett L.A., Wolin S.J., Reiss D. (1987) *Drinking Problems in a Family Context.* Hutchinson, London.

55. Prochaska J.O., DiClemente C.C. (1982) Transtheoretical therapy: toward a more integrative model of change. *Psychother. Theory Res. Pract.,* **19**, 276–288.

56. Connors G.J., Donovan D.M., DiClemente C.C. (2001) *Substance Abuse Treatment and the Stages of Change.* Guilford Press, New York.

57. Miller W.R. (2003) A collaborative approach to working with families. *Addiction,* **98**, 5–6.

58. Gossop M., Marsden J., Stewart D. (2001) *NTORS after Five Years: The National Treatment Outcome Research Study: Changes in Substance Use, Health and Criminal Behaviour During the Five Years after Intake.* National Addiction Centre, London.

59. Copello A., Orford J. (2002) Addiction and the family: is it time for services to take notice of the evidence? *Addiction,* **97**, 1361–1363.

60. Health Advisory Service (1996) *Children and Young People: Substance Misuse Services.* HMSO, London.

61. Stanton M.D., Todd T.C. and Associates (1982) *The Family Therapy of Drug Abuse and Addiction.* Guilford Press, New York.

62. Stanton M.D., Shadish W.R. (1997) Outcome, attrition, and family-couples treatment for drug abuse: a meta-analysis and review of the controlled, comparative studies. *Psychol. Bull.*, **122**, 170–191.
63. Catalano R.F., Gainey R.R., Fleming C.B., Haggerty K.P., Johnson N.O. (1999) An experimental intervention with families of substance abusers: one-year follow-up of the focus on families project. *Addiction*, **94**, 241–254.
64. Santisteban D.A., Coatsworth J.D., Perez-Vidal A., Kurtines W.M., Schwartz S.J., LaPerriere A., Szapocznik J. (2003) Efficacy of brief strategic family therapy in modifying Hispanic adolescent behaviour problems and substance use. *J. Fam. Psychol.*, **17**, 121–133.
65. Smith J., Meyers R., Miller W. (2001) The community reinforcement approach to the treatment of substance use disorders. *Am. J. Addict.*, **10**, 52–59.
66. Copello A., Orford J., Hodgson R., Tober G., Barrett C. on behalf of the UKATT Research Team (2002) Social behaviour and network therapy: key principles and early experiences. *Addict. Behav.*, **27**, 345–366.
67. Fals-Stewart W., Birchler G. (2001) A national survey of the use of couples therapy in substance abuse treatment. *J. Subst. Abuse Treat.*, **20**, 277–283.

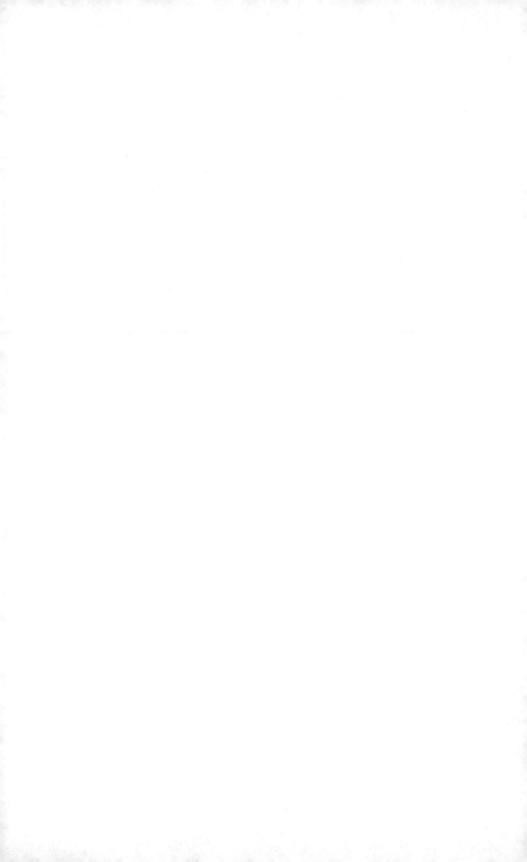

The Role of Family Organizations in Mental Health Care

Margaret Leggatt

World Fellowship for Schizophrenia and Allied Disorders, Victoria, Australia

INTRODUCTION

Family organizations in the area of mental illness have been established in many parts of the world as the result of several factors. In Western countries, the main factor was the move towards treating people in the community as a result of policies of deinstitutionalization. The failure of most societies to provide adequate community facilities for rehabilitation and accommodation left family members as the main source of care and support for their mentally ill relatives. Families were expected to carry out these caring roles without information about the illnesses, without education or training in how to manage, and with little or no emotional support. At the same time, many psychological theories about mental illness blamed parents as having caused mental illness to develop in their offspring. Exclusion and neglect of families proved fertile ground for the development of the family organizations.

In developing countries, the relationship between family caregivers and mental health professionals has been different. The attribution of blame for causing mental illness in their children has not been part of professional–family interactions. The development of family organizations in these countries has been brought about because the burden of caregiving is exacerbated by conditions of extreme poverty combined with much more deeply entrenched stigma and misperception about mental illness.

HISTORICAL OVERVIEW

In the main, family organizations began as small groups of relatives, predominantly parents, meeting together as support for themselves. Because

Families and Mental Disorders. Edited by Norman Sartorius, Julian Leff, Juan José López-Ibor, Mario Maj and Ahmed Okasha. © 2005 John Wiley & Sons Ltd. ISBN 0-470-02382-1

they had been excluded by mental health professionals from participating in treatment and care regimes, the sharing of their 'lived experiences' led to these groups being seen as providing self-help through mutual support.

One of the earliest organizations was Zenkaren, The National Federation of Families with the Mentally Ill in Japan, formed in 1965. The National Schizophrenia Fellowship (NSF) in the United Kingdom (now RETHINK) was formed in 1971 as a result of the overwhelming response from families to a letter written to *The Times* by John Pringle, a father with a son with schizophrenia. A decade later, NSF had more than 100 groups in Britain, and had been a model and inspiration for many sister organizations world-wide, most notably in Australia, New Zealand and Canada. The National Alliance for the Mentally Ill (NAMI) was started in the USA in 1979, when a group of families of persons with mental illness hosted a conference. The idea of a national organization resulted in delegates at this conference agreeing on a name, purpose and funding method. By-laws were drafted, a steering committee was selected, tax-exempt status soon followed, an office was opened in Washington in 1982, and six years later the organization had grown to over 600 groups [1].

In 1982, what is now called the World Fellowship for Schizophrenia and Allied Disorders (WFSAD) was founded in Toronto by representatives of an eight-nation coalition of family organizations from Western, developed countries. The benefits of family support organizations in these countries led them to want to share their experiences, but it was not until 1991 that the WFSAD became seriously involved in family empowerment at the grass-roots level. Prior to this, the role had been as a conduit for information exchange between the countries making up the national membership of the WFSAD.

In December 1992, European organizations developed the European Federation of Associations of Families of People with a Mental Illness (EUFAMI). This comprises 23 family organizations from 19 European countries. The main goals of EUFAMI are stated as: (a) empowerment of family and friends who care for people with mental illness through training and promotion of self-help strategies; (b) mobilization of all available means to combat stigma and discrimination against people with mental illness; and (c) adoption by professionals of standards of best practice in prevention and treatment of mental illness [2].

Johnson [3] surveyed organizations worldwide that were focused on families of people with severe mental illness. Information was obtained from Australia, Bermuda, Belgium, Canada, Germany, India, Ireland, Israel, Japan, the Netherlands, New Zealand, Russia, South Africa, Spain, Sweden, Switzerland, Ukraine, the UK, the USA and Uruguay. Several countries known to have family organizations did not respond—France, Austria, Denmark, Norway, Portugal, Romania and Italy. Many of these groups were small and newly-formed; in most countries they had not achieved the status of a national organization.

Johnson [4] comments on the great differences between nations in how they have organized family groups, with some countries forming national organizations within a few years (France, Ireland, Sweden, Japan, Ukraine and the USA are examples), while other countries have multiple organizations spread throughout the nation (Italy, the Netherlands and Australia with three organizations and Israel with two). Others, such as Russia, have many local organizations, which do not represent the entire nation. Some have local organizations that tend to speak for the rest of the nation.

The development of a national organization is hindered largely because groups are often overwhelmed by problems at the local level and lack resources to develop a national body. It is therefore encouraging that in India, where the WFSAD has helped with financial, educational and moral support, "we see today the founding of a National Federation of the Mentally Ill . . ." [5]. Eight years ago, the WFSAD helped to found two national family organizations in East Africa [6]. Recently, the WFSAD founded a group of 16 family organizations in 12 countries in Central and South America, called the Alianza Latina.

From small beginnings, where groups of family carers came together out of desperation to find some solutions to the problems with which they were confronted, the "family movement" worldwide is becoming a force to be reckoned with, and has impressive achievements to its credit. While reference is made to this force as a movement, from the less powerful "small group" in developing countries to the greater impact of the larger national organization (usually a much older and more established institution in a Western country), it is now clear what the WFSAD, EUFAMI and families of the mentally ill everywhere are concerned about, and what they can achieve.

STRUCTURE AND FUNCTION OF FAMILY ORGANIZATIONS

A review of the mental health literature reveals little that is specific about the family organizations, although occasional vignettes can be found [e.g. 1,3,4,7]. In order to understand more about family organizations, voting members of the WFSAD were sent a questionnaire asking them about their structure, their activities and what they hoped to achieve in the future. Of 22 voting members of the WFSAD, 9 replied. Most of those who did not reply were faced with language barriers. Nevertheless, responses received provide an interesting cross-section of the achievements of small family groups as well as strong national family-driven organizations.

The stated purposes of the organizations varied, but the themes were similar to those of EUFAMI: empowerment of families and consumers, the promotion of mental health through programmes to reduce stigma and discrimination, improvements in quality of life through the provision of better mental health services (particularly community services) and campaigning politically. All organizations were registered with government as not-for-profit organizations.

In all the organizations with the exception of the Russian one, family carers are the pre-eminent members of governing committees, hence the understanding of these bodies as Family Organizations. The Russian organization (in which all members of the governing committee are mental health professionals) is typical of many countries, particularly those in the developing world, where professionals have taken major roles in supporting and helping to develop family support groups. Populations in these countries see doctors particularly as the ones with power and authority to make things happen.

In all the organizations, with the exception of the Kenyan and Russian ones, family carers comprise the substantial majority of members. Several organizations do not seem to have mental health professionals as members. This is interesting in view of the discussion about the relationship between family carer groups, family organizations and mental health professionals that forms the latter part of this chapter.

From a list of activities, organizations were asked to show which ones they provided to family carers. All but one organization reported that they provided information resources/printed materials, advocacy to politicians and anti-stigma projects. All but two provided conferences/seminars, and all but three provided family-led self-help groups, educational courses for family carers, and advocacy on behalf of members (for example, helping someone get treatment). Five out of nine provided a telephone helpline.

As well as services to families, organizations were asked if they provided services to people with mental illness. It was found that five out of nine provided voluntary work, and four out of nine housing/accommodation.

Small family groups have commenced accommodation projects (e.g. in Argentina), while the established family organizations have been responsible for many initiatives in the development of community recreational, rehabilitation and accommodation facilities. For example, from a publicity brochure produced by Zenkaren, it is stated that of 1740 sheltered workshops in Japan, 897 are managed by local family group associations. These facilities function not only as job-training centres, but they also provide people with mental illness with a place to meet where they are able to function as members of a community. It should be pointed out that

Japanese "sheltered workshops" do not match the concept of "sheltered workshop" in other countries. These Japanese enterprises are more like small businesses that employ psychiatrically disabled people.

All organizations reported reliance on funds from private donors (donations, bequests) and membership subscriptions. For India, Kenya, Russia and South America, these were the only sources of funding. For the older, more established and bigger organizations, substantial funds were received from all the sources listed in the questionnaire—private donors and membership subscriptions, as well as government grants, fundraising by members of the organizations, grants from pharmaceutical companies, business and philanthropic concerns.

In the beginning, groups/organizations obtain financial support from their members. As they grow and become recognized (particularly if they provide services for patients/consumers), funds become available from other sources. This is not necessarily the case in developing countries, where conditions of extreme poverty make mental health a very low priority and the needs of family carers are even less recognized. The most distressing aspect of the WFSAD's role is the relentless request for financial support to struggling organizations in developing countries. The WFSAD's workforce is voluntary except for meagre salaries to a small administrative staff.

Questions were asked to find out what the organizations felt were the most important projects in which they were currently engaged, and what the major problems were for them in achieving their objectives. Continuing and expanding the programmes to fulfil the needs of family carers was important in most organizations. These programmes ranged from encouraging the formation of small self-help and support groups to sophisticated, structured family education and training courses.

The overwhelming need to reduce the stigma and discrimination associated with mental illness has resulted in family organizations being responsible for "mental health days", "awareness weeks" and use of the media to promote understanding and more positive images of mental illness. Public/community education still takes many forms, but notable in the responses to this questionnaire were the emphases on political campaigning "to ensure that consumers and carers have access to education and support" (Australia), and "campaigning to government to implement policy changes—again and again' with programmes to "grow our campaigners, members, supporters" (UK). Notable also were educational projects involving "non-traditional partners such as emergency room physicians and police" in the USA and "police sensitization" in India.

Not surprisingly, the most often cited barrier to developing these projects was the lack of funds, with some organizations highlighting the absence of government support or the tightening of government budgets to the mental health area.

Of equal importance as barriers to implementation, were a wide range of issues relating to volunteers (mainly family members) and staff. Organizations needed more volunteers. Many families were either not able to volunteer because of the heavy burden of caring, or did not volunteer because of the stigma associated with such work. In Kenya, the general level of poverty meant that the majority of carers had to spend their time earning a living rather than volunteering. NAMI highlighted the difficulty associated with holding an organization together when "very disparate views are held". This made the setting of a common agenda problematic. SANE (Australia) and Zenkaren (Japan) commented on the shortage of skilled manpower available for carrying out their community mental health projects.

The low priority of mental illness with policy makers in health services, not to mention disagreements about mental health policy in different governmental spheres, hampered effective progress. Behind government indifference lay the persistent feeling that many people in government still did not really understand mental illness.

As family organizations came about because of gaps in service provision, and if they are to continue to grow, it is important to understand what is different and unique to these organizations. Overwhelmingly, all respondents claimed that emotional support was the key function or core aspect of their organization's service to families, and was the major difference between the family organizations and professional services. Only family carers who have experienced the trauma associated with caring for a relative who has a mental illness can understand the emotional impact this has. A quote from NAMI (USA): "You cannot teach what you don't know, or you cannot lead where you will not go."

Another key function was training in illness management, particularly the management of a wide range of behavioural problems that were part of or that arose because of the person's mental illness. Family carers who spend all day every day, month and year coping with mental illness develop expertise in illness management, often through trial and error.

Other kinds of helpful information that respondents reported receiving primarily from the family organizations were good examples of treatment and care leading to recovery (usually due to medication compliance and family support); the everyday dilemmas and conflicts experienced by families sharing their lives with a mentally ill person, and how to bring about conflict resolution; positive ways of asking for help, suggestions for referrals to psychiatrists and for "managing the mental health system", with particular emphasis on how to develop good practices with professionals so that they are responsive to what people want; general and specific information and emotional support through telephone helplines and online sources; and facts about government legislation, benefits and new medicines.

The national family organizations now employ mental health professionals alongside other employees, with a range of different qualifications, and provide a wide range of mental health services. Many have gone through changes where the original family-run programmes to support family carers have been de-emphasized by expansion into other areas of mental health service provision.

FAMILY ORGANIZATIONS: PROCESS AND OUTCOMES

It is obvious that family organizations worldwide play a substantial role in mental health care, but specific outcomes achieved for family carers and their mentally ill relatives are not widely appreciated or known about.

Relevant literature on this subject emanates predominantly from the USA and the UK. It is largely concerned with describing the changing structures and differing processes of the family self-help through mutual support movement from small, local, peer-led groups to programmes that now embrace many combinations of professional mental health workers and family members working together in a variety of different settings. These settings vary from independent family groups in non-mental health community environments to professionally supported and facilitated groups in mental hospitals and community mental health clinics.

Self-Help through Mutual Support

Self-help groups were defined by Katz and Bender in 1979 as "voluntary, small group structures formed by peers who have come together for mutual assistance in satisfying a common need and bringing about social and/or personal change, such as improvement in confidence and the development of problem-solving skills. They develop values through which members may attain an enhanced sense of personal identity. Members of such groups perceive their needs are not being met by existing social institutions" [8].

Since the above description and during the past two decades, there has been a remarkable expansion in the activities of groups devoted to self-help and mutual aid, mainly in Western countries [1,7]. This development is important politically. Implicit in previous welfare programmes and in charitable organizations that rely on volunteers is the one-way giving of handouts to those in need. Self-help through mutual support challenges the "needy" to become self-reliant through utilizing processes that lead to self-empowerment. The popularity and rapid growth of such groups in the mental health field has been attributed to a variety of socio-political and organizational imperatives: deinstitutionalization and the shift to community care, the breakdown of family and community networks, the increasing dissatisfaction of users and carers with inadequate services, and the growing consumer movement and its emphasis on self-empowerment [1].

Self–help through mutual support seeks to re-establish basic core traditions of community and neighbourhood by developing self-reliance in ordinary individuals to manage the exigencies in everyday situations. "Self-help through mutual support is a process wherein people who share common experiences, situations or problems can offer each other a unique perspective that is not available from those who have not shared the experiences" [7].

In the mental health field, self-help groups: (a) provide a safe and simple environment "in stark contrast to professionally led psychotherapeutic groups where the control lies with the trained professional therapist/group leader who manipulates members' reactions to achieve their emotional resolution" [9]; (b) allow families to seek help in a fashion that is comfortable for them [10]; (c) exemplify a democratic philosophy, for example, rotating group leadership, nonhierarchic structure, and the acceptance of troubled, stigmatized behaviour [11]; (d) are "anti-big, anti-bureaucratic, anti-impersonality" [7]; (e) are controlled and governed by the members; and (f) are "non-profit" and "no charge" ("since social support is provided and returned without payment, its demonstrable benefits and low costs are of interest to health policy makers") [12].

While the literature on self-help through mutual support researches the phenomena through studies of self-help groups, the process of self-help can occur in many different formats. Individual peers supporting others through informal sharing of experiences (telephone support or face-to-face meetings) should be available for those for whom groups can be intimidating.

Alternative peer support to that offered in groups may be important for different ethnic communities, for whom even to communicate with one other family can initially be too traumatic. The shame of mental illness precludes anyone else knowing of its presence, even extended family members. Again, different cultures may find groups more acceptable if they acknowledge a strong cultural tradition; for example, "African American families sharing their experiences with other congregants showed that church-based support groups improved their knowledge and morale" [13].

Online support is beginning to be recognized as a self-help mechanism. In an analysis of online support for caregivers of people with a mental illness, Perron [14] found that a "discourse analysis revealed that messages had a primary focus of disclosure and providing information or advice. Discussion of emotions and diagnoses were found in nearly half of the messages."

Self-help through mutual support is organized help; it has to be set up, routinized and provided on a regular basis. It does not "just happen". This makes it different from conventional family, community or neighbourhood support, which tends to occur more spontaneously. This is an important point to remember, because it reflects the nature of mental illness itself. Family carers need to be organized to meet with each other. In many situations, some outside help is needed to support the group until it is able to continue under its own auspices.

Experiential knowledge is one of the criteria for defining self-help groups. "It is an amorphous, changeable entity which does not lend itself to traditional research methodologies; nor does it lend itself to generalizations. Yet it distinguishes self-help groups from other types of helping bodies, and is highly valued by those who participate in those groups" [15]. What is its value relative to other forms of knowledge? Schubert and Borkman [15] suggest that:

- The first component is "wisdom and know-how gained through reflection upon personal lived experience". When self-help group members share their day-to-day experiences, they become aware of "common elements in both problems and attempted solutions while recognizing the uniqueness of their own situations . . . experiential knowledge tends to be specific, pragmatic, somewhat idiosyncratic" and contextual.
- The second component is "belief in the validity and authority of the knowledge gained from an experience". It is "lay knowledge—handed down, common sense knowledge". Persons must believe that the knowledge obtained from their experiences has value and is worth sharing with others. Such sharing enables members of a group to define more clearly the problem they are facing and to evolve guidelines for dealing with it.
- Experiential knowledge is transmitted in small group conversations, telephone calls and informal face-to-face meetings between people who are coping with similar situations.
- Experiential knowledge consists of statements, stories or narratives reflecting some aspect of an individual's experience that she or he values and trusts as knowledge. To an uninvolved observer, much experiential knowledge may sound like or appear to be small talk or everyday conversation.
- Experiential knowledge is contrasted with professional knowledge. "Professional knowledge is information, knowledge and skills developed, applied and transmitted by an established specialized occupation to those who have fulfilled the requirements of a profession. Compared to experiential knowledge it is analytical, grounded in theory or scientific principle, and abstract." Unless professionals have the problem, their

perspective remains based on their training and research. "Professional knowledge is exclusive and private. Professionals are paid help, information flows one-way, helping activities are scheduled, organized and constrained by time" [16].

The "helper/therapy principle" [7] states that those who help others also receive help themselves. In the mental health field, the helpers are also able to see themselves as an example of someone who has come to terms with, and learned the best ways of coping with the same set of problems that are now confronting the recipient of help. This, in turn, instils a sense of hope in the recipients of help. Recipients of help are often then able to become helpers themselves [8].

Family-to-Family Education Programmes

While many family organizations around the world consist mainly of self-help support groups, the larger, established organizations have developed their own impressive family education programmes, such as "Understanding and Coping with Schizophrenia: 14 Principles for the Relatives" [17] and the "Family-to-Family" education programme [18]. The family carers who developed these programmes claim that their experiences have given them the knowledge which mental health professionals do not have—the "personal lived experience" of day-to-day coping. Family "educators" are trained by their peers and give their services voluntarily. These beginnings show a potential resource for mental health services that as yet has not been properly recognized, supported or developed.

The "Family-to-Family" education course describes and then resolves three major problems that arise as the result of mental illness in a family member:

- Mental illness is a trauma, and the effects of trauma are helplessness and isolation. The course provides recognition, understanding and processing of traumatized people's emotional states.
- The course externalizes the harsh, unforgiving messages about mental illness that everyone absorbs—weak character or character defect, bad people, inadequate parenting, bad marriages etc. This is a consciousness-raising exercise aimed at resolving the harmful stereotypes that have been absorbed.
- Personal empowerment is developed. The course emphasizes how to place living with trauma into a life perspective that fosters self-care and self-realization. "It is absolutely certain that this focus on trauma and healing is the most appealing aspect of the course. Family members

overwhelmingly endorse the emphasis on emotional self-disclosure and group affirmation of legitimate feelings, giving the highest content area score to classes focused on learning about feelings and self-care" [19].

A pilot study of "Family-to-Family" [20] found that the 37 participants "demonstrated significantly greater family, community and service system empowerment and reduced displeasure and worry about the family member who had a mental illness. These benefits were sustained at 6 months."

The most sophisticated education and training programmes provided by the well-developed family organizations utilize a volunteer workforce to great effect. These courses include an "empowering call to action" for "constructive political and social change" [18].

Family education and training are still not adequately provided in most countries. These programmes could be developed extensively as they seem to provide the information needed by families of persons with mental illness that is not being given to them by the mental health system.

Mechanisms of Change: The Self-Help Process that Leads to Empowerment

The sharing of knowledge experienced through coping with mental illness and the resulting recognition of one's contribution as a legitimate resource in the treatment and care of a relative are powerful aspects of the self-help through mutual support process. These mechanisms occur within a framework that validates the emotional devastation that family carers experience and that allows the trauma to be worked through in the company of and with the support of other "fellow travellers". Another mechanism for change through the self-help process would seem to be time. "There is a time factor related to benefit, and benefit accrues over time" [10].

Members become better at asserting themselves through gaining confidence, understanding and support. This empowerment of family carers diminishes their burden. Treatment models, with their continuing emphasis on "pathology", often fail to acknowledge the positive skills and strengths of family carers. Continual emphasis on what is wrong is physically and emotionally exhausting, and does little to reverse carers' loss of self-esteem and confidence—a direct consequence for them of mental illness in a close relative.

While a treatment focus is necessary for families to learn how to manage, transition to empowerment through the mechanisms of change within the self-help framework is not often considered by professionals to be part of their responsibility.

Support Groups

While self-help through mutual support typified the commencement style of the earliest family groups, predominantly in Western countries, some of the literature relevant to these developments in mental health now draws a distinction between self-help groups and support groups. In reality, the differences between family self-help through mutual/peer support and the support group is often blurred. Much of the literature has not embraced the emphasis that is developing in some research that wishes to explore these differences.

Family support groups in mental health are often facilitated by professionals: this involvement of professionals seems to be the major emphasis in defining the differences between support and self-help groups. Behavioural and societal changes are subordinate to the goals of emotional support and education for family carers [1]: behavioural change here seems to be referring to the potential of self-help to transform people's world-views about a particular phenomenon.

In family support groups, there is a combination of professional knowledge and skills with exchanges among family group members who share a common problem [16]. Professional-led groups tend to be psychoeducational (giving families information that will help them to understand the "diagnosis"), with the emphasis on improving family competence in order to improve client outcomes, whereas family-led groups focus more on advocacy issues—how to get better help [16]. Professionally led support groups where a professional plans, organizes and facilitates the group are usually more structured, with information, problem-solving and coping techniques as well as support [21].

Support groups with professional involvement may be more common in Eastern societies, whereas the self-help approach occurs more often in Western developed countries. "Published accounts that we have about self-help in other parts of the world suggest that North American groups may be significantly more independent of professionals than those in other countries" [1].

Pickett *et al.* [22] list the following benefits of support groups emerging from their study of attenders and non-attenders of these groups:

- *Relationships:* "improvements in relationships with their ill family member, and a subsequent diminution in family disruption; higher levels of adaptive coping through members providing help to each other...by sharing coping methods, brainstorming solutions to situations, and providing emotional support".
- *Education:* increased knowledge of mental illness and its treatment.

- *Service use:* increased access to services and greater use of community resources; better advocacy for securing care for their ill relatives and bringing about change in mental health services.
- *Support:* decreased isolation through hearing about the experiences of others and the subsequent development of shared responsibilities and helpfulness among group members.
- *Emotional well-being:* significantly less depression and burden in support group participants: "caregivers expressed that the support group offers a place to rehabilitate feelings, not just of resignation but of helplessness, pain, fear and all the rest…a safe, secure atmosphere where their fears and anxieties could be faced and discussed without the need to defend their positions. Caregivers said that they felt that a professional was finally listening to them, hearing their side of things" [21].

Problems with Self-Help through Mutual Support and with Support Groups

Although there are many benefits from self-help through mutual support and support groups, there are issues that need to be examined if the self-help movement in mental health is to expand:

- At the level of small groups, there can be negative effects of group membership: feeling overwhelmed by listening to other people's stories, and realizing more clearly what is wrong with their relative can be very distressing if it is not handled well. This is potentially very damaging for families facing mental illness for the first time/episode [23].
- Reasons for dropping out include not having enough time to attend, the fact that the group is no longer helpful, problems with transportation and parking, inadequate leadership, and lack of comfort with other members [24]. Groups can be too unfocused and can degenerate into complaint meetings expressing nothing but negative feelings. This can be destructive and the cause of family carers not wanting to belong.
- Membership of support groups is deemed not to be representative of family carers as a whole. They are essentially middle class. For example, comparisons of NAMI groups in one state suggest that there are important differences between people who belong to mental health support groups and people who do not. Members are a bit younger, more likely to be parents and more affluent. Their mentally ill relatives have more education, more employment and are less likely to live at home. Members are less likely to be African American. These demographic differences raise the possibility that those not currently part of NAMI may have a different experience of mental illness [25].

- A study that looked at who attends support groups and who does not "found significant differences in socio-demographic characteristics and level of functioning of the relative with mental illness. The support group participants are more likely to be white, educated, middle-aged and middle income. Their relative with mental illness was more likely to be living at home, to have a diagnosis of schizophrenia and to have experienced multiple hospitalizations" [24]. He/she was likely to require more caring, but used mental health services less frequently.
- There is an under-representation of minority cultures.
- Unification of many small groups into a single network that can speak with one voice about national policy can have the detrimental effect of losing the grassroots character, if and when the local groups lose touch with the central organization but tend to be governed by it [7].
- Anti-professional attitudes. There is considerable dissatisfaction expressed by caregivers where they feel excluded by professionals from giving "their side of the story" and the intimate knowledge that they have of their mentally ill relative. This has led to hostilities between family carers and professionals, with families seeing professionals as inadequate, and professionals entrenching their beliefs about "family pathology". Professionals do not receive training about self-help groups and they do not have the opportunities to learn about self-helpers' personal experiences. Professionals frequently question the effectiveness of self-help groups; they can feel threatened by anti-professional attitudes, emotional attacks, challenges to professional "authority" and competition with the professional service monopoly. Thus, despite the potential benefits, few professionals refer their clients to mutual support groups [26].

FUTURE RELATIONSHIPS BETWEEN FAMILY GROUPS, THE FAMILY ORGANIZATION AND MENTAL HEALTH SERVICES

In the development of the "Families as Partners in Care" project, the Board members of the WFSAD endorsed the following statement [27]: "Research findings show that better outcomes are achieved for people with mental illness by involving and working with their family carers in an educational and supportive partnership". This resolution resulted in a strategy plan to implement family intervention programmes where all stakeholders—carers, consumers and clinicians—would work together in partnership.

The first step in bringing about a change in the relationship between self-help support groups and the professional mental health service is to develop an understanding that it is only through partnership that empowerment for family carers and consumers can be achieved most effectively. In the mental health field, families who have been emotionally devastated and sidelined will regain more control over their lives through a partnership with mental health services that values and utilizes the knowledge they have gleaned through their "lived experiences". Rather than operating from an "expert" professional framework that can create dependency, professionals should have a role in encouraging the family carer towards this personal empowerment.

Partnerships imply equality, plus "reciprocity, helpfulness, complementarity, collaboration, understanding and clear roles". "Competition, territorialism, authoritarianism, dominance, non-supportiveness and judgment...are negative qualities to be avoided" [16]. Mutual respect and "open communication" are "interpersonal and human qualities of professionals" that self-helpers would like to find in their professional workers [16].

Other factors that will need to be overcome, if equality is to be achieved, are the negative attitudes that families and professionals have towards each other. This needs to be replaced by mutual respect based on an appreciation of the difficulties all key stakeholders face, whether it is family carers coping with mental illness in a close relative, or professionals working in a system that is under-resourced, full of ethical dilemmas and of relatively low status in the eyes of the community.

Strategies mentioned in the literature [7,28] for professional education and training, in order to appreciate what is important about family self-help and support in mental health care, include the following:

- Professionals need to attend self-help support groups to hear the issues that families see as important and how families interact with each other. This should commence preferably as part of undergraduate training, but should be an integral part of in-service training. Many professionals are unaware of the existence of family groups, or, even if aware, are not familiar with the nature of self-help group interactions. Attendance as "observers" will help them to appreciate the relevance of "experiential" knowledge and know-how, and to recognize the importance of incorporating this knowledge into treatment and care plans. In this way, family carers will become a resource that can and should be highly valued. This will be of benefit to the professional as well as to the consumer.
- Professionals and family carers alike need to be educated to appreciate "professional" and "self-help" models, and to value the strengths and limitations of each. It is not too fanciful to believe that an appreciation of each other's position will alleviate many of the problems that arise through the failure of communication between professionals and family

carers; learning from each other allows common goals to be achieved for the mentally ill person. This will relieve some of the pressures on mental health systems caused by failure of effective communication.

- Some professionals refer some families to the family groups/family organizations some of the time, but this needs to be formalized and to become a regular and accepted part of help and support for many more families than happens at present. There should be follow-up by professionals to see if families have actually taken advantage of what can be offered. "Simply mentioning a group is insufficient. Referrals must be made by informed persons who are positive but realistic about the focal self-help group . . . several partial or full sessions are desirable to impart information about the self-help group and deal with any difficulties experienced by the prospective member in his or her early contacts with the group" [29].

- Other roles for professionals include providing support to the group, information, consultation and a willingness to help start up self-help and support groups. Professionals in some countries have started self-help and support groups, with the idea of withdrawing from the group when it is able to continue without professional assistance. This often proves difficult, as the family members have come to rely on the professional and feel they will not be able to continue without their input. But it is important for professionals to withdraw from leadership to allow for the empowerment process to develop. "If the group is not time-limited, peer leadership (among members) becomes stronger. For professional facilitators, this signals the potential for converting to a consultant role. This transition can be effected through three strategic moves by the practitioner: first, gradually becoming less active in the meetings he or she attends; second, not attending every meeting; and third, meeting with peer group leaders for consultation outside the group's meeting time" [29].

RESEARCH AND EVALUATION

Although research studies previously referred to in this chapter have revealed the benefits of family self-help and support groups, the "structural characteristics, change processes and probable outcomes" of these groups for people who use them are not clearly known or understood [29]. This is another reason why there may be hesitations in properly supporting family organizational initiatives.

Research to date has suffered methodological problems:

- Outcomes have been assessed using traditional "scientific" research methodologies, rather than a methodology devised to explore processes that take place over periods of time, and have outcomes that are less easily quantifiable; research processes that seem essentially more subjective and therefore less scientifically valid. Because research projects that are in-depth and longitudinal are only able to cope with small samples, generalization of the findings can be open to criticism. There is a need to understand what "outcomes" self-help group members want for themselves, and then how these can be measured.

- Samples have been biased. The essential middle-class nature of most family organization members referred to earlier, and the fact that "focus groups" (the basis of many surveys about family groups) are usually carried out with self-selecting participants, has not led to research that understands the range of outcomes for many other family constellations and circumstances, including the huge variety of ethnic characteristics, which are often completely ignored.

- Future research in this area needs to "define more objective measures of benefit rather than relying on the self-report of participants" although "the subjective experience anecdotally reported by the parents cannot be ignored". Research needs to be done to see how the self-help experience can be utilized for "first-episode" families [23]. Kuei-Ru et al. [21] argue for research methodologies to "isolate experimental variables from other confounding influences, balance experimental and control groups in terms of demographic factors but also in terms of caregiving factors". Powell [29] feels that more research needs to distinguish between groups that are professionally facilitated and those that rely only on the "experiential wisdom" of the self-help members.

- Perhaps one of the most useful areas of research would be to explore the factors that prevent even greater participation by individuals from a variety of backgrounds [24]. Winefield and Harvey [30], in their study of the effects of group meetings for family caregivers facilitated by professionals, found that attendance and participation rates were high once subjects were engaged. In spite of extensive publicity about the groups, the number of caregivers who showed interest was relatively small. If engagement with mental health services is difficult, it is likely that engagement of people who do not as yet participate in self-help groups will not increase. Given the benefits of group participation that have been described, it would be of interest to explore in-depth the reasons for non-participation in support systems, and then to determine how greater participation can be achieved. Such an undertaking will need closer collaboration with academic and professional workers than seems possible at present. Self-help support is not a high research priority in mental health.

- Self-help organizations are undertaking research themselves. Such research informs the family organization about its own membership and provides data to policy makers, planners and providers of mental health services about problems and gaps in service provision. More self-help organizations could undertake this kind of research to provide a database for highlighting areas of strength as well as weakness in mental health service delivery.

The role of researchers is to develop valid information about self-help. What seems to be needed now is "a new vision of mutually beneficial relationships between researchers and self-help organizations". This research would lead to "increased professional awareness of self-help groups, to a better balance in the country's service agenda, and to a better use of cost-free services...and it could be used to achieve a better balance between self-help and professional services research" [29].

POLICY ISSUES: SHIFTS IN POWER AND CONTROL, AND RESOURCE ALLOCATION

In advocating for the wider use of the self-help organization, Powell [29] comments:

> The number of people knowing about or using self-help is limited by the prevailing and not often commented on culture of professional privilege...the consequence is a policy imbalance. In the mental health area, state mental health and human service agencies and their federal counterparts allocate the lion's share of their resources to the study and improvement of professional services, apparently little cognizant of the diverse ways by which people get help. The literature mirrors the near monopoly privilege of professionals. Until professionals become more aware of how their privileged position results in ignorance about self-help programs, their clients and patients will be denied access to them. Unless professionals convey this information, clients are unlikely to be sufficiently informed to make a decision about their potential usefulness. Professionals, after all, are well positioned in their roles as acute care specialists or as crisis regulators to open the gates to participation in these services.

Salzer *et al.* [31] continue this theme: "The extent to which professional services are valued relative to layperson-delivered services, even if acknowledged as providing differing benefits, will likely affect the degree to which layperson services like self-help groups are supported throughout the world ... To the extent that a professional-centric attitude interferes with professional support of the self-help movement, valuable allies in the struggle to expand the reach of mental health services will be lost."

Health care policies are including greater participation from consumers and carers in the planning and implementation of mental health services. It will be the consumer and carer voice in decision making that will also help to reduce the power and resource imbalance between self-helpers and professional services. The worry that professionals have about the self-help movement taking away resources from professional services is more than compensated for by the extraordinary influx of resources that accompanies the development of the family organizations. Mental health policies world-wide need to incorporate increased support for the families of patients with mental illness, not only through implementing best practice for families in mental health services, but through the recognition that family groups and the family organizations provide services to families that cannot be provided by mental health professionals.

CONCLUSIONS

Although the growth of the family movement in mental health has been impressive, there are still many countries where informal support for family carers is not known. Even in countries where self-help support groups and organizations have commenced, most still face inadequate understanding of what they do and lack resources to further develop their important functions. Self-help through mutual support is a basic under-utilized resource. In times of increasing pressure on economic resources, it seems foolish not to invest in this low-cost benefit to families everywhere.

What is equally impressive is the increasing desire of family groups and organizations in regional areas to meet with and learn from each other. Families of the mentally ill universally are willing to help other families; they are unconcerned about cultural, social, economic, ethnic, religious, linguistic or any other differentiating characteristic. International confer-ences held by WFSAD, EUFAMI, NAMI and Zenkaren are exhilarating experiences and testimony to the similarity of problematic situations in which families caring for someone with a mental illness find themselves the world over.

The family self-help and support movement has shown that family carers who are part of this movement can go a long way to actively participate to fulfil their own needs. Through these interactions, they are able to learn the best management techniques for difficult behavioural problems in order to cope with the mental illness in a family member. The family organizations have shown how they utilize opportunities for developing leadership and pursuing political action.

But it is not enough. Family carers need a responsive mental health service that provides best practice not only for their mentally ill relatives, but for family carers as well, particularly the vast majority of family carers who do not participate in support groups or a family organization.

Support of the family self-help movement will be a strong force for expansion of personal and social resources for families. It has the capacity to be an added resource for overworked clinicians. It presents innovative challenges for researchers to explore methodologies that uncover in-depth experiences that will better inform policy makers and planners of mental health services.

In turn, families who feel valued by professional services and have learnt to appreciate the difficulties faced by the professional workforce have the incentive to improve mental health care through efficient use of the family organizations' capacity for targeted political advocacy. Self-help combined with clinical help and support will result in empowerment of family carers.

The family movement will grow, slowly and with difficulty, but it is here to stay. It will be less slow and less difficult, if more effective partnerships can be forged with professional workers, researchers, policy makers and planners of mental health services.

REFERENCES

1. Kurtz L.F. (1997) *Self-Help and Support Groups—A Handbook for Practitioners*. Sage, Thousand Oaks, CA.
2. EUFAMI (2001) Breaking the silence. Carers' views on the help given during the first episode of psychosis. A European perspective. www.eufami.org.
3. Johnson D.L. (1994) Families around the world form organizations for the mentally ill. *Innovations Research*, **3**, 25–30.
4. Johnson D.L. (2002) A brief history of the international movement of family organizations for persons with mental illness. In: Lefley H.P., Johnson D.L. (eds) *Family Interventions in Mental Illness: International Perspectives*. Praeger, Westport, CT, pp. 209–220.
5. Froggatt D. (2003) The role of the World Fellowship for Schizophrenia and Allied Disorders (WFSAD) in the development and support of family organizations. Personal communication.
6. Leggatt M. (2002) Families and mental health workers: the need for partnerships. *World Psychiatry*, **1**, 52–54.
7. Riessman F., Carroll D. (1995) *Redefining Self-Help: Policy and Practice*. Jossey-Bass, San Francisco, CA.
8. Leggatt M. (2001) Carer and carer organizations. In: Thornicroft G., Szmukler G. (eds) *Textbook of Community Psychiatry*. Oxford University Press, Oxford, pp. 475–486.
9. Hatzidimitriadou E. (2002) Political ideology, helping mechanisms and empowerment of mental health self-help/mutual aid groups. *J. Commun. Appl. Psychol.*, **12**, 271–285.

10. Citron M., Solomon P., Draine J. (1999) Self-help groups for families of persons with mental illness: perceived benefits of helpfulness. *Commun. Ment. Health J.*, **35**, 15–30.

11. Hodges J.Q., Markward M., Keele C., Evans C.J. (2003) Use of self-help services and consumer satisfaction with professional mental health services. *Psychiatr. Serv.*, **54**, 1161–1163.

12. Lavoie F., Stewart M. (1995) Mutual aid groups and support groups: the Canadian context. *Can. J. Commun. Ment. Health*, **14**, 5–12.

13. Pickett-Schenk S.A. (2002) Church-based support groups for African American families coping with mental illness: outreach and outcomes. *Psychiatr. Rehabil. J.*, **26**, 173–180.

14. Perron B. (2002) Online support for caregivers of people with a mental illness. *Psychiatr. Rehabil. J.*, **26**, 70–77.

15. Schubert M.A., Borkman T. (1994) Identifying the experiential knowledge developed within a self-help group. In: Powell T.J. (ed.) *Understanding the Self-Help Organization: Frameworks and Findings*. Sage, Thousand Oaks, CA, pp. 227–246.

16. Constantino V., Nelson G. (1995) Changing relationships between self-help groups and mental health professionals: shifting ideology and power. *Can. J. Commun. Ment. Health*, **14**, 55–70.

17. Alexander K. (1991) *Understanding and Coping with Schizophrenia: 14 Principles for the Relatives*. Schwartz and Wilkinson, Melbourne.

18. Burland J. (1998) Family-to-family: a trauma and recovery model of family education. *New Directions Ment. Health Serv.*, **77**, 33–41.

19. Pickett S.A., Cook J.A., Laris A. (2000) Brief report. Journey of hope program outcomes. *Commun. Ment. Health J.*, **36**, 413–424.

20. Dixon L., Stewart B., Burland J., Delahunty M., Luckstead A., Hoffman M. (2001) Pilot study of the effectiveness of the family-to-family education program. *Psychiatr. Serv.*, **52**, 965–967.

21. Chou K.-R., Liu S.-Y., Chu H. (2002) The effects of support groups on caregivers of patients with schizophrenia. *Int. J. Nurs. Studies*, **39**, 713–722.

22. Pickett S.A, Heller T., Cook J. (1998) Professional-led versus family-led support groups: exploring the differences. *J. Behav. Health Sci. Res.*, **25**, 437–445.

23. O'Brien P.J. (2002) Reflections of a facilitator for a parent support group in an adolescent in-patient psychiatric program. *Fam. Ther.*, **29**, 141–151.

24. Heller T., Roccoforte J.A., Cook J.A. (1997) Predictors of support group participation among families of persons with mental illness. *Fam. Rel.*, **46**, 437–442.

25. Leighninger R.D., Speier A.H., Mayeux D. (1996) How representative is NAMI? Demographic comparisons of a national NAMI sample with members and non-members of Louisiana mental health support groups. *Psychiatr. Rehab. J.*, **19**, 71–73.

26. Chinman M., Kloos B., O'Connell M., Davidson L. (2002) Service providers' views of psychiatric mutual support groups. *J. Commun. Psychol.*, **30**, 349–366.

27. World Fellowship for Schizophrenia and Allied Disorders (2001) Families as partners in care. An initiative of the WFSAD. A work in progress. www.world-schizophrenia.org.

28. Salzer M., McFadden L., Rappaport J. (1994) Professional views of self-help groups. *Admin. Policy Ment. Health*, **22**, 85–95.

29. Powell T.J. (1994) Self-help research and policy issues. In: Powell T.J. (ed.) *Understanding the Self-Help Organization: Frameworks and Findings.* Sage, Thousand Oaks, CA, pp. 1–19.
30. Winefield H.R., Harvey E.J. (1995) Tertiary prevention in mental health care: effects of group meetings for family caregivers. *Aust. N. Zeal. J. Psychiatry*, **29**, 139–145.
31. Salzer M.S., Rappaport J., Segre L. (2001) Mental health professionals' support of self-help groups. *J. Commun. Appl. Soc. Psychol.*, **11**, 1–10.

Research on Burden and Coping Strategies in Families of People with Mental Disorders: Problems and Perspectives

Elizabeth Kuipers* and Paul E. Bebbington‡

*Institute of Psychiatry, King's College London, London, UK
‡Royal Free and University College London Medical School, London, UK

INTRODUCTION: CARING FOR CARERS

It has been well documented that caring for someone with a severe mental health problem can be bad for the carer's own physical and psychological health [e.g., 1–7]. Caring is an inherently unequal relationship: the person doing the "caring" has more responsibility and has more to do than the person being cared for, who is to some extent dependent. While such relationships can be sources of great joy and satisfaction (rarely documented), they are more likely to lead to what is called the "burden" or impact of care in carers, and to feelings of frustration and guilt in the person requiring it. If caring is prolonged (and in many mental health conditions, it can last until one of the pair dies), problems can be exacerbated; things may not get better with time. A further difficulty is that carers find they have no choice [8,9]. Unlike some other relationships, carers find themselves in this role because of something happening to someone else; a partner, parent, sibling or child is diagnosed with a serious mental health problem.

The issues raised by this situation are common to all mental health conditions; they include the initial confusion and shock, a lack of information, the stigma of psychiatric diagnoses, difficult and embarrassing behaviour problems, poor continuing care for the service user, and usually little or no support for those doing the caring. Care can endure for many years, while carers age and become infirm, and other family roles are neglected. Carers are usually women, and many of them have more than one caring role. In one of our studies, 20% of people looking after someone with a first episode

Families and Mental Disorders. Edited by Norman Sartorius, Julian Leff, Juan José López-Ibor, Mario Maj and Ahmed Okasha. © 2005 John Wiley & Sons Ltd. ISBN 0-470-02382-1

of psychosis had previous experience of caring for someone else with a mental health problem [10].

Even for first-time carers, there are other stresses in life; they may have their own jobs, they may have other children or elderly relatives who also need looking after, they may have unrelated financial or accommodation problems; caring for someone with a mental health problem may be the least of their difficulties. Kwan [11], for instance, reported that negative caregiving experiences affected quality of life less than other everyday stresses.

Research on carers has now spanned more than 50 years, since the middle of the last century when deinstitutionalization first spotlighted the sorts of difficulties that wives had when their husbands were first allowed home from the psychiatric hospital [12]. As is apparent from this volume, the topic has expanded greatly in the interval. A literature search of "carers" and "burden" from 2000 to the end of 2003 elicited nearly 500 entries, which have been scanned for this chapter.

Informal care has been recognized as an important function by the UK government for 20 years, culminating in a national strategy for carers [13]. Indeed, nationally representative data about the extent and nature of caring has been collected every 5 years since 1985 in the British General Household Survey [14]. However, there had been less focus on the care of carers themselves, and thus the General Household Survey in 2000 was augmented to provide data on the mental health of carers aged 16 years or older in England, and the extent to which caring impacted upon their health [15]. While this covered caring of all types, the results cast a particular light on caring for people with mental health problems.

Adults were followed up if they reported in the 2000 General Household Survey that they provided care in an unpaid capacity for a person living in their own or in another private household. Around 2000 carers were identified and interviewed. About one quarter of all the households in the carers' sample contained two or more carers. For the majority of carers, the main or only caring relationship was with an elderly adult: over half of those cared for were over 75 years old. Only 4% of dependants were children aged under 16 years. Most carers were looking after women (68%). They were usually caring for their own relatives: parents, 38%; spouse or partner, 16%; or another relative, 15%. Two thirds (67%) of people being cared for had only physical problems or difficulties, whereas 19% had both physical and mental problems, and 7% were described as being only mentally affected. More than half of carers had been carrying out their role for over 5 years.

Carers were assessed by the well-known Clinical Interview Schedule-Revised (CIS-R) [16]. A total score of 12 or more is conventionally taken as indicating the presence of one of the "common mental disorders". It is interesting that, as a whole, the sample of carers did not appear to have elevated levels of psychiatric disturbance, compared with the results from the British National Survey of Psychiatric Morbidity [17]. However, certain sub-groups did.

There were more mental problems among carers when the person being cared for was younger (under 65 years), particularly the 45 to 64 age group. Carers of spouses or partners were over two and a half times more likely than people looking after parents to have above threshold CIS-R scores, once the other factors had been taken into account. Carers of children were nearly twice as likely to have elevated scores.

However, the interesting finding from our standpoint is that the odds of high symptom scores for carers looking after people who were both physically and mentally affected were double those of carers of people with only physical problems or difficulties. Individuals who took on the main responsibility for someone by themselves were more likely than those who shared or did not have this responsibility to report mental health problems. Carers who lived with the person they looked after all the time were also more likely to have high CIS-R scores. Not surprisingly, the more individuals carers looked after, the more likely they were to report neurotic symptoms.

After logistic regression, a number of features relating to the context of caring relationships seemed to be independently associated with poor mental health in carers. One of these was whether the carer had been allowed to take a break of more than a few hours. Those unable to take a break were more than three times as likely to have high CIS-R scores. Being a carer with a small primary support group (of eight or fewer adults) doubled the odds of a high CIS-R score. Good relationships with family or friends were important for mental health carers. Finally, CIS-R scores were more than twice as likely to be high in carers who felt that the act of caring had had an adverse effect on their relationship with friends, their social life or their leisure activities. These British data are based on caring of all types. However, the findings have clear and general implications for people caring for friends or relatives with mental illness.

In summary, it seems crucial for carers to feel that they can take a break or have some respite, that they are not alone, and that their social support is effective. Likewise, it is important that they do not perceive caring as having had a negative impact on other parts of their life. In other words, it seems important that carers should not be left on their own to do a difficult job and that both practical and emotional forms of support are easily available to them.

METHODOLOGICAL PROBLEMS AND LIMITATIONS

Despite the proliferation of research in this area, there are still significant methodological problems. Some will be discussed now, with particular reference to research in psychosis, which is the area we are familiar with.

Definitions

Since research on caring first started, there has been a lack of consistency in the definitions used, and a wide variety of measures for quantifying the range of difficulties perceived to be associated with the caring role. Platt [18] initially defined burden as "the presence of problems, difficulties or adverse events which affect the life (lives) of the psychiatric patients' significant others (e.g. members of the household and/or the family)". The concept of burden was also reviewed by Schene et al. [19]. As discussed by Kuipers [9], there are many definitions, but in Platt's view they share a common underlying frame of reference: "the effect of the patient upon the family" [20]; the impact of living with a (psychiatric) patient on the way of life or health of family members [21] and "the difficulties felt by the family of a psychiatric patient" [22]. As can be seen, all these definitions take a particular view of the issues; the main emphasis is the effect of the patient on the family system. The problems at this stage are seen to operate in one direction, from the patient to the rest of the family, and the assumption is that the effects will mainly be negative.

Dimensions of Burden

Hoenig and Hamilton [23] made the first attempt to distinguish between two different sorts of burden on relatives, so-called "objective" and "subjective" burden. Objective burden is defined as the kind of disruption to life and routines that can be externally verified, say, by a research interviewer, or by measuring patient disability independently; such items include financial problems, or the amount of care needed by a patient. Subjective burden is more about how these difficulties make the relative feel; as such, it is closely related to such concepts as stress or distress. In most studies the latter are now measured independently, for instance, by establishing General Health Questionnaire (GHQ) levels in carers, or directly assessing levels of depression. Platt et al. [24] also attempted to assess what has been called the "patient relatedness" [see, for instance, 1] of an event: how much a given event is independent of patient difficulties (e.g. unemployment in the carer or accommodation difficulties may not be related to their caring role).

Factors that Influence Burden: General Issues

An article by Lowyck et al. [25] reviews the factors associated with burden in schizophrenia. However, their criticisms also reflect concerns on burden research in other conditions. They point out that there is a lack of consensus on the factors that determine the extent or pattern of burden. They argue that this is due to the range of definitions of burden employed, to the concentration of studies on only one or two variables, and to the lack of a consistent approach to which ones should be prioritized. They also point out that studies vary in the time periods examined. In fact, most studies are cross-sectional, looking at associations at one point in time. Those that are prospective or longitudinal, do so pragmatically. Lowyck *et al.* recommend that the standardization of measures would be helpful, as would some agreement about definitions, and consistency of time periods across studies. Such recommendations are often made, but can hardly be enforced, particularly when studies are set up by a variety of groups and funding bodies, in local circumstances that cannot always be replicated.

The Role of Appraisal

Distinguishing between dimensions of burden relies on individuals being able to separate them. More recent research has made it clear that subjective and objective burden are often not independent [e.g., 26]. How a carer feels about problems, and how cause is attributed, may not be separable from their rating of the impact of the difficulties. It is now accepted that whether an event is problematic depends on an appraisal of resources and coping skills [e.g., 27]. This has complicated the picture. It has become clear that carers' ratings of difficulties cannot be taken as reliable indicators of the situation; one person's insuperable difficulties may be appraised by another as positive. This accounts for at least some of the inconsistencies in studies that only look at difficult symptoms.

Difficult Symptoms

It is the case that all disorders have symptoms or behaviour problems that are regarded as difficult to cope with by carers. In psychosis, poor social functioning causes problems in a variety of cultures [e.g., 28–30], as does disorganization [e.g., 31,32]. Poor insight is also associated with increased burden [e.g., 33,34]. In mania, violence has been identified as burdensome when it is present [35], as it is in psychosis [36]. However, other demographic or organizational factors can also be identified as increasing the level of problems, such as looking after a male [37], or a reduction of hospital admission times [38]. These problems can be apparent in a first episode [39,40] or the first year of caring, and may even be worse then than later on [41]. In dementia, similar issues arise: a variety of symptoms and problems predict carer burden, from depression, delusions and hallucinations to wandering and aggression [e.g., 42,43].

Although all disorders sometimes lead to difficult symptoms and behaviour problems, they are often not directly related to carer burden scores, or they are related in inconsistent ways. When the severity of the patients' symptoms is found to be correlated with greater family burden [e.g., 44], a typical finding is that burden is also correlated with some other linked variable. Thus, Rosenheck et al. [44] found that burden was also associated with higher contact time with carers and increased time in the community. Thus, even though reducing symptoms seemed on the face of it to be helpful, it meant that service users spent more time in the community and with their carers, with the result that burden increased paradoxically. The benefits for carers of improving symptomatology had been cancelled out.

The Role of Coping

Once appraisal and coping started to be used as a model [e.g., 27], a number of studies attempted to relate these factors to burden. The results seem to suggest that measuring burden and symptom severity on their own is not helpful. What has been more useful is an examination of the intervening factors: how are the problems appraised?, how does this relate to coping resource?, how does this in turn relate to carer distress?

In general, results suggest that it is improvements in coping that reduce distress. Schene et al. [45], in a study of 480 Dutch carers, found that problems and distress could be lowered by a combination of reducing patient symptomatology, increasing carers' coping capacities, and decreasing the number of contact hours with the patient. Joyce et al. [46] developed a model of caregiving in which coping and distress were central. Marriott et al. [47] found that improving coping was helpful in an intervention with carers of people with dementia.

The style of coping also appears to be important. Magliano et al. [48] found a reduction of burden over time in relatives who adopted less emotion-focused coping; problem solving is often more productive. Chakrabati and Gill [49] found that problem-focused coping was more common in the caregivers of bipolar patients, and emotion-focused coping (associated with perceptions that nothing can be changed) in carers of people with schizophrenia. The authors suggest that these differences may account for the differences in burden felt by the two groups. Another form of coping that has been found helpful, but can be overlooked, is strength of religious belief: it was found to be a significant predictor of well-being in carers in one study [50], as was prayer in another [31].

Social Networks

However, it is often not possible to change coping style without access to resources. Contextual factors may need to be considered before change can take place. For instance, the social network available to carers and their families appears extremely important.

In a study of 709 patients and their carers in Italy, Magliano *et al.* [51] describe professional and social network support as crucial if burden is to be reduced. They had previously found [48] that burden was reduced not only by improving coping but by practical help to bolster social networks and by an improvement in patient social functioning. Studies in other settings have found similar results [e.g., 52–54]. Joyce *et al.* [46] found that support from confidants improved effective coping. Presumably, when carers are less isolated, and they can call on the resources of a social network, whether informal or professional, their coping resources are likely to increase, and the resulting distress to decrease.

Effects on Different Carers

Until recently, another criticism of carer research was that it concentrated on one main carer, ignoring the effects on the family network as a whole, and on other carers such as siblings, children or grandparents. This is being rectified, though the literature is still small. Ostman and Hansson [55], in a longitudinal study of mental health services in Sweden, showed that where patients had children, only half of them had needs that were met. Healthy spouses often had to give up their jobs and had a higher need of services compared to spouses without children. There is still no literature on the experience of children caring for those with severe mental health problems. While likely to be a small group, the Swedish study suggests that their needs are unduly neglected.

There is now some evidence about the impact on siblings. They are likely to feel guilt, burden and the effects of stigma, though not as much as the primary carer [e.g., 56]. Some carers experience the role differently, and different kinds of carer predominate in different conditions. Typically, spouses or partners are more involved in conditions such as depression and bipolar disorder. In dementia, some carers will be partners, and some will be grown-up children, usually daughters. In contrast, parents, usually mothers, are more likely to be carers for people with schizophrenia and schizoaffective disorder. In anorexia, both parents are likely to be involved. While the patterns of concern vary slightly with the role, in that partners lose their own confidant(e), and parents can mourn the loss of a more competent adult, many of the themes of upset transcend conditions. Anger, loss, grief and guilt are common. Stigma has more recently been identified as being burdensome in its own right [e.g., 57]. Sadly, these perceptions do not appear to have improved much over the past few decades.

Burden across the Life Cycle: Carers Are Not Homogeneous

Lefley [58] has consistently discussed the fact that carers are not a homogeneous group, and that their needs will change over time and over the life cycle. Carers are defined by the role, and do not form a cohesive group. They will start the caring role at different times in their life cycle, and for some it will be a major role, while for others it will be peripheral or rejected altogether. For many, it will be one of multiple care roles, i.e. caring for a child and an elderly parent. In some conditions, such as eating disorders, the role may look like a particularly intense form of parenting, with monitoring of weight and eating times. In other conditions, such as depression, the carer may take over roles such as that of the main earner. In dementia, taking over basic functions such as feeding and cleaning will be required. The carer who has just taken on the role will have different views and needs from someone who has been doing it for 20 years. An elderly carer looking after someone with Alzheimer's disease may feel he has little in common with the parent of a person with newly diagnosed bipolar disorder and comorbid alcohol misuse.

Research into burden often fails to take these facts into account; that samples may not have much in common demographically, and may be opportunistic (e.g. using carers support groups for their sampling) rather than epidemiological. Assumptions made about the needs of one set of carers may not generalize to other groups of carers within conditions, let alone to those coping with other disorders.

PERSPECTIVES

Despite these problems and limitations, there has been some progress. The initial tendency for researchers to focus on blame, implicit in some of the earlier studies, seems to have been replaced more recently with a more balanced view.

Terminology

The use of the word "burden" has itself exaggerated the tendency to understand the issues from only one perspective: that the carer is *burdened* by the role. This belies the reality that many individuals take on such roles willingly, and that there are positives in a caring relationship. Early measures did not consider this possibility. However, measures that can identify positive attributes have of course found them. The Experience of Caregiving Inventory (ECI, 59) was a pioneering attempt in psychosis research to look for good experiences of caregiving, not just negative ones. Szmukler prefers the term "impact of care" to the word "burden", because of the connotations of the latter, and he and colleagues have helped move perceptions of caring away from the purely negative. Other examples of this kind of research support the finding that carers find the role positive. Schwartz and Gidron [60] reported that all of their sample of 93 carers felt they received help and support from their mentally ill adult child, as well as feeling that they had gained important satisfaction from fulfilling their parenting duties and had learnt about themselves. Veltman *et al.* [61] reported carers feeling beneficial effects such as gratification, love, pride and life lessons learned.

Models

Another advance in the last decade has been to think about burden in relation to other measures, and so to increase our understanding of what is entailed.

Burden and its Relationship to Expressed Emotion

Although both developed at around the same time in the 1950s, burden and expressed emotion (EE) research initially took different pathways. Burden focused on carers' difficulties with their role. EE, which is a measure of the quality of a relationship, focused on the interaction between carers and the persons being cared for. EE is a way of using prosodic variables (the tone, pitch and speed of voice) to rate variables such as warmth, criticism and emotional overinvolvement, when relatives are interviewed and describe their relationship with an identified patient. This measure was developed and validated by Brown and Rutter [62], initially to investigate the effects of family atmosphere on people with schizophrenia returning home after a stay in hospital. It has been consistently found that high levels of criticism and overinvolvement ("high EE") are reliable indicators of a stressful relationship, and predict a poor outcome in a range of conditions, initially in schizophrenia [reviewed in 63,64], but more recently in a range of physical health problems, such as obesity, epilepsy and rheumatoid arthritis [reviewed in 65].

When burden and EE were examined together [e.g., 66,67], it became apparent that they were tapping into similar concerns. Those with high ratings on EE were also likely to show high levels of burden. Both seem to be a rating of the appraisal of difficulties, and are associated with increased distress. EE and subjective burden look particularly similar: both seem to be a proxy for upset. They are also related to poor coping strategies such as avoidance, even in first episodes. In the study by Raune *et al.* [40], 46 carers of those with first-episode psychosis were interviewed and rated on burden, EE and coping. High EE was related to higher subjective burden, higher avoidant coping and lower perceived patient functioning. As the authors discuss, why high EE carers appraise their situation as more stressful even at the start of the caring role is an important question. Their greater use of avoidant coping implies theoretically that it might indeed derive from poorer coping skills [e.g., 68,69]. Alternatively, there are suggestions in the literature about other factors that may contribute. These include carer perceptions that difficult behaviour is done on purpose by the patient [e.g., 70], a more negative carer self-concept [71] and less carer empathy [72]. Particular situations may have care impact. Stressful appraisal might be more likely in smaller families [73] and where there are gender-role-based ideas about caring [e.g., 74]. Some patient behaviours (e.g. negative symptoms) lend themselves more easily to carer misinterpretation, or misattribution.

The Role of Attribution

Another strand of research, with particular contributions from Barrowclough and her colleagues, has been concerned with how attribution relates to EE, distress and, by implication, what is usually measured by burden. Barrowclough and Hooley [75] reviewed the evidence on attributions and EE, and came to the conclusion that high criticism relatives (one form of high EE) are particularly likely to have blaming attributions about patients, and to hold them responsible for their difficulties. These attributions are seen as increasing the likelihood of relapse in patients, mediated through controlling behaviour in relatives that may serve to distress patients and reduce their self-esteem. "An argument can be made for the development and evaluation of interventions designed to help relatives adopt less blaming and more flexible beliefs about the nature of patients' problems" [75]. If burden, EE, attribution and distress in carers are all linked via coping, this gives pointers to how such distress might be alleviated.

Illness Perception

A further important association is with another form of attribution, the illness perceptions of carers. These have clear relevance to the other factors being measured in burden research. Illness perceptions have been looked at in physical illness for some time [reviewed in 76] using the self-regulatory model of Levanthal *et al.* [77]. A specific measure, the Illness Perception Questionnaire (IPQ, 78), arose directly out of an interest in carer attributions following the occurrence of serious health problems, such as myocardial infarction. Interestingly enough, with carers of people with such problems, it has been found that their perception of the illness affects the well-being both of the patient and of themselves. The parallels are obvious. This work is now being extended to carers' perceptions of severe mental illness. Barrowclough *et al.* [79] found that carer functioning, the carer–patient relationship and patient illness characteristics were associated with different dimensions of illness perception. Carer distress and burden, EE and patient functioning were all measured. They found that "problems with carer well-being were mainly related to perceptions of the magnitude of illness consequences for themselves" [79]. More critical relatives perceived themselves to have less control over the illness and a more chronic time line, and perceived a greater number of symptoms.

One of the interesting features of considering burden as a facet of illness perceptions in other illnesses that require a change of lifestyle, is that it normalizes carer reactions. It enables us to identify the changes required separately from the stigma surrounding mental health issues. If carers' reactions to a heart attack can affect how both carers and patients feel and cope with the difficulties, carers' reactions to a diagnosis of a severe mental health problem may appear in a new light—not as pathological, or as a need to blame the identified patient, but as something that both parties have to deal with, and where recovery can be facilitated if both sides can react in optimal ways.

We are now at a stage where burden can be seen in the context of an event that needs to be dealt with (objective burden). The situation has to be appraised by the carer (attribution, illness perceptions, EE), then coping resources must be mobilized (social network, confidants, practical and emotional problem solving, information and support from services). The resulting distress and perceived burden can then be minimized (difficult symptoms reduced, optimal recovery encouraged, carer distress and depression identified and treated as necessary).

INTERVENTIONS

While there is a literature on interventions for carers, it is noticeable that burden is rarely documented as improved. This is probably because, until recently, most interventions were aimed at improving patient outcomes, and carer outcomes have tended to be assessed as a secondary outcome, certainly not as a primary outcome in their own right. While distress can be reduced, particularly if coping is improved, burden usually remains unchanged [e.g. 80]. Other studies have shown no changes at all [e.g. 81]. One of the few investigations to aim specifically at reducing carer distress was a small study ($n = 29$) of carers of people with Alzheimer's disease randomly allocated to an interview control group or individual family intervention [47]. Interventions consisted of carer education, stress management and training in coping skills. Significant reductions in distress and depression were reported in the carer intervention group, accompanied by reductions in patient behavioural disturbance. Specific intervention focused on the needs of this particular carer group. Helping them to understand, reappraise and cope differently with the caring role appeared to be effective. The authors describe the intervention as a direct attempt to help carers cope better with their own emotional state and to have a clear perspective on how best to deal with difficult and challenging behaviour. According to the authors [47], this reduced carer subjective burden and improved feelings of being able to cope.

This is an interesting result. Most studies have not sought to improve carer distress directly and, when they have, it has usually been as part of a package of care aimed at improving patient outcomes. It may thus be the case that the burden of care does not itself lessen while caring continues, but that, as in other stressful situations, if appraisal and coping can be improved and resources put in place to reduce isolation and provide social support, the distress of the caring role can be reduced. If caring is seen as potentially depressogenic, at least for some people, then interventions that treat this depression and deal with the difficulties, while not denying their reality, may be helpful. If in the process carers can feel better and cope more effectively, their very consistency is likely to reduce behavioural difficulties, which are often the most stressful part of symptom presentation. This in turn will improve carer appraisal and outcome as part of a virtuous circle.

There is an argument that we should stop the kind of burden research that just focuses on difficulties, which are after all well attested, and overly negative. Perhaps instead we should look more specifically at the kinds of difficulties individual carers have at their particular stage of caring and at their time of life. If we can assess this more accurately, individualized care to meet their current needs might in fact be helpful.

It seems likely that while caring continues, carers may not "get better". This phrasing is in any case overly pathologizing and probably unrealistic. The stress associated with long-term care needs to be recognized. Interventions that carers ask for include information in order to understand and appraise problems accurately, support that allows for some time off such as respite care, social support to reduce isolation, assistance with problem solving to deal with the current difficulties, and care that continues to be available across the life span and as needs change.

CONCLUSIONS

More precise models integrating burden research into a more general understanding of how problems are dealt with seem to have been helpful and, if developed further, would allow for more specific testing of hypotheses about the relationships between appraisal, attribution, illness perceptions, coping and distress. It would be beneficial if the focus were to move away from cross-sectional studies, of which there are many, to longitudinal studies, in order to study how variables change over time. Once this is more clearly established, we can look at intervention studies that focus on carer needs and on improving distress for those with high levels. Research on the positives of the caring role would also be helpful, particularly across different conditions.

Finally, research that involves the patients' perspective is almost totally absent. To our knowledge, only one study has compared carer and patient perspectives [79] and this was a focus on illness perceptions. Beyond the anecdotal we know very little about what it is like to be cared for, and how this might be improved for both carer and recipient. We do know that people who are diagnosed with mental illness feel stigmatized, feel guilty about being looked after, and sometimes feel infantilized by the amount of care they receive. Further, if carers foresee more negative consequences for a patient, the patient is more likely to rate the relationship as less positive [79]. Additionally, many users worry about how they will manage when their carer is too old or infirm to maintain the caring role.

Research taking a more balanced view of everyone's perspective would be a step forward. Future research should aim to move away from blame and try to be specific about the sort of caring that improves recovery, while enhancing well-being for all involved.

REFERENCES

1. MacCarthy B., Lesage A., Brewin C.R., Brugha T.S., Mangen S., Wing J.K. (1989) Needs for care among the relatives of long-term users of day care. A report from the Camberwell High Contact Survey. *Psychol. Med.*, **19**, 725–736.
2. Wagner A.W., Logsdon R.G., Pearson J.L., Teri L. (1997) Caregiver expressed emotion and depression in Alzheimer's disease. *Aging Ment. Health*, **1**, 132–139.
3. Harvey K., Burns T., Sedgewick P., Higgitt A., Creed F., Fahy T. (2001) Relatives of patients with severe psychotic disorders: factors that influence contact frequency: report from the UK 700 trial. *Br. J. Psychiatry*, **178**, 248–254.
4. Treasure J., Murphy T., Szmukler T., Todd G., Gavan K., Joyce J. (2001) The experience of caregiving for severe mental illness: a comparison between anorexia nervosa and psychosis. *Soc. Psychiatry Psychiatr. Epidemiol.*, **36**, 343–347.

5. Tarrier N., Barrowclough C., Ward J., Donaldson C., Burns A., Gregg L. (2002) Expressed emotion and attributions in the carers of patients with Alzheimer's disease: the effect on carer burden. *J. Abnorm. Psychol.*, **111**, 340–349.

6. Jungbauer J., Mory C., Angermeyer M.C. (2002) Does caring for a schizophrenic family member increase the risk of becoming ill? Psychological and psychosomatic troubles in caregivers of schizophrenia patients. *Fortschr. Neurol. Psychiatrie*, **70**, 548–554.

7. Wittmund B., Wilms H.U., Mory C., Angermeyer M.C. (2002) Depressive disorders in spouses of mentally ill patients. *Soc. Psychiatry Psychiatr. Epidemiol.*, **37**, 177–182.

8. Kuipers E., Leff J., Lam D. (2002) *Family Work for Schizophrenia: A Practical Guide*, 2nd edn. Gaskell, London.

9. Kuipers E. (2001) The needs of carers. In: Thornicroft G. (ed.) *Measuring Mental Health Needs*, 2nd edn. Gaskell, London, pp. 342–362.

10. Kuipers E., Raune D. (2000) EE and burden in first onset psychosis. In: Birchwood M., Fowler D., Jackson C. (eds) *Early Interventions in Psychosis*. John Wiley & Sons, Chichester, pp. 128–140.

11. Kwan T. (2001) Quality of life in family caregivers of persons with schizophrenia. *Dissertation Abstracts Int.*, **61**(8-B), 4078.

12. Yarrow M.R., Schwartz C.G., Murphy H.S., Deasy L.C. (1955) The psychological meaning of mental illness in the family. *J. Soc. Issues*, **11**, 12–24.

13. Department of Health (1999) *Caring about Carers: A National Strategy for Carers*. The Stationery Office, London.

14. Rowlands O., Parker G. (1998) *Informal Carers 1995 General Household Survey (Supplement A)*. The Stationery Office, London.

15. Singleton N., Maung N.A., Courie A., Sparks J., Bumpstead R., Meltzer H. (2002) *Mental Health of Carers*. The Stationery Office, London.

16. Lewis G., Pelosi A., Araya R.C., Dunn G. (1992) Measuring psychiatric disorders in the community: a standardized assessment for use by lay interviewers. *Psychol. Med.*, **22**, 465–486.

17. Singleton N., Bumpstead R., O'Brien M., Lee A., Meltzer H. (2001) *Psychiatric Morbidity Among Adults Living in Private Households, 2000*. The Stationery Office, London.

18. Platt S. (1985) Measuring of the burden of psychiatric illness in the family: an evaluation of some rating scales. *Psychol. Med.*, **15**, 383–393.

19. Schene A.H., Tessler R.C., Gamache G.M. (1994) Instruments measuring family or caregiver burden in severe mental illness. *Soc. Psychiatry Psychiatr. Epidemiol.*, **29**, 228–240.

20. Goldberg D.P., Huxley P. (1980) *Mental Illness in the Community*. Tavistock, London.

21. Brown G.W. (1967) The family of the schizophrenic patient. In: Copen A.J., Walk A. (eds) *Recent Developments in Schizophrenia*. Royal Medico-Psychological Association, London, pp. 43–59.

22. Pai S., Kapur R.L. (1981) The burden on the family of a psychiatric patient: development of an interview schedule. *Br. J. Psychiatry*, **138**, 332–335.

23. Hoenig J., Hamilton M.W. (1966) The schizophrenic patient in the community and his effect on the household. *Int. J. Soc. Psychiatry*, **12**, 165–176.

24. Platt S., Weyman A., Hirsch S. (1983) *Social Behaviour Assessment Schedule (SBAS)*, 3rd edn. NFER-Nelson, Windsor.

25. Lowyck B., De Hert M., Peeters E., Gilis P., Peuskens J. (2001) Can we identify the factors influencing the burden on family members of patients with schizophrenia? *Int. J. Psychiatry Clin. Pract.*, **5**, 89–96.
26. Cuijpers J., Stam H. (2000) Burnout among relatives of psychiatric patients attending psychoeducational support groups. *Psychiatr. Serv.*, **51**, 375–379.
27. Folkman S., Lazarus R.S. (1985) If it changes it must be a process: study of emotion and coping during three stages of a college examination. *J. Personal Soc. Psychol.*, **48**, 150–170.
28. Hasui C., Sakamoto S., Sugiura T., Miyata R., Fujii Y., Koshiishi F., Kitamura T. (2002) Burden on family members of the mentally ill: a naturalistic study in Japan. *Compr. Psychiatry*, **43**, 219–222.
29. Wong D. (2000) Stress factors and mental health of carers with relatives suffering from schizophrenia in Hong Kong: implications for culturally sensitive practices. *Br. J. Soc. Work*, **30**, 365–382.
30. Volterra V., Ruggeri M., De Ronchi D., Antonelli A., Belelli G., Mastrocola A., Veronesi S. (2002) Practical and emotional family burden relating to psychopathology and social functioning of chronic psychotic patients in some Italian community-based psychiatric services (CPSS). *Minerva Psichiatrica*, **43**, 85–99.
31. Shibre T., Kebede D., Alem A., Negash A., Deyassa N., Fekadu A., Fekadu D., Jacobsson L., Kullgren G. (2003) Schizophrenia: illness impact on family members in a traditional society—rural Ethiopia. *Soc. Psychiatry Psychiatr. Epidemiol.*, **38**, 27–34.
32. Wolthaus J.E.D., Dingemans P.M.A.J., Schene A.H., Linszen D.H., Wiersma D., Van Den Bosch R.J., Cahn W., Hijman R. (2002) Caregiver burden in recent-onset schizophrenia and spectrum disorders: the influence of symptoms and personality traits. *J. Nerv. Ment. Dis.*, **190**, 241–247.
33. Sakai Y., Kim Y., Akiyama T., Kurita H. (2002) Burden on the families of patients with schizophrenia: relations to patients' and families' awareness of mental disorder. *Clin. Psychiatry (Japan)*, **44**, 1087–1094.
34. Thompson M.Y. (2002) Awareness of schizophrenia and caregiver burden. *Dissertation Abstracts Int.*, **62**(12-B), 5982.
35. Dore G., Romans S.E. (2002) Impact of bipolar affective disorder on family and partners. *J. Affect. Disord.*, **67**, 147–158.
36. MacInnes D.L., Watson J.P. (2002) The differences in perceived burdens between forensic and non-forensic caregivers of individuals suffering from schizophrenia. *J. Ment. Health*, **11**, 375–388.
37. Thornicroft G., Leese M., Tansella M., Howard L., Toulmin H., Herran A., Schene A. (2002) Gender differences in living with schizophrenia: a cross-sectional European multi-site study. *Schizophr. Res.*, **57**, 191–200.
38. Lauber C., Eichenberger A., Luginbuhl P., Keller C., Rossler W. (2003) Determinants of burden in caregivers of patients with exacerbating schizophrenia. *Eur. Psychiatry*, **18**, 285–289.
39. Tennakoon L., Fannon D., Doku V., O'Ceallaigh S., Soni W., Santamaria M., Kuipers E., Sharma T. (2000) Experience of caregiving: relatives of people experiencing a first episode of psychosis. *Br. J. Psychiatry*, **117**, 529–533.
40. Raune D., Kuipers E., Bebbington P. (2004) Expressed emotion at first-episode psychosis: investigating a carer appraisal model. *Br. J. Psychiatry*, **184**, 321–326.
41. Lowyck B., De Hert M., Peeters E., Wampers M., Gilis P., Peuskens J. (2002) Burden on the family: a study of 120 relatives of schizophrenic patients in Belgium. *Tijdschr. Psychiatrie*, **44**, 151–159.

42. Donaldson C., Tarrier N., Burns A. (1997) The impact of the symptoms of dementia on caregivers. *Br. J. Psychiatry*, **170**, 62–68.
43. Donaldson C., Tarrier N., Burns A. (1998) Determinants of carer stress and Alzheimer's disease. *Int. J. Geriatr. Psychiatry*, **13**, 248–256.
44. Rosenheck R., Cramer J., Jurgis G., Perlick D., Xu W., Thomas J., Henderson W., Charney D. (2000) Clinical and psychopharmacologic factors influencing family burden in refractory schizophrenia. *J. Clin. Psychiatry*, **61**, 671–676.
45. Schene A.H., van Wijngaarden B., Koeter M.W. (1998) Family caregiving in schizophrenia: domains and distress. *Schizophr. Bull.*, **24**, 609–618.
46. Joyce J., Leese M., Kuipers E., Szmukler G., Harris T., Staples E. (2003) Evaluating a model of caregiving for people with psychosis. *Soc. Psychiatry Psychiatr. Epidemiol.*, **38**, 189–195.
47. Marriott A., Donaldson C., Tarrier N., Burns A. (2000) Effectiveness of cognitive–behavioural family intervention in reducing the burden of care in carers of patients with Alzheimer's disease. *Br. J. Psychiatry*, **176**, 557–562.
48. Magliano L., Fadden G., Economou M., Held T., Xavier M., Guarneri M., Malangone C., Marasco C., Maj M. (2000) Family burden and coping strategies in schizophrenia: 1-year follow-up data from the BIOMED I study. *Soc. Psychiatry Psychiatr. Epidemiol.*, **35**, 109–115.
49. Chakrabati S., Gill S. (2002) Coping and its correlates among caregivers of patients with bipolar disorder: a preliminary study. *Bipolar. Disord.*, **4**, 50–60.
50. Rammohan A., Rao K., Subbakrishna D.K. (2002) Religious coping and psychological wellbeing in carers of relatives with schizophrenia. *Acta Psychiatr. Scand.*, **105**, 356–362.
51. Magliano L., Marasco C., Fiorillo A., Malangone C., Guarneri M., Maj M. (2002) The impact of professional and social network support on the burden of families of patients with schizophrenia in Italy. *Acta Psychiatr. Scand.*, **106**, 291–298.
52. Ohaeri J.U. (2001) Caregiver burden and psychotic patients' perception of social support in a Nigerian setting. *Soc. Psychiatry Psychiatr. Epidemiol.*, **36**, 86–93.
53. Macmaster S.A. (2001) Differences in the well-being of family caregivers of adults with mental illness and a co-occurring substance abuse disorder. *Dissertation Abstracts Int.*, **62**(1-A), 331.
54. Bischel S.L. (2001) Collaboration and congruence between family member and case manager perceptions in the treatment of individuals with schizophrenia. *Dissertation Abstracts Int.*, **62**(2-A), 771.
55. Ostman M., Hansson L. (2002) Children in families with a severely mentally ill member. Prevalence and needs for support. *Soc. Psychiatry Psychiatr. Epidemiol.*, **37**, 243–248.
56. Jewell T.C. (2000) Adult siblings of people with serious mental illness: the relationship between self-and-sibling-care beliefs and psychological adjustment. *Dissertation Abstracts Int.*, **60**(11-B), 5776.
57. Ryder A.G., Bean G., Dion K.L. (2000) Caregiver responses to symptoms of first-onset psychosis: a comparative study of Chinese- and Euro-Canadian families. *Transcult. Psychiatry*, **37**, 255–265.
58. Lefley H.P. (2003) Changing caregivers needs as persons with schizophrenia grow older. In: Cohen C.I. (ed.) *Schizophrenia into Late Life: Treatment, Research and Policy*. American Psychiatric Publishing, Washington, DC, pp. 251–268.

59. Szmukler G.I., Burgess P., Herrman H. (1996) Caring for relatives with serious mental illness: the development of the Experience of Caregiving Inventory. *Soc. Psychiatry Psychiatr. Epidemiol.*, **31**, 137–148.
60. Schwartz C., Gidron R. (2002) Parents of mentally ill adult children living at home: rewards of caregiving. *Health Social Work*, **27**, 145–154.
61. Veltman A., Cameron J.I., Stewart D.E. (2002) The experience of providing care to relatives with chronic mental illness. *J. Nerv. Ment. Dis.*, **190**, 108–114.
62. Brown G.W., Rutter M.L. (1966) The measurement of family activities and relationships. *Hum. Relat.*, **19**, 241.
63. Bebbington P., Kuipers L. (1994) The predictive utility of EE in schizophrenia: an aggregate analysis. *Psychol. Med.*, **24**, 707–718.
64. Butzlaff R.L., Hooley J.M. (1998) Expressed emotion and psychiatric relapse: a meta-analysis. *Arch. Gen. Psychiatry*, **55**, 547–552.
65. Weardon A.J., Tarrier N., Barrowclough C., Zastowny T.R., Rahill A.A. (2000) A review of expressed emotion research in health care. *Clin. Psychol. Rev.*, **20**, 636–666.
66. Smith J., Birchwood M., Cochrane R., George S. (1993) The needs of high and low expressed emotion families: a normative approach. *Soc. Psychiatry Psychiatr. Epidemiol.*, **28**, 11–16.
67. Scazufca M., Kuipers E. (1996) Links between EE and burden of care in relatives of patients with schizophrenia. *Br. J. Psychiatry*, **168**, 580–587.
68. Barrowclough C., Tarrier N., Johnston M. (1996) Distress, expressed emotion, and attributions in relatives of schizophrenia patients. *Schizophr. Bull.*, **22**, 691–702.
69. Scazufca M., Kuipers E. (1999) Coping strategies in relatives of people with schizophrenia before and after psychiatric admission. *Br. J. Psychiatry*, **174**, 154–158.
70. Hooley J.M., Campbell C. (2002) Control and controllability: beliefs and behaviour in high and low expressed emotion relatives. *Psychol. Med.*, **32**, 1091–1099.
71. Hooley J.M., Hiller J.B. (2000) Personality and expressed emotion. *J. Abnorm. Psychol.*, **109**, 40–44.
72. Giron M., Gomez-Beneyto M. (1998) Relationship between empathic family attitude and relapse in schizophrenia: a 2-year follow-up prospective study. *Schizophr. Bull.*, **24**, 619–627.
73. Leff J., Wig N., Bedi H., Menon D.K., Kuipers L., Korten A., Ernberg G., Day R., Sartorius N., Jablensky A. (1990) Relatives' expressed emotion and the course of schizophrenia in Chandigarh. A two-year follow-up of a first-contact sample. *Br. J. Psychiatry*, **156**, 351–356.
74. Bentsen H., Boye B., Munkvold O.G., Notland T.H., Lersbryggen A.B, Oskarsson K.H., Ulstein I., Urem G., Bjorge H., Berg-Larson R. (1996) Emotional over-involvement in parents of patients with schizophrenia or related psychosis: demographic and clinical predictors. *Br. J. Psychiatry*, **169**, 622–630.
75. Barrowclough C., Hooley J.M. (2003) Attributions and expressed emotion: a review. *Clin. Psychol. Rev.*, **23**, 849–880.
76. Weinman J., Heijmans M., Figueiras M.J. (2003) Carer perceptions in chronic illness. In: Cameron L.B., Leventhal H. (eds) *The Self-Regulation of Health and Illness Behaviour*. Routledge, London, pp. 207–219.
77. Leventhal H., Nerenz D.R., Steele D.F. (1984) Illness representations and coping with health threats. In: Baum A., Singer J. (eds) *Handbook of Psychology and Health* vol. 4. Lawrence Erlbaum Associates, Hillsdale, NJ, pp. 219–252.

78. Weinman J., Petrie K., Moss-Morris R., Horne R. (1996) The Illness Perception Questionnaire: a new method for assessing the cognitive representation of illness. *Psychol. Health*, **11**, 431–445.
79. Barrowclough C., Lobban F., Hatton C., Quinn J. (2001) An investigation of models of illness in carers of schizophrenic patients using the Illness Perception Questionnaire. *Br. J. Clin. Psychol.*, **40**, 371–385.
80. Barrowclough C., Tarrier N., Lewis S., Sellwood W., Mainwaring J., Quinn J., Hamlin C. (1999) Randomised controlled effectiveness trial of a need-based psychosocial intervention service for carers of people with schizophrenia. *Br. J. Psychiatry*, **174**, 505–511.
81. Szmukler G., Kuipers E., Joyce J., Harris T., Leese M., Maphosa W., Staples E. (2003) An exploratory randomised controlled trial of a support programme for carers of patients with psychosis. *Soc. Psychiatry Psychiatr. Epidemiol.*, **38**, 411–418.

11

Research on Family Interventions for Mental Disorders: Problems and Perspectives

Ian R.H. Falloon

University of Auckland, Auckland, New Zealand

INTRODUCTION

The role of patients' families in the clinical management of mental disorders has always courted controversy. Even today, in most mental health services, family members are regarded as potential sources of abuse that may have contributed to the onset, or at least to the severity, of mental disorders. Fortunately, the impact of high-quality social psychiatric research has helped clarify these issues and has highlighted the potential benefits of family care, as well as areas where interventions may assist family members to become more effective and efficient in their roles [1]. Almost all national and international treatment guidelines that have been published in the past decade have made specific reference to the need for services to include family members (and/or close friends) as key team members in the continued care of patients with serious mental disorders. In this chapter we will endeavour to summarize the evidence upon which such recommendations have been made, examine its validity, and point out areas where further high-quality research may be needed.

THE GOALS OF FAMILY INTERVENTIONS

Before we can consider the evidence of the benefits of any intervention, it is essential to define the goals that we hope to achieve through its use. In common with most psychosocial interventions, family strategies have had a

Families and Mental Disorders. Edited by Norman Sartorius, Julian Leff, Juan José López-Ibor, Mario Maj and Ahmed Okasha. © 2005 John Wiley & Sons Ltd. ISBN 0-470-02382-1

wide variety of goals, some very modest, others highly ambitious. The most common goals include:

- provision of housing, protection and financial assistance;
- supervision of nutrition and self-care;
- advocacy and empowerment of patients and family;
- interpersonal support for patients;
- interpersonal support for carers;
- companionship for patients and supervision of daily occupational and leisure activity;
- reduction in time patients spend in face-to-face contact with carers;
- supervision and assistance with medication;
- monitoring early warning signs;
- management of stress for all family/household members;
- enhancement of relationships between patients and family;
- enhancement of relationships between all family members;
- improved understanding about mental disorders and their treatment;
- monitoring symptoms and early warning signs of major episodes;
- assistance in crisis management;
- assistance in social and work skills training;
- assistance in psychological strategies;
- helping patients and carers clarify and achieve their personal goals.

OUTCOME ASSESSMENT

With such a variety of potential goals, it is clear that the interventions are likely to be heterogeneous, and require a range of measures to establish their efficacy. Many studies have addressed several of these goals, but have only measured outcomes of one issue, such as the utilization of hospital care. For this reason, interventions that may have been highly effective at achieving their goals have been considered ineffective at achieving goals that were not among their key targets. This heterogeneity largely invalidates the use of meta-analytic approaches to examine the overall results of the extensive body of outcome research that has been conducted over the past three decades.

The early research on outcome focused on enhancing the supportive role of family members towards the patient and one another. It was based upon the social research studies suggesting that stressful social environments and difficulties coping with stressful life changes were among the strongest predictors of recurring and persisting courses of major mental disorders, particularly the functional psychoses [2,3]. A wide variety of intervention strategies were employed that aimed not merely to reduce major psychotic episodes, but also to provide a comprehensive programme of psychosocial rehabilitation, while moderating stress associated with caregiving roles of family members [4]. Secondary findings were apparent improvements in adherence to medication and to ancillary work and social rehabilitation programmes, and suggestions of overall reduced costs to the community [5].

Recent studies have tended to focus on specific components in briefer, less comprehensive programmes, often attempting to relieve the stress on key carers, or merely attempting to improve adherence to medication through highly structured group education [6]. Such adjunct education should not be considered in the same light as the more comprehensive approaches, no more than adding a medication to counter a side effect should be considered comparable with the core pharmacotherapy of any major disorder. Unfortunately, several reviews have not made clear distinctions between the different types of family intervention programmes, thereby leading to somewhat confusing conclusions [7].

In the next section we will summarize the outcome research in specific mental disorders, and on specific outcome measures. We will attempt to answer the following questions: Do family-based interventions work? If so, for what disorders, or targeted problems and goals are they most useful? What formats produce the best results?

FAMILY INTERVENTIONS FOR SCHIZOPHRENIA

Family Education Strategies

More than 40 studies have evaluated a variety of mental health education programmes aimed at enhancing the knowledge and understanding of family caregivers of patients with major mental disorders, mainly, but not exclusively, schizophrenia. These studies have seldom lasted more than 3 months and consisted of 10–12 sessions, usually interactively didactic in nature [8]. The reported results have invariably been positive, with outcomes including enhanced knowledge about mental illness and its treatment, improved adherence to medication, more positive attitudes towards caregiving roles and improved coping abilities. Direct patient benefits in terms of reduced clinical and social morbidity have been less evident, but these have not usually been the primary targets of the education. High quality randomized controlled studies with standardized measures and follow-up assessments are few [9–13].

Comprehensive Family-Based Interventions

While optimal drug therapy remains the cornerstone of the long-term clinical management of psychotic disorders, additional benefits have been reported when optimal pharmacotherapy has been integrated with family-based treatments [14–16]. The family strategies attempt to reduce the impact of environmental stresses on the biologically vulnerable individual while promoting social functioning in the community. Two major types of strategies have been developed along these lines. The first, carer-based stress management, derived from cognitive–behavioural therapy, seeks to enhance the problem-solving efficiency of the patient and his or her social support system and to actively promote the achievement of personal goals [17]. The second, sometimes termed psychoeducation, aims to teach care-givers stress reduction skills, and to increase tolerant attitudes and non-confronting coping skills towards behavioural problems associated with both residual positive and negative symptoms [1,18]. It may be noted that these aims are contrasting, with the stress management approach encouraging patients to tackle and overcome the stresses they find when trying to achieve their chosen life goals, whereas the second approach advocates a more gradual re-entry process, where goals are often restructured by the therapists to less ambitious objectives that are less likely to cause stress. Recurrences and exacerbations of symptoms are expected in the first approach, and are considered opportunities to strengthen coping abilities and to understand better the vulnerability/stress concepts. Such an approach has much in common with the desensitization *in vivo* methods used in cognitive–behavioural management of anxiety, or teaching patients to live a full life with diabetes. This training in managing a biomedical vulnerability involves teaching patients and their caregivers to monitor early warning signs of major episodes and provide assertive crisis care at the earliest sign of an impending exacerbation.

To date, 44 published and unpublished controlled studies have assessed the outcome of comprehensive family-based interventions applied over periods of 3 months to 4 years. Three quarters of the studies were of a high quality from a methodological standpoint. The results of these strategies have shown that major psychotic episodes and consequent crisis management in hospital can be reduced by around 50% when they are combined with optimal drug treatment. However, only the stress management approach has shown consistent benefits in terms of improved social functioning, reduced family burden and continued benefits once the intensive phase of education and training has been completed. All these studies will not be reviewed here but the key research findings and issues will be discussed [see 16 for further details].

It should be noted that a much lower proportion of the psychoeducation studies used adequate research methodology. The results of these two contrasting approaches have often been pooled in meta-analyses, compromising the basic need for homogeneity for this method of summarizing data across studies, and often leading to confusing results [6,7]. However, the benefit of comprehensive approaches is clearly observed, and does not require sophisticated statistical methods. The clearest benefits indicate a consistent added reduction in the frequency of major psychotic episodes or hospital admissions of around 50%, when compared with optimal drug treatment and supportive case management. Undoubtedly some, but not all, of this benefit can be attributed to the improved efficiency of medication management associated with the health education component that is a key aspect of the comprehensive methods. At present too few studies have attempted to unbundle the comprehensive programmes in order to explore the benefits of the individual components [19,20]. However, it is clear that not all patients and their families need long-term complex family programmes to achieve stable recovery from clinical and social morbidity, just as not all need continued antipsychotic medication. However, further research is needed to help us select accurately those who will benefit from less-intensive interventions of all kinds.

Remission of Residual Symptoms

A further aim of stress management approaches is to minimize psychotic and non-psychotic symptoms that may persist after a major psychotic episode [21]. The benefits of stress management strategies in reducing this residual psychopathology, and thereby enhancing the trend towards full remission of schizophrenia, have been assessed in 14 studies. These studies compared rating scales of psychopathology at the beginning of the study with the ratings obtained a year later. In 13 of these studies, an overall trend towards recovery was observed, both with experimental and control treatments [22–34]. Zhang *et al.* [35] noted this trend only for those patients receiving the stress management who did not have any symptom exacerbations. Three studies that used blind assessors to conduct standardized interviews of psychopathology before treatment and at 24 months showed that almost two thirds of cases receiving the family-based approach achieved full remissions of both psychotic and deficit schizophrenic symptoms at two years [22,32,34]. One study observed significant effects of family treatment on negative symptoms [36]. Future research should focus on remission and recovery, not merely relapse and rehospitalization. There seems to be an exciting possibility that stress management approaches may not merely reduce the rates of recurrent major episodes, but may contribute to full and lasting recovery from all psychotic and negative symptoms for a substantial proportion of people experiencing schizophrenic disorders.

Social Outcome

Recovery of premorbid expectations of social functioning may be more difficult to achieve than clinical remission. Fourteen studies have employed standardized assessments of social functioning, although in three the methods lacked adequate scientific rigour, and one proved too complex to include [37]. Six of the ten remaining studies showed significantly greater benefits for stress management strategies [22,24,25,34,35,38], one a clear trend [30] and three showed no significant benefits when compared with drug treatment and case management [19,26,27]. Thus, despite the difficulties of measuring gains on inventories that include a broad range of areas of social functioning, many of which are not personally relevant to every patient, advantages for the family-based approaches are evident [15].

Family Benefits

An important goal of family interventions is to enhance family functioning and to reduce stresses, particularly those associated with caring for the patient. A mean reduction in the stress of caregiving of 40% was reported in five studies that examined this outcome [22,28,30,34,35]. This was contrasted with a reduction of 12% in the drugs and case management conditions. Six of the eight studies that compared family stress management with case management showed significant advantages for the stress management approach [22,24,25,31,34,35]. The self-help multiple-family group approach of Buchkremer et al. [27] showed no change in a measure of family problems associated with the patient's illness, but was associated with increased warmth and reduced hostility towards the patient.

Measures of family stress varied across all studies. This makes direct comparisons difficult. In addition, stress associated with the patient's mental disorder is difficult to distinguish from other stress that caregivers may be experiencing. Family systems theorists have constantly pointed out the phenomenon of scapegoating, whereby a person seeks out one major stress factor and attributes all his or her stress as deriving from that person or issue. An epidemiological study of all long-term care cases in one location indicated that, even when all forms of evidence-based treatment were provided, including continued home-based family cognitive–behavioural strategies, key carers still experienced half the stress in their lives associated with the patient and his mental disorder [39]. This field is likely to benefit considerably from refinement of measures of family stress and burden. It is also worth noting again that most of these methods do not seek to minimize stress levels, but rather to enable people to cope more efficiently with all sources of stress as they progress towards their personal life goals.

Economic Benefits

Improvements in clinical, social and family functioning would be expected to reduce the need for intensive medical and social care and thereby produce economic benefits for service providers. Six studies have reported such benefits, albeit in relatively unsophisticated assessments of costs [22, 25,28,40–42]. It is important to note that no study showed that the addition of family approaches costs more to the services. In most instances the cost savings to the services of integrating family assistance in this way are substantial. Further, the additional cost to the family was usually minimal, particularly as most treatment sessions can be arranged flexibly to minimize loss of earnings or the cost of transport. It seems evident that overall costs to services of family approaches, even those provided in patients' homes, are an excellent investment when they halve the number of major episodes that require intensive care. However, most savings that arise from such interventions are related to less use of crisis services and hospital care. These savings are not always readily transferred to the community-based services, at least not until hospital units can be closed, so that the financial benefits may be more theoretical than practical.

Enduring Benefits

The duration over which stress management strategies were applied varied from 6 months to 4 years, with most providing this treatment for 9–12 months. It was apparent that benefits endured, and trends towards clinical and social recovery continued, when the treatment approach was continued without major modifications throughout the study period [22,30,31,34,36,41, 43]. When treatment ceased at the end of the study period, it was noted that the stress of impending termination of a successful treatment programme may contribute to an excess of episodes at this period [37].

Withdrawal of intensive training in stress management was not usually associated with an immediate cessation of apparent clinical benefits. All 4 studies that followed up cases for at least 4 years have shown long-term evidence of clinical benefits [43–46]. One study of a multi-family problem-solving approach that was continued for 4 years showed a rehospitalization rate four times lower than treatment as usual [43]. However, the methodology of these long-term follow-up studies is less than optimal and it is clear that for individual cases the benefits tend to diminish once active treatment is stopped. As with all major health problems, comprehensive treatment needs to be continued until all residual impairments, disabilities and handicaps have been resolved, and then followed by monitoring of early signs of recurrences and the provision of booster treatment when this is indicated. Studies of long-term optimal programmes of this nature are essential [47].

Comparative Benefits of Stress Management Approaches

Whereas it is clear that brief mental health education has limited overall benefits, it is not clear which combination of ingredients, or setting of comprehensive treatment, is most effective and efficient. The effect sizes of clinical benefits of the key combinations of interventions suggest that long-term educational or systemic approaches may be less efficacious than those using problem solving and cognitive–behavioural methods [48]. Although a carer-based approach has been strongly advocated, there is also strong support for long-term individual approaches that use similar stress management methods. In one study that compared individual and family-based approaches, 38% of patients receiving family treatment had a major episode of psychosis, affective disorder, or had withdrawn from treatment by 24 months, compared to 28% of those allocated to supportive case management, and only 13% of those receiving intensive individual stress management training [49,50]. These advantages continued to the end of the third year. The improvement in clinical scales of residual symptoms were greatest with the family approach, but social functioning benefits were mainly in the first year, whereas those of the intensive individual approach continued to increase throughout the 3 years. In this study, patients expressed low satisfaction with the family treatment, and were highly satisfied with the individual approach, which had 73% more sessions (2.4 per month over the 36 months versus 1.4). Unlike their earlier studies, Hogarty's Pittsburgh group did not find any significant added benefits after 24 months of combined family and individual strategies. Similar conclusions have been drawn by other reviewers [53]. Of course, not all adult patients live together with, or in close contact with, their families. For this reason it may be important to extend research to non-family carers, such as close friends or housemates in residential settings, where the same stress management principles and treatment strategies may be expected to have similar validity.

A study of a cohort of patients who were receiving assertive community treatment found that the addition of crisis family treatment could prevent major episodes as effectively as continuous multi-family treatment, but it was less successful in achieving social benefits, particularly in the field of employment [30].

In common with most psychotherapy and pharmacotherapy research, a major deficit in this body of research has been the limited ability to measure emotional, cognitive and behavioural changes in families that consistently predict patient outcomes. Several studies have employed the expressed emotion (EE) index as a measure of positive change in the family atmosphere [20,52–54]. Others have used direct observation of family problem solving [22,28,55,56]. At best, the association between clinical and social outcome and these measures of change in the family patterns of interaction has been modest. All are complex measures that lack the precision needed to use them as criteria for family educational programmes. In the absence of a highly predictive criterion for therapists to aim at, the next best thing is to ensure that they follow the treatment manuals closely. However, the few studies that have employed such process measures have also failed to impress [22,57]. However, the vulnerability stress theory posits a multifactorial biological and psychosocial interaction, and measures of only one facet, stress management of key caregivers, or even of the broader social support system, are unlikely to capture the majority of the variance associated with the course of major mental disorders. Although it is clear that these approaches make a major difference, the precise mechanisms remain largely unknown, but offer the prospect of an exciting innovative field of biosocial research.

Single-Family versus Multi-Family Groups

A series of eight studies that compared stress management conducted predominantly in multi-family groups with that conducted mainly in single-family sessions showed a mean advantage of only 2% greater clinical success for the single-family approach in the first year of treatment [19,30, 33,41,43,58–60]. Two further studies have compared a multiple family group with a medication and case management control. The first study of self-help relatives' groups did not involve the patients and showed a higher rate of hospital admissions than the control condition [27], while the second showed reduction in service use, including hospital admissions, associated with multi-family treatment [61]. McFarlane *et al.* [41] have shown that there may be advantages for the multi-family approach when it is used as a long-term maintenance strategy, but this important work has not yet been replicated fully, although two other studies that used multi-family approaches in the second year of the programmes showed excellent maintenance of clinical benefits [22,60]. The complex methodology of the comparative studies prevents any clear conclusions about the relative merits of these approaches, particularly when the strategies used have been different in quality as well as intensity in the single- and multiple-family settings. Although multi-family strategies may appear more cost-effective, it is important that all costs are considered, not merely the time spent conducting the treatment sessions, before concluding that this strategy should be the method of choice for services, where cost is an over-riding concern. It is unlikely that any one training format will meet the needs of all cases, and a comprehensive service will include single-family and multi-family approaches.

Integration with Social and Work Skills Training Strategies

The addition of skills training strategies to assist patients to cope more effectively with stresses in community settings outside the family ambit appears to add benefits to methods that focus on stress within the patient's family. Five studies that combined social skills training strategies with carer-based stress management have shown the best one-year clinical outcomes to date [20,22,24,53,62]. Only 19% of patients receiving this integrated approach had poor outcomes during the first year of treatment. The precise manner in which these strategies are integrated has not been studied. In some programmes the social and work skills training has been an integral part of the family problem solving sessions, in others the two approaches are conducted in separate sessions. It is evident that the benefits of conducting social skills training for schizophrenia without the collaborative support of key caregivers appear rather limited [63].

Integration with Other Cognitive–Behavioural Strategies for Residual Symptoms

Cognitive–behavioural strategies have proven beneficial for resolving residual psychotic, deficit, affective and anxiety symptoms, all of which are common in functional psychotic disorders [20,22]. These strategies have been demonstrated as highly efficacious when studied in non-schizophrenic populations [64]. To date there have been no controlled studies that have compared family programmes that include such strategies with those that use only generic problem solving methods. One study that employed a wide range of cognitive–behavioural strategies showed an improvement in the rates of affective and anxiety episodes in the second year of treatment and a substantial proportion of cases in remission from all psychiatric symptoms [22].

Does Family-Based Stress Management Reduce the Level of Medication Needed to Prevent Recurrences?

Most attempts to lower dosages of antipsychotic drugs well below those deemed clinically optimal have done this in a double-blind manner, and have not used the graduated withdrawal methods considered pharmaco-logically safe. It is, therefore, not surprising that they have proven relatively unsuccessful. Despite this, a study by Hahlweg *et al.* [28] showed a rela-tively low rate of major episodes with a targeted dose strategy throughout the period that regular family stress management sessions were conducted. The National Institute of Mental Health (NIMH) Treatment Strategies study partially replicated this finding, suggesting that family-based strategies with early detection of potential exacerbations may enable lower doses of medication to be used without increasing the risk of major episodes [60]. Although the results of this study have been portrayed as demonstrating that adding family interventions to optimal drug treatment has no benefits, it should be noted that the two-year rehospitalization rate of 19% for cases receiving standard medication doses plus the cognitive–behavioural family approach for the first year is the second lowest reported in the literature. However, the 31% rate for the continuous educational multi-family educational approach was not statistically different. Further sophisticated studies of the synergistic effects of biomedical and psychosocial strategies may help in the refinement of these strategies, including the as yet unresolved issue of how and when to withdraw medication once stable recovery has been achieved.

Family Interventions and Early Intervention

It has been suggested that family stress management strategies are not effective for patients in their first episode of schizophrenia [65]. This conclusion appears to have been based on a single study where all cases received a basic course in family stress management during their hospital admission for an initial psychotic episode [66]. At discharge, patients were randomly assigned to continued family intervention or to individual case management. In the following 12 months, 16% of patients receiving the continued family intervention had major episodes compared to 15% of those who received individual case management. The remarkable feature here was the effectiveness of the individual approach as a maintenance strategy following the brief family stress management. A more clearly controlled study that compared similar family and individual approaches over 24 months of continued treatment showed consistent benefits for the family intervention [32]. The better prognosis for first-episode cases and low numbers reduced statistical significance. However, most studies have found that first-episode cases have shown the greatest benefits from the family methods [67]. The optimal treatment for early cases of schizophrenia has not yet been established and requires further well-controlled research. It is likely that a proportion will show maximum benefits from simpler education programmes [35], but others will need more extensive work to achieve and sustain full recovery. In the absence of the ability to predict outcomes of individual cases, it would not seem wise to eliminate the use of those family interventions that have proven efficacy in reducing clinical and social morbidity [45].

FAMILY INTERVENTIONS FOR BIPOLAR DISORDER

The educational and stress management strategies that have been developed for schizophrenia have been applied more recently to bipolar disorder. The main difference is that most bipolar subjects are married, so that the key caregivers are usually spouses.

Educational Approaches

A series of studies has examined the benefits from educational strategies aimed to improve the understanding of patients and their key caregivers about vulnerability and stress factors, the recognition of early signs of recurrences, and the benefits of treatment, albeit mainly pharmacotherapy [68–72]. The results of these strategies show improved acceptance of medication prophylaxis and some reduction in morbidity, particularly when they extended beyond a few simple didactic sessions to include concepts of stress management and detection of early signs of impending major episodes. However, the methodology and heterogeneity of these studies make it difficult to draw any firm conclusions.

Family-Based Stress Management

The results of the published studies of family-based stress management approaches for bipolar disorder have been mixed [73]. Clarkin et al. [74] found no reductions in major episodes after 9 sessions of education and communication training with couples, whereas Miklowitz and Goldstein [75], Miklowitz et al. [76] and Rea et al. [77] found reductions in major episodes after 24 months of a 9–12 month approach that focused on stress management through structured problem solving training. It is evident that the complexity of bipolar disorder, especially in terms of the two contrasting types of episodes, necessitates extensive education before patients and families can understand the disorder and its biomedical and psychosocial aspects. This would seem to suggest that longer and more intensive interventions may be necessary for lasting benefits even for first-episode cases [78]. A major pragmatic study is underway to examine this issue in a large cohort [79].

FAMILY INTERVENTIONS FOR DEPRESSIVE DISORDERS

Despite substantial evidence for the association between family and marital factors and the onset and course of major depressive disorders [80], most psychosocial strategies have focused on stress and vulnerability from the individual perspective. There is limited evidence that family or marital strategies achieve somewhat greater benefits than the individual cognitive–behavioural or interpersonal approaches, particularly where marital conflict is an ongoing major stressor [82–89].

Preliminary studies of family interventions for adolescent depression have also shown potential benefits [90,91].

Lack of supportive relationships has been implicated in the aetiology and course of depressive disorders in women. Recent efforts to remedy this have shown promise in preventing post-natal depression [92] and in chronic depression [93]. The latter study focused on developing close friendships as an alternative to family or marital support. This wider social perspective of close relationships may be a more fruitful way of conceptualizing family interventions, particularly in societies where stable families relationships are relatively uncommon, with divorce and relocation interfering with traditional interpersonal support systems.

Early intervention using a carer-based approach when depressive symptoms first emerge may prove highly efficacious in preventing major affective episodes, associated social morbidity and potential suicide risk [94]. While offering considerable promise, the family interventions in depression are highly variable in treatment goals and strategies, and few high-quality studies have been conducted. Further carefully controlled studies are essential to enable carer-based approaches to be targeted with greater precision to the specific problems associated with major affective disorders.

EFFECTIVENESS OF FAMILY APPROACHES IN ROUTINE CLINICAL PRACTICE

One major concern is the ability to replicate the benefits of controlled trials in routine clinical practice. In this field there has been a tendency to dilute the methods, using merely part of the intervention programmes, often only the mental health education component. As would be predicted, these studies have limited benefits, mainly improved adherence to medication [6]. However, substantial clinical and social benefits are generally less than those associated with more comprehensive programmes applied over longer periods.

However, a series of comprehensive field trials have been completed, with almost all reporting successful replication of the controlled trial results [35,37,95–100]. One exception to this was an Australian study that attempted to train mental health professionals, mainly social workers, to use both cognitive–behavioural family interventions as well as more complex cognitive methods [101]. There have been few efforts to measure the competence of therapists in these approaches, so that it has not been clear what specific skills professionals need to acquire before they can achieve optimal results [102]. Despite a consensus that few mental health services are organized in a way that facilitates working with families, it is not clear what alternative management structures are needed. Clarification of these issues should be based on sound research, rather than speculation.

CONCLUSIONS

It can be concluded that there is substantial high-quality research evidence to suggest that strategies that enhance the competence of the informal care units (usually consisting of partners, parents or close friends) in the day-to-day care for people with major mental disorders have a clinically significant impact on the course of these disorders. This evidence is strongest for schizophrenia and bipolar disorder. The greatest benefits appear to be in the long-term prevention of major recurrences associated with comprehensive methods that integrate carers into the therapeutic team through education and training in stress management strategies. Continued professional support and supervision of the programmes are associated with a fall-off in gains, albeit not as rapid as one might expect. Unfortunately, many studies have focused on relapse and rehospitalization as end points. This has led to the conclusion that family interventions merely delay recurrent episodes rather than prevent them. However, there is reason to believe that those strategies that have proven effective in delaying one episode may prove even more effective in delaying the next when they are refined with continued experience and training. We do not abandon pharmacotherapy at the first recurrence of a disorder, nor should we abandon family stress management. All evidence-based interventions are far from perfect, and refinement is constantly needed. The multi-family group setting has shown promise as a maintenance strategy, but replications are required, and it is unlikely that any one format will fit all cases. However, the education, communication and problem-solving strategies are highly flexible and can be readily adapted to a variety of settings, including poorly resourced services in developing countries. Further studies need to explore methods of maintaining and extending benefits over much longer periods than the current body of research has examined to date [47].

Comorbidity of psychosis with substance abuse, depression and anxiety is an unresolved issue of considerable importance. Promising early studies suggest that integrating specific cognitive–behavioural strategies for these problems with family interventions may prove effective, but high-quality replications are urgently needed. The cognitive–behavioural family approach facilitates this integration, and recently a series of educational guidebooks have been produced for both professionals and consumers that incorporate all the evidence-based cognitive–behavioural strategies within the family problem-solving framework [103].

Although straightforward education about mental disorders and their biomedical and psychosocial treatment is a valuable component of all evidence-based family approaches, and appears to improve adherence to treatment programmes, when applied alone it does not seem sufficient to reduce the risk of major episodes or of continuing clinical or social morbidity. Services should be encouraged to view brief psychoeducational programmes as no more than an initial phase in the development of more substantive programmes that are clearly highly cost-effective, but require an initial investment of slightly greater professional time and skill. Despite many suggestions that brief education alone may have maximal benefits for patients living in supportive, low-stress households, controlled studies need to demonstrate this. Unfortunately, the ability to assess household stress usually requires extensive and highly skilled assessment using the EE index. This assessment adds considerably to the cost of the intervention programme. Clinical assessments used in both cognitive–behavioural and systemic family and couple therapies may be able to determine more accurately the strengths and weaknesses of patients' personal support networks and target the specific education and problem-solving skills that may be enhanced by different strategies over different time periods, including the various phases of each patient's disorder. In the absence of research to guide us in the choice of strategies, it may be important to resist the push to consumer choice, especially if the consumer is ill-informed and emotionally involved in the stress of caring for a disabled loved one. However, the views of consumers, especially those who are well informed, are of enormous value, and indeed were one of the major factors in the initial and continuing development of this field [8].

In addition to the benefits in terms of improved prognosis, there is growing evidence that social morbidity is reduced, particularly when treatment continues for at least two years and integrates personal goal setting and aspects of social and work skills training. Benefits from these approaches are also evident for the carers themselves, with reduced stress associated with their caregiving roles. However, even with these family programmes, the stress associated with continued family care of chronic cases remains considerable [39]. Family care is an incredibly valuable therapeutic resource, but it should not be expected that all families will be able to provide long-term management for disabled patients. Efforts to develop similar therapeutic programmes in a variety of non-familial residential services must be given a high priority. However, care should be taken to involve families in the continued treatment programmes even when patients no longer reside in the family home. It is a foolish mistake to think that, once a relative is no longer living in the family household, the family have no further stress associated with that person's mental disorder and treatment. Of course, the stress factors may change, but are seldom eliminated [104].

Despite the clear evidence of efficacy and efficiency, relatively few services have incorporated these carer-based strategies into their routine practice [105]. This problem is shared with most non-commercial advances in clinical practice. In addition to adequate training in educational and psychological strategies, assertive management of services is needed to ensure that the efforts of key caregivers of all patients are fully integrated into clinical programmes at all times. Of course these caregivers are not always relatives. However, almost all patients have somebody who cares for them, or at least somebody who cares about them. These people may be friends, neighbours, work colleagues, or even hairdressers, barmen, fitness instructors or shop assistants. Although the caring bonds between family members are often lifelong, patients who do not enjoy continued care from their close relatives may be able to identify alternative caregivers, who may be available and willing to assist with these education-based programmes. In countries where relatively few adults live with relatives, such as Sweden, the term "resource group" has been used to describe a patient's interpersonal support group, which includes not only any caring relatives, but also friends and associates who provide a similar day-to-day problem solving resource [106]. There is no reason to believe that the stress management approaches that have proven so useful for family units should not show similar benefits with non-family resource groups. Further research with these groups is needed.

A final caveat: it must be pointed out that the controlled research studies of family approaches have shown consistent clinical, social, family and economic benefits when compared to pharmacotherapy and case management alone. But few studies have compared them with well-matched individual or group educational or cognitive–behavioural methods. The few studies that have done so, have produced contrasting results [51]. More well-controlled comparisons of family and non-family interventions are likely to enhance our understanding of the processes that lead to long-term recovery from major mental disorders.

The highly consistent positive results of family interventions have led many observers to suggest that further research is not needed. While it is undoubtedly true that further high-quality replications are not required, this chapter underscores the numerous deficiencies in our understanding, which have stalled progress towards the refinement of these strategies, that are a vital ingredient for improved quality of mental health care.

REFERENCES

1. Leff J., Vaughn C. (1985) *Expressed Emotion in Families*. Guilford Press, New York.
2. Vaughn C., Leff J. (1976) The measurement of expressed emotion in the families of psychiatric patients. *Br. J. Soc. Clin. Psychol.*, **15**, 157–165.
3. Miklowitz D.J., Goldstein M.J., Nuechterlein K.H., Snyder K.S., Mintz J. (1988) Family factors and the course of bipolar affective disorder. *Arch. Gen. Psychiatry*, **45**, 225–231.
4. Lam D.H. (1991) Psychosocial family intervention in schizophrenia: a review of empirical studies. *Psychol. Med.*, **21**, 423–441.
5. Falloon I.R.H., Roncone R., Held T., Coverdale J.H., Laidlaw T.M. (2001) An international overview of family interventions: developing effective treatment strategies and measuring their benefits to patients, carers, and communities. In: Lefley H.P., Johnson D.L. (eds) *Family Interventions in Mental Illness: International Perspectives*. Greenwood, Westport, CT, pp. 3–23.
6. Pekkala E., Merinder L. (2001) Psychoeducation for schizophrenia (Cochrane Review). In: *The Cochrane Library*, Issue 3. Update Software, Oxford.
7. Pharoah F.M., Mari J.J., Streiner D. (2000) Family intervention for schizophrenia. *Psychiatry Res.*, **30**, 141–148.
8. Solomon P. (1996) Moving from psychoeducation to family education for families of adults with serious mental illness. *Psychiatr. Serv.*, **47**, 1364–1370.
9. Atkinson J.M., Coia D.A., Gilmour W.H., Harper J.P. (1996) The impact of education groups for people with schizophrenia on social functioning and quality of life. *Br. J. Psychiatry*, **168**, 199–204.
10. Birchwood M., Smith J., Cochrane R. (1992) Specific and non-specific effects of educational intervention for families living with schizophrenia: a comparison of three methods. *Br. J. Psychiatry*, **160**, 806–814.
11. Merinder L.B., Viuff A.G., Laugesen H.D., Clemmensen K., Misflet S., Espensen B. (1999) Patient and relative education in community psychiatry: a randomised controlled trial regarding its effectiveness. *Soc. Psychiatry Psychiatr. Epidemiol.*, **34**, 287–294.
12. Solomon P., Draine J., Mannion E. (1996) The impact of individualized consultation and group workshop family education interventions in ill relative outcomes. *J. Nerv. Ment. Dis.*, **184**, 252–255.
13. Szmukler G.I., Herrman H., Colusa S., Benson A., Bloch S. (1996) A controlled trial of a counselling intervention for relatives with schizophrenia. *Soc. Psychiatry Psychiatr. Epidemiol.*, **31**, 149–155.

14. Huxley N.A., Rendall M., Sederer L. (2000) Psychosocial treatments in schizophrenia: a review of the past 20 years. *J. Nerv. Ment. Dis.*, **88**, 187–201.

15. Pilling S., Bebbington P., Kuipers E., Garety P., Geddes J., Orbach G., Morgan C. (2002) Psychological treatments in schizophrenia: I. Meta-analysis of family intervention and cognitive behaviour therapy. *Psychol. Med.*, **32**, 763–782.

16. Falloon I.R.H. (2003) Family interventions in mental disorders: efficacy and effectiveness. *World Psychiatry*, **2**, 20–28.

17. Falloon I.R.H., Boyd J.L., McGill C.W. (1984) *Family Care of Schizophrenia: A Problem-Solving Approach to the Treatment of Mental Illness.* Guilford Press, New York.

18. Anderson C.M., Reiss D.J., Hogarty G.E. (1986) *Schizophrenia and the Family.* Guilford Press, New York.

19. Hornung W.P., Holle R., Schultze-Mönking H., Klingberg S., Buchkremer G. (1995) Psychoedukativ-psychotherapeutische Behandlung von schizophrenen Patienten und ihren Bezugspersonen. Ergebnisse einer 1-jahres-Katamnese. *Nervenartz*, **66**, 828–834.

20. Tarrier N., Barrowclough C., Vaughn C., Bamrah J.S., Porceddu K., Watts S., Freeman H. (1988) The community management of schizophrenia: a controlled trial of a behavioural intervention with families to reduce relapse. *Br. J. Psychiatry*, **153**, 532–542.

21. Shepherd M., Watt D., Falloon I., Smeeton N. (1989) *The Natural History of Schizophrenia*, Psychological Medicine Monograph no. 16. Cambridge University Press, Cambridge.

22. Falloon I.R.H., Associates (1985) *Family Management of Schizophrenia: A Study of Clinical, Social, Family, and Economic Benefits.* Johns Hopkins University Press, Baltimore, MD.

23. Zastowny T.R., Lehman A.F., Cole R.E., Kane C. (1992) Family management of schizophrenia: a comparison of behavioral and supportive family treatment. *Psychiatr. Q.*, **63**, 159–186.

24. Veltro F., Magliano L., Falloon I.R.H., Morosini P.L., Capocascale F., Fasulo E., Russo M.C. (1996) Behavioural family therapy for patients with schizophrenia: a randomised controlled trial. Presented at the Congress of the World Association for Psychosocial Rehabilitation, Rotterdam, 21–24 April.

25. Xiong W., Phillips M.R., Hu X., Wang R., Dai Q., Kleinman J., Kleinman A. (1994) Family-based intervention for schizophrenic patients in China. A randomised controlled trial. *Br. J. Psychiatry*, **165**, 239–247.

26. Randolph E.T., Eth S., Glynn S.M., Paz G.G., Leong G.B., Shaner A.L., Strachan A., Van Wort W., Escobar J.I., Liberman R.P. (1994) Behavioural family management in schizophrenia: outcome of a clinic-based intervention. *Br. J. Psychiatry*, **164**, 501–506.

27. Buchkremer G., Schultze-Mönking H., Holle R., Hornung W.P. (1995) The impact of therapeutic relatives' groups on the course of illness of schizophrenic patients. *Eur. Psychiatry*, **10**, 17–27.

28. Hahlweg K., Durr H., Müller U. (1995) *Familienbetreuung schizophrener Patienten.* Psychologie Verlags Union, Weinheim.

29. Telles C., Karno M., Mintz J., Paz G., Arias M., Tucker D., Lopez S. (1995) Immigrant families coping with schizophrenia. Behavioral family intervention v. case management with a low-income Spanish-speaking population. *Br. J. Psychiatry*, **167**, 473–479.

30. McFarlane W.R., Dushay R.A., Stastny P., Deakins S.M., Link B. (1996) A comparison of two levels of family-aided assertive community treatment. *Psychiatr. Serv.*, **47**, 744–750.

31. Zhang M., He Y., Gittelman M., Wong Z., Yan H. (1998) Group psychoeducation of relatives of schizophrenic patients: two-year experiences. *Psychiatry Clin. Neurosci.*, **52**(Suppl. 3), 44–47.

32. Grawe R.W., Widen J.H., Falloon I.R.H. (2002) Early intervention for schizophrenic disorders: implementing optimal treatment strategies in clinical services. In: Kashima H., Falloon I.R.H., Mizuno M., Asai M. (eds) *Comprehensive Treatment of Schizophrenia*. Springer-Verlag, Tokyo, pp. 290–297.

33. Montero I., Asencio A., Hernandez I., Masanet M.J., Lacruz M., Bellver F., Iborra M., Ruiz I. (2001) Two strategies for family intervention in schizophrenia: a randomised trial in a Mediterranean environment. *Schizophr. Bull.*, **27**, 661–670.

34. Sungur M.Z., Guner P., Ustun B., Cetin I., Soygur H. (2003) Optimal treatment project for schizophrenia: results from a randomized, controlled, longitudinal study. *Seishin Shinkeigaku Zasshi*, **105**, 1175–1180.

35. Zhang M., Yan H., co-authors (1993) Effectiveness of psychoeducation of schizophrenic patients: a prospective cohort study in five cities of China. *Int. J. Ment. Health*, **22**, 47–59.

36. Dyck D.G., Short R.A., Hendryx M.S., Norell D., Myers M., Patterson T., McDonell M.G., Voss W.D., McFarlane W.R. (2000) Management of negative symptoms among patients with schizophrenia attending multiple-family groups. *Psychiatr. Serv.*, **51**, 513–519.

37. Hogarty G.E., Anderson C.M., Reiss D.J., Kornblith S.J., Greenwald D.P., Ulrich R.F., Carter M. (1991) Family psychoeducation, social skills training, and maintenance chemotherapy in the aftercare of schizophrenia. II. Two-year effects of a controlled study on relapse and adjustment. *Arch. Gen. Psychiatry*, **48**, 340–347.

38. Barrowclough C., Tarrier N., Lewis S., Sellwood W., Mainwaring J., Quinn J., Hamlin C. (1999) Randomised controlled effectiveness trial of a needs-based psychosocial intervention service for carers of people with schizophrenia. *Br. J. Psychiatry*, **174**, 505–511.

39. Falloon I.R.H., Magliano L., Graham-Hole V., Woodroffe R.W. (1996) The stress of caring for disabled patients in a community rehabilitation service. *J. Nerv. Ment. Dis.*, **184**, 381–384.

40. Held T. (1995) *Schizophreniebehandlung in der Familie*. Lang, Frankfurt am Main.

41. McFarlane W.R., Link B., Dushay R., Marchal J., Crilly J. (1995) Psychoeducational multiple family groups: four-year relapse outcome in schizophrenia. *Fam. Process*, **34**, 127–144.

42. Tarrier N., Lowson K., Barrowclough C. (1991) Some aspects of family interventions in schizophrenia. II: Financial considerations. *Br. J. Psychiatry*, **159**, 481–484.

43. McFarlane W.R., Lukens E., Link B., Dushay R., Deakins S.A., Newmark M., Dunne E.J., Horen B., Toran J. (1995) Multiple-family groups and psychoeducation in the treatment of schizophrenia. *Arch. Gen. Psychiatry*, **52**, 679–687.

44. Hornung W.P., Feldman R., Klingberg S., Buchkremer G., Reker T. (1999) Long-term effects of a psychoeducational psychotherapeutic intervention for schizophrenic outpatients and their key-persons—results of a five-year follow-up. *Eur. Arch. Psychiatry Clin. Neurosci.*, **249**, 162–167.

45. Linszen D., Dingemans P., Lenior M. (2001) Early intervention and a five-year follow up in young adults with a short duration of untreated psychosis: ethical implications. *Schizophr. Res.*, **51**, 55–61.

46. Tarrier N., Barrowclough C., Porceddu K., Fitzpatrick E. (1994) The Salford family intervention project: relapse rates of schizophrenia at five and eight years. *Br. J. Psychiatry*, **165**, 829–832.

47. Falloon I.R.H., the Optimal Treatment Project Collaborators (1999) Optimal treatment for psychosis in an International Multisite Demonstration Project. *Psychiatr. Serv.*, **50**, 615–618.

48. Held T., Falloon I.R.H. (1999) Family therapy of schizophrenia. *Keio J. Med.*, **48**, 151–154.

49. Hogarty G.E., Kornblith S.J., Greenwald D., DiBarry A.L., Cooley S., Ulrich R.F., Carter M., Flesher S. (1997) Three-year trials of personal therapy among schizophrenic patients living with or independent of family, I: Description of study and effects on relapse rates. *Am. J. Psychiatry*, **154**, 1504–1513.

50. Hogarty G.E., Greenwald D., Ulrich R.F., Kornblith S.J., DiBarry A.L., Cooley S., Carter M., Flesher S. (1997) Three-year trials of personal therapy among schizophrenic patients living with or independent of family, II: Effects on adjustment of patients. *Am. J. Psychiatry*, **154**, 1514–1524.

51. Pitschel-Walz G., Leucht S., Bauml J., Kissling W., Engel R.R. (2001) The effect of family interventions on relapse and rehospitalization in schizophrenia—a meta-analysis. *Schizophr. Bull.*, **27**, 73–92.

52. Leff J., Kuipers L., Berkowitz R., Eberlein-Fries R., Sturgeon D. (1982) A controlled trial of social intervention in the families of schizophrenic patients. *Br. J. Psychiatry*, **141**, 121–134.

53. Hogarty G.E., Anderson C.M., Reiss D.J., Kornblith S.J., Greenwald D.P., Javna C.D., Madonia M.J. (1986) Family psycho-education, social skills training and maintenance chemotherapy in the aftercare treatment of schizophrenia. *Arch. Gen. Psychiatry*, **43**, 633–642.

54. Linszen D.H., Dingemans P.M., Nugter M.A., Van der Does A.J., Scholte W.F., Lenior M.A. (1997) Patient attributes and expressed emotion as risk factors for psychotic relapse. *Schizophr. Bull.*, **23**, 119–130.

55. Bellack A.S., Haas G.L., Schooler N.R., Flory J.D. (2000) Effects of behavioural family management on family communication and patient outcomes in schizophrenia. *Br. J. Psychiatry*, **177**, 434–439.

56. Simoneau T.L., Miklowitz D.J., Richards J.A., Saleem R., George E.L. (1999) Bipolar disorder and family communication: effects of a psychoeducational treatment program. *J. Abnorm. Psychol.*, **108**, 588–597.

57. Weisman A., Tompson M.C., Okazaki S., Gregory J., Goldstein M.J., Rea M., Miklowitz D.J. (2002) Clinicians' fidelity to a manual-based family treatment as a predictor of the one-year course of bipolar disorder. *Fam. Process*, **41**, 123–131.

58. Leff J., Berkowitz R., Shavit N., Strachan A.S., Glass I., Vaughn C. (1989) A trial of family therapy v. a relatives group for schizophrenia. *Br. J. Psychiatry*, **154**, 58–66.

59. Roncone R., Morosini P.L., Falloon I.R.H., Casacchia M. (2002) Family interventions in schizophrenia in Italian mental health services. In: Kashima H., Falloon I.R.H., Mizuno M., Asai M. (eds) *Comprehensive Treatment of Schizophrenia*. Springer-Verlag, Tokyo, pp. 284–289.

60. Schooler N.R., Keith S.J., Severe J.B., Matthews S.M., Bellack A.S., Glick I.D., Hargreaves W.A., Kane J.M., Ninan P.T., Frances A., *et al.* (1997) Relapse and

rehospitalisation during maintenance treatment of schizophrenia. *Arch. Gen. Psychiatry*, **54**, 453–463.

61. Dyck D.G., Hendryx M.S., Short R.A., Voss W.D., McFarlane W.R. (2002) Service use among patients with schizophrenia in psychoeducational multiple-family group treatment. *Psychiatr. Serv.*, **53**, 749–754.

62. Wallace C.J., Liberman R.P. (1985) Social skills training for patients with schizophrenia: a controlled clinical trial. *Psychiatry Res.*, **15**, 239–247.

63. Pilling S., Bebbington P., Kuipers E., Garety P., Geddes J., Martindale B., Orbach G., Morgan C. (2002) Psychological treatments in schizophrenia: II. Meta-analyses of randomised controlled trials of social skills training and cognitive remediation. *Psychol. Med.*, **32**, 783–791.

64. Andrews G. (1996) Talk that works: the rise of cognitive behaviour therapy. *Br. Med. J.*, **313**, 1501–1502.

65. Birchwood M., McGorry P., Jackson H. (1997) Early intervention in schizophrenia. *Br. J. Psychiatry*, **170**, 2–5.

66. Linszen D., Dingemans P., Van der Does J.W., Nugter A., Scholte P., Lenior R., Goldstein M.J. (1996) Treatment, expressed emotion and relapse in recent onset schizophrenic disorders. *Psychol. Med.*, **26**, 333–342.

67. Falloon I.R.H., Monterno I., Sungur M., Mastroeni A., Malm U., Economou M., Grawe R., Harangozo J., Mizuno M., Murakami M., *et al.* (2004) Implementation of evidence-based treatment for schizophrenic disorders: two-year outcome of an international field trial of optimal treatment. *World Psychiatry*, **3**, 104–109.

68. Van Gent E.M., Zwart F.M. (1991) Psychoeducation of bipolar-manic patients. *J. Affect. Disord.*, **21**, 15–18.

69. Clarkin J.F., Glick I.D., Haas G.L., Spencer J.H., Lewis A.B., Peyser J., DeMane N., Good-Ellis M., Harris E., Lestelle V. (1990) A randomized clinical trial of inpatient family intervention: V. Results for affective disorders. *J. Affect. Disord.*, **18**, 17–28.

70. Glick I.D., Burti L., Okonogi K., Sacks M. (1994) Effectiveness in psychiatric care. III: Psychoeducation and outcome for patients with major affective disorder and their families. *Br. J. Psychiatry*, **164**, 104–106.

71. Honig A., Hofman A., Rozendaal N., Dingemans P. (1997) Psychoeducation in bipolar disorder: effect on expressed emotion. *Psychiatry Res.*, **72**, 17–22.

72. Wang X., Wang F., Ma A., Guan L., Fu W., Liu X., Sun S., Li J. (2000) A controlled study of family education for bipolar disorders. *Chinese Ment. Health J.*, **14**, 399–401.

73. Huxley N.A., Parikh S.V., Baldessarini R.J. (2002) Effectiveness of psychosocial treatments in bipolar disorder: state of the evidence. *Harvard Rev. Psychiatry*, **8**, 126–140.

74. Clarkin J.F., Carpenter D., Hull J., Wilner P., Glick I. (1998) Effects of psycho-educational intervention for married patients with bipolar disorder and their spouses. *Psychiatr. Serv.*, **49**, 531–533.

75. Miklowitz D.J., Goldstein M.J. (1990) Behavioral family treatment for patients with bipolar affective disorder. *Behav. Modif.*, **14**, 457–489.

76. Miklowitz D.J., Richards J.A., George E.L., Frank E., Suddath R.L., Powell K.B., Sacher J.A. (2003) Integrated family and individual therapy for bipolar disorder: results of a treatment development study. *J. Clin. Psychiatry*, **64**, 182–191.

77. Rea M.M., Tompson M.C., Miklowitz D.J., Goldstein M.J., Hwang S., Mintz J. (2003) Family-focused treatment versus individual treatment for bipolar

disorder: results of a randomized clinical trial. *J. Consult. Clin. Psychol.*, **71**, 482–492.

78. Falloon I.R.H., Pellegrini E., Mastroeni A., Galetti F., Roncone R., Casacchia M. (2002) Integrated biomedical and psychosocial treatment for bipolar disorder: a review. *Psychiatr. Networks*, **5**, 8–27.

79. Sachs G.S., Thase M.E., Otto M.W., Bauer M., Miklowitz D., Wisniewski S.R., Lavori P., Lebowitz B., Rudorfer M., Frank E., *et al.* (2003) Rationale, design, and methods of the systematic treatment enhancement program for bipolar disorder (STEP-BD). *Biol. Psychiatry*, **53**, 1028–1042.

80. Keitner G.I., Miller I.W. (1990) Family functioning and major depression: an overview. *Am. J. Psychiatry*, **147**, 1128–1137.

81. Friedman A.S. (1975) Interaction of drug therapy with marital therapy in depressive patients. *Arch. Gen. Psychiatry*, **32**, 619–637.

82. Jacobson N.S., Dobson K., Fruzzetti A.E., Schmaling K.B., Salusky S. (1991) Marital therapy as treatment for depression. *J. Consult. Clin. Psychol.*, **51**, 547–557.

83. Beach S.R., O'Leary K.D. (1992) Treating depression in the context of marital discord: outcome and predictors of response of marital therapy versus cognitive therapy. *Behav. Ther.*, **23**, 507–528.

84. Jacobson N.S., Fruzzetti A.E., Dobson K., Whisman M., Hops H. (1993) Couple therapy as a treatment for depression: II. The effects of relationship quality and therapy on depressive relapse. *J. Consult. Clin. Psychol.*, **61**, 516–519.

85. Waring E.M., Chamberlaine C.H., McCrank E.W., Stalker C.A., Carver C., Fry R., Barnes S. (1988) Dysthymia: a randomised study of cognitive marital therapy and anti depressants. *Can. J. Psychiatry*, **33**, 96–99.

86. Waring E.M., Chamberlaine C.H., Carver C.M., Stalker C.A. (1995) A pilot study of marital therapy as a treatment for depression. *Am. J. Fam. Ther.*, **23**, 3–10.

87. Teichman Y., Bar-el Z., Shor H., Sirota P., Elizur A. (1995) A comparison of two modalities of cognitive therapy (individual and marital) in treating depression. *Psychiatry Interpers. Biol. Processes*, **58**, 136–148.

88. Emanuels-Zuurveen L., Emmelkamp P.M. (1997) Spouse-aided therapy with depressed patients. *Behav. Modif.*, **21**, 62–77.

89. Leff J., Vearnals S., Brewin C.R., Wolff G., Alexander B., Asen E., Dayson D., Jones E., Chisholm D., Everitt B. (2000) The London Depression Intervention Trial. Randomised controlled trial of antidepressants v. couple therapy in the treatment and maintenance of people with depression living with a partner: clinical outcome and costs. *Br. J. Psychiatry*, **177**, 95–100.

90. Diamond G.S., Reis B.F., Diamond G.M., Siqueland L., Isaacs L. (2002) Attachment-based family therapy for depressed adolescents: a treatment development study. *J. Am. Acad. Child Adolesc. Psychiatry*, **41**, 1190–1196.

91. Kolko D.J., Brent D.A., Baugher M., Bridge J., Birmaher B. (2000) Cognitive and family therapies for adolescent depression: treatment specificity, mediation, and moderation. *J. Consult. Clin. Psychol.*, **68**, 603–614.

92. Misri S., Kostaras X., Fox D., Kostaras D. (2000) The impact of partner support in the treatment of postpartum depression. *Can. J. Psychiatry*, **45**, 554–558.

93. Harris T., Brown G.W., Robinson R. (1999) Befriending as an intervention for chronic depression among women in an inner city. 1: Randomised controlled trial. *Br. J. Psychiatry*, **174**, 219–224.

94. Falloon I.R.H., Shanahan W., Laporta M. (1992) Prevention of major depressive episodes: early intervention with family-based stress management. *J. Ment. Health*, **1**, 53–60.

95. Amenson C.S., Liberman R.P. (2001) Dissemination of educational classes for families of adults with schizophrenia. *Psychiatr. Serv.*, **52**, 589–592.

96. Berglund N., Vahlne J.O., Edman A. (2003) Family intervention in schizophrenia—impact on family burden and attitude. *Soc. Psychiatry Psychiatr. Epidemiol.*, **38**, 116–121.

97. Bertrando P., Bressi C., Clerici M., Beltz J., Donatini L., Cazzullo C.L., Pagani C., Brambilla F., Nahon L., Cecchin G., *et al.* (1989) Terapia familiare sistemica ed emotività espressa nella schizofrenia cronica. Uno studio preliminare. *Attraverso lo Specchio*, **25**, 511–562.

98. Brooker C., Falloon I., Butterworth A., Goldberg D., Graham-Hole V., Hillier V. (1994) The outcome of training community psychiatric nurses to deliver psychosocial intervention. *Br. J. Psychiatry*, **165**, 222–230.

99. Brooker C., Tarrier N., Barrowclough C., Butterworth A., Goldberg D. (1992) Training community psychiatric nurses to undertake psychosocial intervention: report of a pilot study. *Br. J. Psychiatry*, **160**, 836–844.

100. Kavanagh D.J., Piatkowska O., Clark D., O'Halloran P., Manicavasagar V., Rosen A., Tennant C. (1993) Application of a cognitive–behavioural family intervention for schizophrenia in multi-disciplinary teams: what can the matter be? *Aust. Psychol.*, **28**, 181–188.

101. Xiang M., Ran M., Li S. (1994) A controlled evaluation of psychoeducational family intervention in a rural Chinese community. *Br. J. Psychiatry*, **165**, 544–548.

102. Falloon I.R.H., McGill C.W., Matthews S.M., Keith S.J., Schooler N.R. (1996) Family treatment for schizophrenia: the design and research application of therapist training models. *J. Psychother. Pract. Res.*, **5**, 45–56.

103. Optimal Treatment Project (2000) *Pathways to Recovery from Mental Disorders: From Caring to Curing: A Guidebook for Consumers and their Families and Friends.* Advanced Research Institute for Evidence-based Education and Treatment, Perugia.

104. Laidlaw T.M., Coverdale J.H., Falloon I.R.H., Kydd R.R. (2002) Caregivers' stresses when living together or apart from patients with chronic schizophrenia. *Commun. Ment. Health J.*, **38**, 303–310.

105. Lehman A.F., Steinwachs D.M. (1998) At issue: translating research into practice: the Schizophrenia Patient Outcomes Research Team (PORT) treatment recommendations. *Schizophr. Bull.*, **24**, 1–9.

106. Malm U., Ivarsson B., Allebeck P., Falloon I.R.H. (2003) Integrated care in schizophrenia: a 2-year randomized controlled study of two community-based treatment programs. *Acta Psychiatr. Scand.*, **107**, 415–423.

From Burden to Empowerment: The Journey of Family Caregivers in India

Radha Shankar* and Kiran Rao‡

*Malar Hospitals, Chennai, India
‡National Institute of Mental Health and Neurosciences, Bangalore, India

INTRODUCTION

In a recent ethnographic study on the involvement of families in Indian psychiatry, Nunley [1] attempted to answer the important question of whether the international expansion of biomedical psychiatry beyond the boundaries of Europe and USA would have the potentially negative consequence of devaluation or exclusion of families from the treatment process. The author concluded that biomedical advances notwithstanding, Indian psychiatrists extolled the benefits of involving families in the delivery of psychiatric care, especially for persons suffering from major mental illness [2,3]. However, the study was unable to inform whether families were seen simply as reasonably "competent providers of care" or as a "valuable and enduring resource" that needed to be supported and guided through programmes of constructive collaboration. We would like to suggest that the report in fact implies a paradoxical situation in which the involvement of families is ostensibly welcomed by the medical establishment, but the failure of the system to comprehensively understand the difficult circumstances under which families get involved, and respond constructively to these situations, in fact devalues the contribution of families. A historical review of family professional relationships suggests that the early attempts to meaningfully acknowledge the contribution of family carers have not received due attention in contemporary practice.

In 1967, Chacko [4] published a seminal article on the family participation in the treatment and rehabilitation of the mentally ill. In the period preceding this publication, significant innovations in practice had been

Families and Mental Disorders. Edited by Norman Sartorius, Julian Leff, Juan José López-Ibor, Mario Maj and Ahmed Okasha. © 2005 John Wiley & Sons Ltd. ISBN 0-470-02382-1

undertaken in large hospitals in India, as reported by Vidyasagar [5] and Narayanan *et al.* [6]. The authors described the manner in which the services of families were comprehensively utilized in the care, recovery and after-care of patients whom they had accompanied to these hospitals for management of a psychotic condition. These reports highlighted the fact that the involvement of relatives in the treatment process while the patient was admitted in the hospital not only facilitated their acceptance of the person recovering from mental illness, but also the return of the patient to their home in the community. The authors detailed the practical reasons which made it imperative to proactively engage Indian carers in the treatment of persons with major mental illness. Most of these issues are still valid today, and include the modest mental health infrastructure in the country, and the preference of families to be involved in the care of their mentally ill relative.

It is not only interesting, but also significant, to note that these experiments were published during a period when the Western literature was dominated by views of family therapists who stressed that family pathology had an aetiological role to play in the causation of major mental illness. Clinical practice therefore recommended that minimizing the involvement of, or altogether excluding, families would in fact facilitate recovery in patients with major mental illness.

It was only during the next decade, coinciding with the process of deinstitutionalization, that reports recognizing the role of families as a key resource in the care of the mentally ill began to emerge from the Western world [7]. In sharp contrast to that period of blaming and excluding natural caregivers, the past twenty years have been characterized by a major shift in the conceptual framework, followed by rigorous research in the form of randomized controlled trials of formal family psychoeducation, which represents a collective designation for interventions that combine the imparting of information with therapeutic elements. Numerous reviews have demonstrated both the efficacy and the effectiveness of these approaches [8–10]. Natural carers are now increasingly recognized as partners in the care of persons with major mental illness, especially as the locus of care is primarily in the community. Although there is criticism that adoption of evidence-based family interventions is still not universal [11,12], trends in the literature suggest that family work has begun to be incorporated into the therapeutic repertoire of Western clinical practice.

Historically, and in contrast to their Western counterparts, Indian caregivers have never been systematically excluded from the treatment process of people with major mental illness: yet it remains a very great and unfortunate paradox that they have not received the benefits of evidence-based family interventions recommended by numerous expert guidelines and consensus statements. It is more than three decades since the pioneering reports on family intervention practices appeared in the Indian literature, and the major responsibility for providing care continues to be assumed by the primary kin network. However, systematic guidance to families to optimize their caregiving ability is not offered in routine clinical practice.

In this chapter, we will discuss the pressing imperative to include purposive, regular and goal-oriented psychoeducation programmes in the therapeutic encounters between health professionals and natural caregivers in the Indian context. The evidence to support our discussion is derived from illness- and family-related studies, societal and cultural variables, and the realities of the mental health infrastructure and the delivery system. We will also review contemporary literature on family interventions in India and discuss issues that could inform on developing models which are appropriate for the Indian context. Finally, a description of the fledgling family movement and its implications for the service delivery system will be presented.

WHY FAMILY INTERVENTIONS IN A FAMILY-CENTRIC CULTURE?

Family-centric cultures by definition presuppose a good deal of involvement by the primary kin network in the lives of people with major mental illness. Is there a need to conceptualize and implement formal programmes of intervention in a culture where family engagement in the caregiving process is robust? Is this in fact an artificial intervention premised on current opinions prevailing in the Euro-American world? We would like to suggest that it is precisely the family centredness of low-income countries such as India that demands proactive approaches of working with carers of people with major mental illness. A consideration of the issues detailed below will illustrate our observation.

A Sustainable Paradigm of Community Care Requires Family Interventions

The mental health infrastructure in India is not only minimal in absolute terms, but its limitations can be even more accurately assessed when seen against the population of this large country. Services are largely urban, and comprise approximately 18 000 beds in 37 state run hospitals, and a small but undetermined number of beds in the private sector. However, most state and teaching hospitals and the private sector have departments of psychiatry which offer ambulatory, outpatient care. Rehabilitation and after care facilities are also very few in number and basic in the services they offer [13]. There is a paucity of trained personnel, with the number of mental health professionals not exceeding 5000. For a population of over one billion, both settings and service providers are grossly inadequate. The disparity between needs and available services led policy makers in India to conclude that "not more than 10% of those requiring urgent mental health care" were receiving help from the existing services [14]. This indicates that a large part of the mental health care has been, and is, taking place in the community, resulting in the family being the primary care provider. This scenario is quite different from what happened in the West, where the locus of care shifted to the community only as a result of the deinstitutionalization movement.

The National Mental Health Programme was devised by policy planners in India to bridge the large gap between demand and supply, and seeks to deliver mental health care through the decentralized, community-based primary health care network. However, the definition of community care needs to be clarified. In many developed countries, treatment and psycho-social interventions in the community are delivered through teams, which include an array of trained nurses, rehabilitation specialists, cognitive therapists, social workers, occupational therapists and psychiatrists [15]. In India, as in most other low-income countries, such resources simply do not exist, and the term "community care" often translates into patients remaining outside hospitals, but with their families [16]. Also, it is important to highlight that implicit in the National Health policy is that while the state will attempt to deliver mental health services through non-institutional decentralized approaches, the *locus of care will continue to be with the family*. If natural caregivers are therefore required to provide ongoing, sustainable care in the community for persons with major mental illness, it becomes absolutely critical to optimize their caregiving ability with programmes of formal support and guidance.

The Course of Illness Demands Family Interventions

Interestingly, in spite of the inadequate mental health services, the course and outcome of schizophrenia in India have been found to be relatively good. Three large-scale international collaborative studies conducted by the World Health Organization (WHO)—the International Pilot Study on Schizophrenia (IPSS), the Determinants of Outcome of Severe Mental Disorders (DOSMD) and the International Study of Schizophrenia (ISoS)—convincingly demonstrated that persons with schizophrenia did better in

India and other developing countries, when compared to their Western counterparts [17]. This better course and outcome have not only been extensively documented, but have raised questions as well [18]. Do these findings, dubbed by Kleinman [19] as "the single most provocative datum to emerge" in this area, suggest that interventions that could moderate the course and outcome of major mental illness may not be necessary in developing countries? It would be instructive to study other literature from India.

The Indian Council of Medical Research [20] reported on a 5-year follow-up study of 326 newly diagnosed patients with schizophrenia. The second year follow-up revealed that 43% of patients had experienced a relapse. These figures had risen to 64% at the end of 5 years. Relapse prevention has been an important goal of working with families, and is often used as an outcome measure for evaluation of interventions. More importantly, the study identified factors that could discriminate between good and bad outcome and these included medication compliance, absence of dangerous behaviour, rise in socio-economic level, and living conditions in which the patient was not subject to avoidance by his network. Comprehensive interventions with families provide carers with a range of options and skills by which the good outcome factors can be optimized. Thara *et al.* [21] and Eaton *et al.* [22], while reporting on a 10-year follow-up of first-episode Indian patients, have also highlighted the importance of early therapeutic interventions, including family interventions, by demonstrating that the prevalence of positive and negative symptoms in schizophrenia stabilized in the first 2 years of the illness. Research therefore suggests that reduction in relapses and early therapeutic interventions are in fact as important in the Indian context as anywhere else in the world.

Using Intensive Family Involvement to Optimize Outcomes is Good Economics in a Developing Country

Two cross-cultural studies reported on age- and gender-matched samples of patients with chronic schizophrenia living in the UK and the USA and compared their living experiences with those from India [23,24].

Analysis of several illness, social and occupational parameters revealed significant differences, including the fact that less than 50% of patients in the Western world lived with their families, while the comparable figure in India was 98.3%. Overall, the data suggested that Indian patients were more socially reintegrated than their Western counterparts. Indian patients not only tend to live with natural caregivers, but both research evidence and clinical practice suggest that the primary kin network has a pre-eminent role in decisions about both the manner and timing of help seeking, as well as withdrawing from the treatment process.

It is the family, on recommendations of the larger social network of relatives and friends, which decides whether the patient will seek help from the psychiatrist or faith healer [1,25]. To a large extent, this is influenced by the family's explanatory model for the illness. Relatives who believe in the supernatural causation of schizophrenia initially consult indigenous healers, while those who perceive schizophrenia as a medical problem consult practitioners of modern medicine [26]. Various roles in providing care are assumed by different people, both family members and friends [27]. The modalities of treatment to be used, including the purchase and supervision of medication and experimentation with alternative treatments, are also invariably decided by the primary network. Long-term studies have shown that caregivers are called upon to provide support to their patients not only during the period of the acute illness, but also in the aftercare and recovery process, including housing and financial support to those who are not employed.

What implications does this intensive involvement of families have on the mental health delivery system? We believe that this natural preference of families to be involved in the care of their mentally ill kin should be utilized in a focused and goal-oriented manner to assist a poorly funded mental health system to deliver optimal mental health care.

Xiong et al. [28] reported on a formal and structured family intervention programme in an outpatient setting in a large state hospital in China. The authors described a typical institution as being characterized by heavy caseloads, brief therapeutic encounters between the psychiatrist and the patient, primarily on an ad-hoc as and when required basis, predominance of the biomedical model and the near absence of psychosocial inputs. The study revealed that 90% of Chinese patients lived with their families, and that both outpatient consultations and follow-up work with the mentally ill almost routinely involved family members. The description of living arrangements of patients and the treatment conditions that obtain in ambulatory settings, more particularly the brief medical inputs given in follow-up care in China, accurately captures the prevailing situation in India as well. The findings of this study therefore become very important to both social planners and clinicians. First, the study has demonstrated the effectiveness of family interventions in a routine, busy, impersonal clinical setting, dominated by the biomedical approach. Second, the salient finding that these psychosocial programmes were cost effective, and the savings could be substantial, is the first definitive evidence of its kind in a low-income country and could have major implications for policy and programme planning. To summarize, we believe that the observations from Xiong et al.'s study [28] have equal if not more validity in India, and require urgent replication and strategic dissemination.

The Consequences of Providing Care are Distressful: Family Interventions in India are Therefore Ethical

Do families just represent a low-cost, plentiful resource in the community who are necessary to offset the limitations of a poorly funded mental health system? In this section we will present evidence to suggest that families need to be perceived as much more than a locus for interventions in the community, and that it is both necessary and ethical to offer programmes of support and guidance to carers.

That Indian families face several adverse consequences while caring for their mentally ill relative is exemplified by the fact that one of the earliest burden questionnaires to measure both subjective and objective burden was developed in India [29]. Studies carried out with family caregivers in different parts of the country at various points in time have revealed similar findings, indicating the consistency with which certain areas are experienced as causing distress. Burden has been perceived by family members mainly in issues related to finance, disruption of family leisure activities and family interaction, and these studies have also documented a negative impact on physical and mental health of caregivers [30–34]. Some research has suggested that the burden faced by urban families was greater than that faced by their rural counterparts [35], while other authors have reported the converse [31]. However, families in both rural and urban areas experience burden in caring [36].

A high level of stress, anxiety and depression among family carers was reported by Sovani [37]. The study by Marimuthu *et al.* [38] suggested that 30% of caregivers met the criteria for psychiatric morbidity. However, Chakrabarti *et al.* [39] did not find a significant impact of the caregiving role on the relatives' emotional and physical health. In support of this finding, Roychaudhuri *et al.* [40] observed that, despite high levels of burden, caregivers reported subjective well-being scores in the normal range, indicating that they possessed considerable coping resources.

Caregiving is provided mainly by parents and spouses [41] and is gendered, with women being the primary care providers [42]. Not much attention has been paid to the impact of caregiving on the marital relationship. Vijayalakshmi and Ramana [43] found that spouses often took over the breadwinner's role, and other family members, especially children, took over the index patient's responsibilities. Mahendru [44] found that 40% of the spouses of male patients with schizophrenia had a neurotic illness and Mahendru *et al.* [45] reported that spouses experienced high degrees of psychiatric morbidity and less participation in social activities than spouses in the control group. Spouses also reported greater emotional burden in the study by Rammohan *et al.* [41].

Duration of the illness correlates positively with burden, with longer duration of illness associated with greater burden [46]. However, the nature of symptoms seems to be more important in determining the extent of burden. Ranganathan *et al.* [47] reported that overt psychopathology, such as disruptive behaviour of the patient, problems with personal care and embarrassing behaviour, was associated with higher levels of burden.

The study by Raj *et al.* [48] suggested that caregivers experienced similar levels of distress associated with positive and negative symptoms immediately after an illness exacerbation. However, follow-up assessments after a period of stabilization revealed greater burden with negative symptoms. This finding must be understood in the context that having an acute relapse or exacerbation does not translate into immediate hospitalization for the patient, and it is not uncommon for families to provide domiciliary care for an acutely disturbed patient.

Medical treatment for people with major mental illness is provided both in state-run facilities, which are subsidized, and in the private sector on a fee for service basis. Insurance or co-payment is negligible. Therefore, families can also experience severe financial stressors.

Deficits in activity and self-care related behaviours were also reported by Gopinath and Chaturvedi [49] to be most troublesome to caregivers. The authors commented that in India it is quite natural to worry about an individual who does not do work or earn or is slow and inactive, whereas families may believe that aggressive or psychotic features are caused by supernatural forces and are not part of the illness. Certain patient characteristics are associated with greater burden for the family caregiver: these include caring for individuals who are younger, male, unemployed or low wage earners [40,50].

Chakrabarti and Kulhara [51] assessed family burden in a number of different psychiatric illnesses (schizophrenia, affective disorders) and argued that there is a need to distinguish between the extent of burden and its pattern. They concluded that it is the quality of burden that merits further investigation, because it may yield useful insights into how mental illness affects families across different social, cultural and ethnic groups.

Family interventions in developed countries were initially premised on their ability to reduce relapses and improve the functioning of the patient. The family was seen primarily as an adjunct to the mental health system, and little or no attention was paid to family burden or to the requirements and expectations of carers from the mental health system [52]. In an era of evolving interventions, the needs of patients and families are seen in the main as highly interrelated, and families are now regarded as equal partners in care [53]. The trends in literature also reflect this perception, and family focused issues are being addressed more proactively in intervention programmes than has been the case in the past [54,55].

The plethora of studies that have been reviewed suggests that caregiver burden has been among the most well-researched topics in the Indian psychiatry literature, leaving no doubt about the extent and nature of distress experienced by relatives, and the importance of finding comprehensive, widespread and practical solutions to the consequences of caregiving. All this has been addressed in editorials in the professional literature [56] and practice guidelines [57]. Yet translation into programmes of action or remediation unfortunately continues to be sporadic and slow. We believe that this could have a very negative impact on the community care of people with major mental illness, as will be outlined in subsequent sections.

INEFFECTIVE COPING BY CARERS MAY IMPACT BOTH THE ILLNESS AND CAREGIVER BURDEN

How do family members, especially the primary care providers, cope with the consequences of ongoing, long-term involvement in the lives of patients with major mental illness?

Bhargava *et al.* [58] reported that family carers mostly used adaptive coping strategies such as positive communication and social involvement with the patient. However, denial emerged as a significant coping strategy adopted by parents in the study by Rammohan *et al.* [41]. The authors also identified negative distraction as the predominant strategy employed by spouses and reported that the presence of denial in coping emerged as a significant predictor of caregiver burden.

Chakrabarti and Gill [59] compared coping styles of caregivers of patients with bipolar disorder and schizophrenia. They found that a variety of strategies, both problem- and emotion-focused, were used by relatives. Emotion-focused strategies were more commonly used by families of patients with schizophrenia, and problem-focused coping strategies by caregivers of bipolar patients. These differences appeared to be associated with differences in caregiver burden and appraisal between the two groups.

An attempt to understand coping behaviours by caregivers of patients with chronic schizophrenia was undertaken by Chandrasekaran *et al.* [42]. Using the family coping questionnaire of Magliano *et al.* [60], the authors identified resignation as the predominant coping strategy. Over 60% of relatives (primarily women and parents) had never made any attempt to find out information about the illness or its management. Resignation also showed correlation with caregiver burden and negative symptomatology. The authors explained this passive attitude as part of a culturally sanctioned fatalism towards life that encourages Indians to accept tribulations with a sense of resignation [61]. However, they cautioned that this passivity on the part of the caregivers could have an adverse impact on the clinical and social outcome of the illness. It is interesting to note that Birchwood and Cochrane [62], in their study on coping behaviour in British families, also raised the issue of whether a disengaged/resigned style of coping by relatives could have a negative impact on the social functioning of patients with schizophrenia.

Since magico-religious beliefs are an important element in the explanatory model of the illness, the use of religious coping and its relationship with psychological well-being in a sample of primary caregivers of persons with schizophrenia were explored by Rammohan et al. [63]. Results indicated that 97% of the caregivers reported belief in God, and that their religious beliefs and practices helped them deal with the stress of the situation. Common religious practices like lighting a lamp or praying to God were the most frequently adopted religious rituals. Strength of religious belief, rather than religious practices, emerged as a significant contributor to psychological well-being.

Coping styles of family caregivers have not received adequate attention. Research in this area is especially important to understand the culture-specific ways in which family members in India have been dealing with this stress. Adaptive methods contributing to well-being can then be enhanced and strengthened as part of intervention programmes, while maladaptive ones can be modified through psychoeducation. The attitudes of mental health professionals have also mirrored those of their Western counterparts, with religious beliefs and practices being largely ignored or being viewed as a cause of delay in seeking psychiatric help.

OPTIMAL PROFESSIONAL SUPPORT REQUIRES SENSITIVITY TO CAREGIVER NEEDS

Nagaswami et al. [64] observed that the urgency to "find a job" and be gainfully employed was the most important felt need for both the patient and family. A focus on meaningful employment or productive activity for the mentally ill person has been a consistent finding in most of the studies designed to elicit needs. Gopinath et al. [65] reported that family carers were keen to obtain a short duration of activity therapy for their patients with schizophrenia as they perceived them to be employable. As early as 1989,

Sethi highlighted the need to reduce disability through day care centres and sheltered workshops [3].

Job placement for the ill relative was also a major concern reported by Shankar and Kamath [66] in their study of caregivers. Elangovan *et al.* [67] explored the needs of patients diagnosed as suffering from chronic schizophrenia and bipolar disorder and found that both groups of patients expressed a primary need to participate in meaningful daytime activities. Relatives wanted more rehabilitation facilities that would enable patients to become productive members [68]. These consistent findings related to employment, income generation and productive activities are not surprising in a low-income country with negligible welfare and social security benefits, since caring for a non-contributory member adds to the already heavy burden of existential stressors. Articulating the needs from an urban caregiver's perspective, Srinivasan [69] stated that training for the patient in daily living skills and vocational activities and day care facilities are of high priority. Selected groups of families are now expressing a different set of needs. Members of the primary kin network are seeking more information about the illness, medication management and other modalities of treatment. A need for specific guidance on how to handle the patient's symptoms and their own distress has also been expressed by caregivers. In keeping with trends in the Western literature, family carers have concerns about the well-being of their patient after their lifetime, and want these issues to be addressed by professionals [37,68,70].

In contrast, Shankar and Kamath [66] found that family members of patients attending an urban rehabilitation centre showed little interest in seeking information about the illness, but were willing to listen to advice that would be beneficial to the patient. Of these families, only 30% wanted emotional support from mental health professionals. The majority chose to discuss problems with other family members and friends, and reported adequate support from these sources.

The 1985 study by Nagaswami *et al.* [64] observed that, if patients were engaged in income generating activities and their families received adequate support, residential care for patients was not articulated as a perceived need by carers. This is in contrast to reports from the West. Fifteen years later, and perhaps reflecting both the changing demography and the perceptions of family groups, Srinivasan [69], a carer herself, stated that good residential facilities are a felt need in urban areas. Kulhara *et al.* [70] reported that both patients and their family carers expressed the need for welfare benefits for individuals with psychiatric disability.

Needs assessments are extremely important, and interventions with families should be driven by the expressed needs of caregivers. However, we would like to caution against the generalizability of results obtained from these studies, and draw attention to the observation made by Shankar and Kamath [66] that needs of carers and patients often reflect a complex amalgam of the family's perceptions of the illness and expectations of cure, education, socioeconomic level and the support system available to the patient and the carers.

Murthy [71] suggested that Indian families have been seen primarily as a substitute for professional care, and not as an essential component of mental health care. Efforts have not been made to understand their needs, to provide support and skills training and to help families in networking. He concluded that, in order to prevent families from abandoning their mentally ill relatives, it becomes even more important to develop and implement family-based interventions in this low-income country.

INDIAN SOCIETY IS CHANGING: PROFESSIONAL INPUTS HAVE NOT KEPT PACE

Leff *et al.* [72] have suggested that traditional joint families that exist in developing countries allow for diffusion of burden in families caring for the mentally ill. Also, the tolerant attitudes of families in India, which is a function of a family-centric culture, could be responsible for mediating the good course and outcome of major mental illness. Reviews of the role of the family in relation to mental health have found that the nuclear family structure is more likely to be associated with psychiatric disorders than the joint family [2,73]. The joint family is seen as a source of social and economic support [2], and is known for its tolerance of deviant behaviour [74], and its capacity to absorb additional roles. Chandrashekar *et al.* [35] reported that fewer rural families sought hospitalization when compared to urban families.

However, we would like to examine the changing structure and function-ing of the contemporary Indian family and its impact on caregiving for people with major mental illness. This will also support our proposition that, even in cultures which are family oriented and therefore assumed to be tolerant and accepting, it is not possible for carers to provide care without active programmes of support and guidance.

In response to the commonly held belief about the existence and role of traditional extended families in developing countries, Pearson and Lam [16] observed that "it is a common misconception that Chinese people live in large extended families and if this has ever been true, it is certainly not true now". This statement also applies to the situation in India, because traditional joint family structures, where family members stay together with their spouses and children, have been significantly replaced in urban areas by "new order" nuclear families. This is consequent to industrialization, urbanization, migration from rural to urban areas, education of women and their entry into paid work [74]. More importantly, the family system has become a highly differentiated and heterogeneous social entity in terms not only of structure, but also of pattern, role relationships, obligations and values. Therefore, generalizations need to be made with a degree of circumspection. What impact does changing demography have on the capacity of carers to provide long-term support to psychiatric patients?

In the context of the transitional changes in Chinese society, Pearson and Lam [16] observed that "in countries with low income levels and numerous existential stressors, changes in family structure may make the care giving burden even more onerous". This has been vividly illustrated by an important epidemiological study carried out by the Indian Council of Medical Research [75], which revealed large numbers of patients with psychoses who were untreated and severely disabled. What was striking was that the patients and their families lived in an urban metropolis, and there were several treatment facilities in the vicinity. In a subsequent analysis of this group of patients, Padmavathi *et al.* [76] found that the larger the family, in terms of it being an extended or joint family, the more it was able to compensate for a dysfunctional member in terms of having fewer expectations, and this seemed to be the crucial factor related to the non-treatment of the patient with major mental illness. Gopinath *et al.* [65] reported that patients who hailed from larger families and had a better educational status tended to discontinue attending a day hospital facility within three months. However, the impact of non-compliance with the rehabilitation programme on the disability of the patient was not assessed.

Bharat [73] has suggested that there is an urgent need to look beyond the narrow confines of the structure and incorporate a much broader matrix of functional and attitudinal elements in order to assess the capacity of the family to provide care. Nunley [1] has reported that the presence of family burden and distress and no respite from the caregiving role may also harm the patient.

More than three decades ago, Bhaskaran [77] observed that, in the majority of the patients living in a mental hospital, the patient–family relationship was almost non-existent, with more than 75% having no contact with any family member. He reported that the burden of care for a chronic illness, the reduced work output of the patient and the stigma attached to mental illness were the main reasons for the "unwanted patient". Gupta *et al.* [78] reported that, although 70% of the patients in the Agra mental hospital had one or more family members, more than half of them had not had a visit from a relative in the previous two years. Surveys of the mental hospitals have also shown that large numbers of long-stay patients have practically no contact with the family [13]. Although the numbers of patients residing in long-term care institutions without contact with their families is relatively small compared to those living with families, Thangarajan [79], in her study of perceptions of urban carers, has shown that families do not feel that hospitals are part of their network of help. Yet families wanted help from the professional system, to provide sustained care to individuals with major mental illness.

Lefley [53] has addressed the problems of ageing caregivers in the Western world who were involved in the care of their adult mentally ill children, and highlighted the severe stress faced by this population. In drawing attention to the needs of urban families, Srinivasan [69] has argued that current sociological and demographic changes taking place in Indian society have a direct bearing on family needs and hence treatment policies. These changes, which include the shrinking size of families, particularly in urban areas, influx of the traditional female caregivers into the workforce, and migratory movements among the younger generation, have left older caregivers without a second generation of support. Issues of community care and support for patients without families are beginning to emerge. This situation will become even more critical and acute in the years to come, due to the changing demography and pattern of caregiving, and the limited guidance offered by the mental health delivery system.

CULTURE IS NOT STATIC: FAMILY-CENTRIC SOCIETIES ALSO NEED FAMILY INTERVENTIONS

Although the structure of family systems is changing rapidly in India, sociologists [80] have proposed the concept of "functional jointedness" between the constituents of the new-order nuclear family, so that close ties are maintained, although the members may not live under the same roof. This promotes a strong family orientation among the constituents. Also the differential weight given to the independence and dependence construct in developing countries is highly germane to the aftercare support given by families, and the manner in which they define their role and their expectations of patients [80].

It could therefore be inferred that these cultural values and beliefs prevalent in India translate into the practice of kin support, and a defined obligation towards a family member. The study by Thangarajan [79] supports this view, because economically underprivileged Indian caregivers reported a sense of obligation to care for their mentally ill relative. Pearson and Lam [16], reporting on the needs of Chinese caregivers, have also highlighted that they were deeply influenced by their sense of family duty to the blood connection, and the traditional belief that family members should care for each other. This is in contrast to reports that Western caregivers prefer not to have a direct day-to-day caregiving role; instead, they would expect that their role remain adjunctive to the comprehensive services that should be offered by the professional mental health system [81].

Does this then suggest that family interventions may not be necessary in family-centric cultures? While these values, beliefs and practices of kin obligation and interdependence define the basic cultural orientation in India as being family-centric, we would like to suggest that a broader perspective of culture, as elaborated by Lopez *et al.* [82], would be more appropriate to contemporary prevailing realities of India.

These authors argue that older views of culture, which focused primarily on the psychological dimensions, and regarded culture as residing largely within individuals, are narrow and limited. Culture is not merely a set of practices that are predicated upon a set of values and beliefs, but must include social perspectives. It is more accurately reflected by the ongoing interactions between group values, norms and experiences on the one hand, and individual innovations and life histories on the other. The social perspective of culture must include understanding the life experiences of people through assessment of their daily routine. This will help capture what is important to people and how they prioritize their activities.

Nunley [1] observed that "Patrilocal joint family continues to be valorized as a cultural ideal". But in the relentless social transformation of India, does an ideal joint family exist? Contemporary understandings of Indian culture must incorporate multidimensional perspectives, and combine them to optimize therapeutic encounters. For example, a sociologist would argue that carer-based interventions must recognize that families are shrinking, and would therefore have limitations in meeting all their kinship obligations. This then necessitates greater professional support for the patient. However, when viewed from the psychological viewpoint, culturally congruent interventions should attempt to strengthen the affective relationships between existing kin. This would be perceived as appropriate for a family-centric culture, and could help offset the impact of the reduction of available carers.

A number of studies have documented that Indian families visit religious shrines in the hope of curing mental illness [e.g. 61,83–85]. However, Tewari *et al.* [84] reported that only 10% of the family caregivers of persons with major mental illness perceived magico-religious treatment to be helpful. Healer consultations were perceived to be useful by one third of the patients in the study by Campion and Bhugra [83]. On the other hand, Raguram *et al.* [85] reported that the majority of the caregivers were satisfied with the improvement shown by the patient as well as with their experience at the temple. However, the research also suggests that most of them discontinued such treatment by the time of their seeking help in a hospital setting [63,83], suggesting a shift and acceptance of a medical model of treatment. It is interesting to note that, in their pathway to care study, Banerjee and Roy [26] found that those who initially consulted indigenous healers took a shorter time to contact the referral centre while those who had consulted physicians took significantly longer.

Hence, the literature suggests that, while religion and cultural practices are important in the lives of carers and patients, models of causation, help seeking and treatment do not remain fixed and immutable. Culture, therefore, is not impervious to change. In fact, Lopez *et al.* [82] suggest that to recognize the dynamic and changeable nature of culture will help clinicians develop more realistic and meaningful interventions with families.

It is often easy to conclude that, in the Indian context, family involvement in patient care is a preference. However, it is also well known that families in India have limited choices or alternatives, on account of the minimally resourced mental health infrastructure and the absence of social security benefits. Would Indian caregivers continue with this extensive and intensive involvement with their mentally ill relative if affordable alternatives were available? Finding answers to this question becomes even more critical in the face of rapid social change and the redefinition of social obligations that may accompany this change. To summarize, we would like to suggest that perceptions that suggest a limited role for formal family interventions in a family-centric society are based on a narrow stereotype of culture that does not reflect contemporary realities. The issue needs to be addressed through multidisciplinary research that incorporates clinical, sociological and anthropological perspectives.

FORMAL FAMILY INTERVENTIONS IN INDIA AND IMPLICATIONS OF THE RELEVANT EVIDENCE

The pioneering attempts at formal family interventions in India, more than four decades ago, have been described in an earlier section. The Indian literature has subsequently carried eclectic descriptions of formal and structured programmes with carers. Interventions comprising educational sessions have been reported by Sovani [37], Prema and Kodandaram [86] and Shankar and Menon [87]. The interventions were carried out in a group format, and assessments revealed a reduction in both negative attitudes to the illness, as well as caregiver distress and burden.

Samuel and Thyloth [27] have discussed the substantial contribution of psychoeducational family programmes and medication management in the prevention of relapse among patients with chronic schizophrenia.

In 1988, Verghese [88] formally evaluated an intervention programme with family carers staying along with their patient in hospital. He concluded that family participation in all aspects of treatment led to an improvement in attitude towards the mentally ill individual.

The suggestion that co-resident relatives might require systemic interventions which focus on improvement of communication and regulation of affect has emerged from the work of Verghese *et al.* [89] in a specialized centre for family work. The authors cautioned that relatives need to be supported before their resilience breaks down or they become dysfunctional.

An intervention with 8–10 families using the focus group technique was attempted by Sarkar *et al.* [90]. The authors reported that the therapeutic processes perceived as helpful by the participants included intra-group interactions, sharing of emotions and psychoeducation about the illness.

The only randomized controlled trial of family interventions was reported by Pai and colleagues [29,91,92]. The authors compared routine hospital care offered to patients with major mental illness with home-based care delivered by a psychiatric nurse. A six-month follow-up indicated that the home intervention group showed higher improvements in symptoms, better social functioning and reduced burden for carers. At the end of two years, the experimental group maintained a better clinical status and fewer hospital admissions. However, differences in social functioning and caregiver burden between the experimental and control group were insignificant, suggesting that, in a chronic and disabling illness, family interventions may need to be augmented with approaches that have a more direct focus on the functioning of the patient.

Sharma *et al.* [93] reported that, in long-term illnesses with multiple deficits such as schizophrenia, day care facilities not only provide respite to the family but could also improve the social and occupational functioning of the patient. The impact of day care on co-resident relatives was the focus of a study by Rao *et al.* [94]. The authors suggested that day care reduced the financial burden on the family, improved family leisure time activities and decreased the physical and mental health problems of the family. The report concluded that, in urban areas, this was a viable method to maintain chronic patients within the family and in the community.

The favourable assessments of educational interventions in the Indian context are in contrast to Western reports, which suggest that brief programmes that are limited to the provision of illness-related information inputs have minimal impact on caregiver distress, as well as on the course and outcome of illness [95].

We would like to suggest that the studies evaluating educational and family groups have lacked methodological rigour, making them difficult not only to replicate, but also to help identify the critical and effective elements of the intervention. More importantly, most of these studies were carried out in specialized research and teaching institutions. Therefore, effectiveness in routine clinical settings, like the outpatient services of large state hospitals and community clinics, needs to be established.

While we have presented empirical evidence to justify the imperative to offer programmes of guidance and support to Indian caregivers, a clear understanding of the conceptual and operational elements and strategies to implement such interventions in clinical settings is lacking. What guidance does the literature provide on this issue? In 1991, Lam [95] wrote about the lack of clarity in identifying "what works and what doesn't in family interventions". More than a decade later, the evidence to identify both the effective and the essential elements of family intervention programmes is still limited. However, meta-analyses of psychoeducational studies [96,97] reveal that the components of effective programmes include a long duration, inclusion of the patient in some phases of the intervention, and information and education about the illness provided within a supportive framework. The intervention modality, defined by the format, is of secondary importance, suggesting that common therapeutic factors underlie the various approaches.

A large body of rigorously researched interventions has been developed for caregivers in the Western world. Should clinicians in developing countries adapt or adopt these empirical models? Related questions include what the goals of family work in the Indian context are, and what factors will define the content, format and delivery of family interventions in a country with a poorly resourced mental health system. Additionally, what are the practical issues that will drive the implementation of evidence based research interventions in routine clinical settings so that the needs of the vast majority of caregivers are met?

It is an enormous challenge to find answers to these questions, and we will review some of the relevant issues.

DEFINING THE CONCEPTUAL FRAMEWORK FOR FAMILY WORK: REDUCTION OF RELAPSE THROUGH EXPRESSED EMOTION BASED INTERVENTIONS

Relapse prevention has been an important goal of working with families, and is often used as an outcome measure for evaluation of interventions. A large body of family intervention literature from the West has reported on attempts to decrease relapse rates either through the reduction of high expressed emotion (EE) in caregivers or minimizing face-to-face contact between high EE caregivers and the patients. Leff *et al.* [72] studied the impact of EE in Indian caregivers on the course and outcome of schizophrenia. The authors drew attention to the very low EE ratings recorded at intake, and the fact that these ratings were not related to family structure (either joint or nuclear). Follow-up assessments at the end of the first year revealed a highly significant reduction in each of the components of the EE index, including the composite ratings. These findings have not been reported in any of the earlier assessments on Anglo-Saxon caregivers. Over 40% of the 78 relatives who comprised the research sample scored zero in all scales of the EE index at the end of the first year, and the authors stressed that the remarkable change in ratings demanded an explanation.

Bebbington and Kuipers [98] conducted an aggregate analysis of the predictive utility of EE in schizophrenia and concluded that the relationship between EE and relapse was robust in most parts of the Western world. In India, the findings fell short of significance because so few families were rated as high EE on the Camberwell Family Interview Schedule.

In a study on Mexican American immigrant caregivers, Jenkins and Karno [99] have documented EE scores that were significantly lower than those reported in Anglo-Saxon families. The authors also drew attention to the fact that high contact time between the high EE relative of Mexican American origin and the patient was not related to outcome, either as an additive or interactive factor with medication. This is in direct contrast to findings with Euro-American caregivers. It was hypothesized that high contact time would buffer the impact of the high EE relative by exposure to low EE relatives. Low contact time would in fact be culturally atypical.

Studies on EE in non-Anglo-Saxon cultures have been critiqued for several methodological shortcomings. More importantly, Jenkins and Karno [99] have questioned the validity of transposing scales which measure cultural idioms and patterns of communication and emotional expressions within Euro-American families to different cultures, and link them to the prediction of relapse. In the absence of new research evidence that clarifies both the validity and the constituents of the EE index in non-Anglo-Saxon cultures, family interventions premised on the reduction of EE ratings in caregivers may not be entirely suitable for the Indian context.

HETEROGENEITY IN CARERS AND SERVICE SETTINGS AND LIMITED ENGAGEMENT IN TREATMENT

India is a vast multilingual country with a striking diversity, not only in education and socio-economic levels of the carers, but also in the service settings where interaction takes place between the mental health system and the patients. Families come into contact with professional care providers in settings that range from primary health centres, to the large state hospitals, to the clinics of private practitioners. Carers and patients also receive therapeutic inputs from health care professionals with varying degrees of specialization. These include the non-specialized primary care workers, general practitioners, psychiatric specialists and even super-specialists who work in family units in large teaching institutions. Professional services are sought in a variety of situations, ranging from crisis help, to rehabilitating a relative who appears to be dull and apathetic. Within this complex scenario, there is the diversity of Indian families in terms of socio-economic status, residence in rural or urban areas, literacy levels, social expectations from the patients, illness conceptions and the changing obligation to care for their mentally ill relative. In this large and pluralistic country, adherence to any one conceptual or service delivery model may have very limited usefulness.

Non-specialist personnel provide inputs in the primary care settings. Therefore, basic programmes of psychoeducation necessarily have to be simple, in order to be delivered by this group of professional workers. Pai and Kapur [91], in a detailed analysis of their pioneering work with family carers, have attempted to identify the key intervention components which were associated with the better outcome in the experimental group. These were not sophisticated cognitive and behavioural approaches which require specialized training, but simple elements like continuity of care, emotional support and practical advice to carers and patients which ensured medication compliance. Interventions also have to be tailored to the social and educational background of the family, because socio-economic realities are also likely to influence service utilization and participation in programmes.

While the large state hospitals have trained personnel, staggering caseloads leave little time for psychosocial interventions. The randomized controlled intervention reported in India by Pai and Kapur [91] was carried out in a busy outpatient setting of a large state hospital. The experimental group had an average of 21 personalized contacts with professionals in their homes over a two-year period. This is in contrast to the routine care group, who visited the hospital on four occasions for brief consultations in an impersonal setting. Xiong et al. [28] have reported that the experimental group, in their successful intervention study, had an average of 8.1 visits to the clinic per year, each of which lasted 45 minutes.

How is this achieved in the face of large caseloads and few personnel? The Chinese study suggests that it is possible with adequate training of personnel to deliver 45 minutes of optimal interaction with each family enrolled in a family intervention programme. Given a baseline frequency of four visits per year in India, how do we increase the attendance of carers and patients at the treatment facility so that they benefit from purposive interventions? We would like to draw attention to the report of Thangarajan [79], who cited caregivers as perceiving the hospital as not part of their support network and suggested that this issue needs to be addressed.

Non-engagement by caregivers in lengthy structured interventions has been reported in the Western literature [100]. In the Chinese study, 18% of caregivers who met the criteria for enrolment refused to participate. It is important to point out that 79% of the treatment group in China was covered by insurance. Subsequently, non-compliance rates in the intervention ranged from 27% for individual family sessions to 32% for family group meetings, which are higher than those reported in Western studies. Although treatment in state hospitals in India is highly subsidized, we could anticipate a similar situation in this low-income country with several social and economic stressors and negligible insurance coverage. Also the issue of stigma as a potential barrier to participating in lengthy interventions has not been explored. In a study that has relevance to the issue of non-engagement, Xiang *et al.* [101] reported that families failed to cooperate with plans drawn up for the community care of the patient due to the following reasons: lack of confidence in the treatment, failure to understand mental illness as a disease that requires treatment, and stigma. We would like to suggest that a variety of social, economic and cultural factors, as well as tangible and intangible barriers within the health delivery system itself, are likely to have an impact on non-engagement and non-compliance by carers and patients in professional interventions. Each of these issues merits discussion, and needs to be addressed through research. We will, however, limit our review to the role and importance of cultural congruence in family interventions.

INCORPORATING A CULTURAL PERSPECTIVE

The need to develop culturally syntonic interventions is a recurring theme, not only in sociological and anthropological literature, but also in writings of interest to clinicians. The manner in which the family identifies, ascribes meaning to and responds to behavioural changes in its kin is likely to impact not only the help-seeking behaviour, but also the willingness to provide care and support in the restitution process. Therefore, the experiences and interpretations of psychiatric conditions by users (families and patients) have a substantive role to play in the development of meaningful health delivery systems, as only those services that are perceived as compatible with the users' beliefs are likely to be utilized. Both Kleinman [102] and Littlewood [103] have argued that an understanding of the local health culture (specifically, the interpretative and pragmatic elements used by people to deal with mental health problems) should be incorporated into programme planning that aims to optimize carer and community participation. The authors have cautioned that innovative psychosocial interventions that are influenced by biomedical concepts should work in synergy with traditional caregiving practices. A striking example of a psychosocial approach that has incorporated a cultural perspective has been provided by Xiong and others [28] in China. In their description of content, format and delivery of the interventions, the authors highlighted the importance of first dealing with the reluctance of Chinese caregivers to participate in talking therapies. This is consequent to the perception that family matters should not be discussed with outsiders, as well as their expectations of the therapeutic encounter with the psychiatrist to be brief and medically oriented. In keeping with the suggestion that interventions should support pragmatic elements used by people to cope, the subsequent interventive inputs were designed not to make the patient independent of the family, but instead become a reasonably productive member who is supported within the kin network. However, the authors stress that further exploration of social and cultural issues needs to be undertaken to impact the problems of non-compliance in the intervention.

In contrast, Lopez *et al.* [82], working with immigrant Hispanic caregivers, challenged the perceptions of families attributing supernatural causes to dysfunctional behaviours, and emphasized the biological basis for mental illness. The authors also encouraged families to be active participants in treatment, to overcome the traditional acceptance of the physician's authority.

We would suggest that a culturally syntonic model for India would need to be based on a broader definition of culture. The elements in this model would include understanding supportive ethno-psychiatric conceptions of illness and would not negate them by the biomedical orientation of the professional. A broader definition of culture will help clinicians appreciate the changing meaning of kin relations and develop a balanced appraisal of kin obligations of carers towards their relative. Finally, such a definition will encourage traditional methods of religious coping that are not maladaptive. Importantly, the health care system needs a comprehensive understanding of the economic, political and historical factors that are defining both the normative behaviours and the emotional climate of contemporary society, so that family carers do not become victims of cultural stereotypes that require them to provide kin support without respite or guidance.

In summary, practical and economic reasons, including the modest mental health infrastructure in the country and the paucity of trained mental health professionals, will require that Indian families remain involved in the care of their mentally ill relative. From a public health perspective, there is an imperative to proactively support the primary kin network in the process of caring. At the level of the individual caregiver and patient, the issue becomes not only more critical but also ethical. Research initiatives based on culturally congruent, socially appropriate and cost-effective models with widespread applicability are urgently needed. In the interim, it may be required to use a combination of didactic, non-formal techniques and structured comprehensive lengthy interventions that represent a judicious blend of evidence-based approaches and the needs of patients and their families [104].

THE FAMILY MOVEMENT IN INDIA: A STORY OF UNFULFILLED PROMISES OR GREAT EXPECTATIONS FOR THE FUTURE?

There have been different social forces contributing to the growth of patient and family organizations in various parts of the world. In many Western countries, some carers came together as an angry backlash against a system that initially blamed them for causing mental illness, and then expected them to provide community care for their mentally ill kin without adequate support [105]. In some countries, the adversarial relationship with professionals notwithstanding, the prime reason to organize into groups was for mutual support and subsequently to advocate for better services. In Japan the family organization was founded in response to a critical debate on the mental health law, which aimed at placing patient management under police control. Although family groups have evolved against differing historical backgrounds and have grown in response to context-specific issues, we would like to share the observation of Lefley and Johnson [106], who wrote that "the emergence of such groups in many parts of the world, together with the political influence of some of these organizations, is rather a remarkable phenomenon given the former powerlessness of this constituency".

The past fifteen years have seen the emergence of a fledgling family movement in India. Beginning with the first family group in the city of Chennai, which was catalysed by mental health professionals, the country today has over fifteen family organizations. The groups are involved in diverse activities, including the conduct of education programmes for carers, setting up income generating activities for patients, creating awareness in the community about mental health issues, and managing transitional living facilities. Mental health advocacy is now emerging on the active agenda of some groups. Two national conferences for carers have been held in 2001 and 2003. Family carers from different parts of this vast country came together in what can be described as a modest but pioneering initiative, culminating in the creation of an apex body of family organizations.

In his overview of international family organizations, Johnson [107] indicates that some have matured to the point of developing their own education programmes. More importantly, many family groups have grown remarkably in a short span of time. This is reflected in national organizations with hundreds of thousands of members, capable of influencing mental health policy.

Has the family movement in India achieved a critical mass and momentum by which it can really make a difference to the planning, delivery and evaluation of mental health services? Do family groups have the capability to impact the lives of patients and carers other than the small numbers of individuals who are associated with them?

A critical appraisal of Indian family organizations reveals that they are, in the main, small, urban and middle class in their orientation. The constituents are often elderly caregivers, and attracting active participation by younger relatives remains a challenge for most groups. Members are often involved in the care of a patient who may not have made a satisfactory recovery. Therefore, primary caregiving duties have to be balanced with organizational work. Clear-cut action agendas in family groups are still evolving, and constituents may have differing expectations from the organization. In the current scenario, many Indian family organizations comprise a few committed individuals who take on the organizational tasks, while most others remain passive participants. The absence of a clear-cut second rung of committed members leaves these groups vulnerable to a vacuum in leadership. Lastly, and perhaps of great significance, is the collaboration between mental health professionals and family groups, with practically all groups working closely with one or more health professionals. However, it is still not clear whether this new development is welcomed across India, in all service settings, by professionals from differing orientations.

Family groups worldwide are confronted with several challenges impacting their effectiveness and continued growth. Fund raising and financial sustenance are an ongoing struggle. Fledgling organizations may find it difficult to maintain their commitment and focus, especially when much of the work is voluntary and unpaid, and they require nurture and support. For established groups, the main challenge is to maintain the momentum of their work, and meet the growing expectations of their members.

In low-income countries these problems will be particularly acute. In addition, stigma will constitute a big barrier to meaningful participation by large numbers of caregivers. However, it is important for India to focus on the psychological issues that can influence the growth, and define the direction of the family movement.

Srinivasan [69] has pointed out that, in a traditional hierarchical society, the relationship between the authority figures, represented by the mental health system, and the patient and carer is like that of "the tutor and the taught". Most families therefore tend to be deferential, and accept the wisdom of the professional unquestioningly. In most Western countries, advocacy and lobbying by carers seek to influence mental health policy and services, as well as legislation. In India, these issues have long been the exclusive domain of professionals. Given the nature of professional–family interaction, the possibility and implications of a Western-style advocacy movement in India cannot be clearly delineated.

The passive acceptance of suffering as preordained and linked to one's fate and destiny is commonly referred to as "karma", and regarded as part of Indian culture. In the context of caregivers and the family movement, Srinivasan [69] suggests that this belief translates into the entrenched perception that actions by families cannot make a difference. This can create a psychological barrier to carers joining family groups.

In 1991, Shankar and Kamath [66] reported on the "cure versus care" dichotomy wherein caregivers stressed that it was the duty of professionals to cure their patient, while providing care was the role they assigned to themselves. We would like to suggest that while this perception may be linked to tolerance and acceptance, it also fosters a climate of passive caring. Family groups provide illness experiences and facilitate self-help initiatives. Since many relatives unquestioningly accept their duty to care, the rationale for more informed and proactive caregiving that is advocated by these encounters may have limited appeal to Indian carers.

Lastly, in this heterogeneous country, caste and community groupings still define the contours and constituents of the non-kin network. Can the experience of pain and suffering, and a common goal for better treatment for their relative, translate into a binding force that holds vastly different caregivers together in family organizations? The issue is still evolving.

We have given a detailed and comprehensive account of the difficult circumstances under which most Indian caregivers provide support. Hence, the emergence of family groups in India is a remarkable phenomenon. There is immense potential for family–professional collaboration to bring about structural and qualitative changes in the mental health care system. However, this requires not only a long-term commitment, but also a substantial reorientation in the attitudes and role definitions of all stakeholders. Will this be possible in this hierarchical society? There are no ready answers.

FUTURE DIRECTIONS

In 1982, Kapur and colleagues carried out the first randomized controlled intervention with families in India. A decade later, Kapur [108] asserted:

"Pious statements about the wonderful Indian family will just not do." This statement reflected not only an assessment about the changing social fabric of India, but also concerns about the failure of the mental health system to build on the findings that derived from his seminal study. On the other hand, Lefley [109] rhetorically asked: "What is it that keeps the Indian family still so involved and committed to its caregiving role?" and then proposed that it could be several things all at the same time—a culturally determined worldview and expectations regarding relations and obligations of kinship, an explanatory model of mental illness that is benign, as well as cultural variations in the expression of emotions. We would like to suggest that both these observations have identified the service delivery, research and training agenda in the area of family care for people with major mental illness.

Both basic and applied research will help develop appropriate and comprehensive models of family work that will suit the needs of this pluralistic society. Multidisciplinary, collaborative studies integrating anthropological, sociological, clinical, economic and operational perspectives are needed in place of fragmented approaches. We believe that such research will also provide inputs to social planners on future policy and programme needs, not just for people with psychoses but also for community mental health. While the focus of this chapter has been on family work in schizophrenia, models of family work are also needed for other chronic disorders such as bipolar illness.

Echoing the needs and sentiments of caregivers, Srinivasan [69] observed that mental health professionals need training in family education, as much as families need education about the illness. It is essential to sensitize professionals and equip them with skills to deliver family interventions. However, the country has a well-documented shortage of mental health workers.

What needs to be done to achieve a critical mass of trained personnel capable of delivering family interventions? We would like to suggest that alternative manpower resources be actively considered, in the process of capacity building: these include community-based rehabilitation workers and experienced and articulate family members themselves.

Studies have consistently demonstrated that clinical status and level of functioning of the patient is the strongest predictor of burden in the caregiver. Therefore, offering family intervention programmes without adequate treatment and rehabilitation services for people with mental illness is likely to make little difference to caregiver burden.

Urban areas require vocational and skills training facilities. In rural areas the vocational needs of patients must be met through community resources. Also, the small but growing demand for respite short-term and long-term residential care can no longer be ignored. It is suggested that many of these initiatives can take place in the non-governmental sector or in the form of public–private collaboration. However, the state must assume primary social responsibility to provide care for families with limited social and economic resources.

In conclusion, we would like to emphasize that in India it is a genuine, mutually respectful partnership between families and professionals that is most likely to impact mental health policy, programmes, legislation, stigma and research.

A vision for the family movement in India would see families changing from passive carers to informed carers, from receiving services to proactive participation, from suffering stigma to fighting stigma. And it is the responsibility of the mental health system to facilitate this journey of caregivers from burden to empowerment.

REFERENCES

1. Nunley M. (1998) The involvement of families in Indian psychiatry. *Cult. Med. Psychiatry*, **22**, 317–353.
2. Sethi B.B., Chaturvedi P.K. (1985) A review and role of family studies and mental health. *Indian J. Soc. Psychiatry*, **1**, 216–230.
3. Sethi B.B. (1989) Family as a potent therapeutic force. *Indian J. Psychiatry*, **3**, 22–30.
4. Chacko R. (1967) Family participation in the treatment and rehabilitation of the mentally ill. *Indian J. Psychiatry*, **9**, 328–333.
5. Vidyasagar (1971) *Innovations in Psychiatric Treatment at Amritsar Hospital— Report in a Seminar on the Organization and Future Needs of Mental Health Services*. World Health House, New Delhi.
6. Narayanan H.S, Embar P., Reddy G.N.N. (1972) Review of treatment in family wards. *Indian J. Psychiatry*, **14**, 123.
7. Goldstein M.J., Rodnick E.H., Evans J.R., May P.R., Steinberg U.R. (1978) Drug and family therapy in the aftercare of acute schizophrenics. *Arch. Gen. Psychiatry*, **35**, 1169–1177.
8. Dixon L.B., Lehman A.F. (1995) Family interventions for schizophrenia. *Schizophr. Bull.*, **21**, 631–643.
9. Fadden G.B. (1998) Family intervention. In: Brooker C., Repper J. (eds) *Serious Mental Problems in the Community: Policy, Practice and Research*. Baillière Tindall, London, pp. 159–183.
10. Fadden G.B. (1998) Research update: psychoeducational family interventions. *J. Fam. Ther.*, **20**, 293–309.
11. Lehman A.F., Steinwachs D.M., the co-investigators of the PORT project (1998) Translating research into practice: the Schizophrenia Patient Outcomes Research Team (PORT) treatment recommendations. *Schizophr. Bull.*, **24**, 1–10.
12. Dixon L.B., Lyles A., Scott J., Lehman A.F., Postrado L., Goldman H., McGlynn E. (1999) Services to families of adults with schizophrenia: from treatment recommendations to dissemination. *Psychiatr. Serv.*, **50**, 233–238.
13. National Human Rights Commission (1999) *Quality Assurance in Mental Health*. National Human Rights Commission, New Delhi.

14. Directorate General of Health Services (1982) *National Mental Health Program for India*. Ministry of Health and Family Welfare, New Delhi.
15. Falloon I.R.H., the Optimal Treatment Project Collaborators (1999) Optimal treatment for psychosis in an international multisite demonstration project. *Psychiatr. Serv.*, **50**, 615–618.
16. Pearson V., Lam P.C.W. (2002) On their own: caregivers in Guangzhou, China. In: Lefley H.P., Johnson D.L. (eds) *Family Interventions in Mental Illness: International Perspectives*. Praeger, Westport, CT, pp. 171–183.
17. Kulhara P., Chakrabarti S. (2001) Culture and schizophrenia and other psychotic disorders. *Psychiatr. Clin. North Am.*, **24**, 449–464.
18. Edgerton, R.B., Cohen A. (1994) Culture and schizophrenia: the DOSMD challenge. *Br. J. Psychiatry*, **164**, 222–231.
19. Kleinman A. (1988) *Rethinking Psychiatry*. Free Press, New York.
20. Indian Council of Medical Research (1988) *Report on the Multicentre Study of Factors Associated with the Course and Outcome of Schizophrenia*. Indian Council of Medical Research, New Delhi.
21. Thara R., Henrietta M., Joseph A., Rajkumar S., Eaton W.W. (1994) Ten-year course of schizophrenia—the Madras longitudinal study. *Acta Psychiatr. Scand.*, **90**, 329–336.
22. Eaton W., Thara R., Federman B. (1995) Structure and course of positive and negative symptoms in schizophrenia. *Arch. Gen. Psychiatry*, **52**, 127–134.
23. Dani M.M., Thienhaus O.J. (1996) Characteristics of patients with schizophrenia in two cities in the US and India. *Psychiatr. Serv.*, **47**, 300–301.
24. Sharma V., Murthy S., Kumar K., Agarwal M., Wilkinson G. (1998) Comparison of people with schizophrenia from Liverpool, England and Sakalwara, Bangalore, India. *Int. J. Soc. Psychiatry*, **44**, 225–230.
25. Chadda R.K., Agarwal V., Singh M.C., Raheja D. (2001) Help seeking behaviour of psychiatric patients before seeking care at a mental hospital. *Int. J. Soc. Psychiatry*, **47**, 71–78.
26. Banerjee G., Roy S. (1998) Determinants of help-seeking behaviours of families of schizophrenic patients attending a teaching hospital in India: an indigenous explanatory model. *Int. J. Soc. Psychiatry*, **44**, 199–214.
27. Samuel M., Thyloth M. (2002) Caregivers' roles in India. *Psychiatr. Serv.*, **53**, 346–347.
28. Xiong W., Phillips M., Xiong H., Wang R., Dai Q., Kleinman J., Kleinman A. (1994) Family-based intervention for schizophrenic patients in China: a randomised controlled trial. *Br. J. Psychiatry*, **165**, 239–247.
29. Pai S., Kapur R.I. (1981) The burden on the family of a psychiatric patient. Development of an interview schedule. *Br. J. Psychiatry*, **138**, 332–335.
30. Muralidhar D., Shariff I.A. (1981) Obstacles in the way of readjustment of the mental patient in the family. *J. Rehabil. Asia*, **22**, 37–41.
31. Moily S., Murthy R.S., Nagarajaiah B., Sekar K., Puttamma M., Kumar K.V., Hiremath S.B. (1997) Burden in families with schizophrenic patients in a rural community. *Indian J. Psychiatry*, **39**, 48.
32. Jose S. (2000) A study of family burden associated with schizophrenic patients. *Behav. Scientist*, **1**, 59–63.
33. Kataria D., Bhargava S.C., Vohra A.K. (2002) A correlational study between psychiatric disability and family burden in schizophrenia. *Indian J. Psychiatry*, **44**, 54.

34. The Mission Report (2003) *Priorities for Mental Health Sector Development in Gujarat*. Department of Health and Family Welfare, Government of Gujarat, Gandhinagar.
35. Chandrashekar C.R., Rao N.V.S.S.R., Murthy R.S. (1991) The chronic mentally ill and their families. In: Bharat S. (ed.) *Research on Families with Problems in India*, vol. 1. Tata Institute of Social Sciences, Bombay, pp. 113–120.
36. Mubarak Ali R., Bhatti R.S. (1988) Social support system and family burden due to chronic schizophrenia in rural and urban background. *Indian J. Psychiatry*, **30**, 349–353.
37. Sovani A. (1993) Understanding schizophrenia: a family psychoeducational approach. *Indian J. Psychiatry*, **35**, 97–98.
38. Marimuthu C., Prashanth N.R., John H.J.K., Russell P. (2000) Mental health of primary caregivers: what do we know? *Indian J. Psychiatry*, **42**.
39. Chakrabarti S., Raj L., Kulhara P., Avasthi A., Verma S.K. (1995) A comparison of the extent and pattern of family burden in affective disorders and schizophrenia. *Indian J. Psychiatry*, **37**, 105–112.
40. Roychaudhuri J., Mondal D., Boral A., Bhattacharya D. (1995) Family burden among long-term psychiatric patients. *Indian J. Psychiatry*, **37**, 81–85.
41. Rammohan A., Rao K., Subbakrishna D.K. (2002) Burden and coping in caregivers of persons with schizophrenia. *Indian J. Psychiatry*, **44**, 220–227.
42. Chandrasekaran R., Sivaprakash B., Jayestri S.R. (2002) Coping strategies of the relatives of schizophrenic patients. *Indian J. Psychiatry*, **44**, 9–13.
43. Vijayalakshmi B., Ramana K.V. (1987) Use of culture-specific coping structures by the families of mentally ill patients. *Indian J. Soc. Work*, **48**, 163–169.
44. Mahendru R.K. (1996) Mental morbidity and personality pattern in the spouses of schizophrenic patients. *Indian J. Psychiatry*, **38**, 14–15.
45. Mahendru R.K., Singh V., Sachan S.N. (1997) A study of psychiatric morbidity in the spouses of schizophrenic patients. *Indian J. Psychiatry*, **39**, 48.
46. Vohra A.K., Garg S., Gaur D.R. (2000) A study of burden on families of schizophrenia and depressive disorder. *Indian J. Psychiatry*, **42**, 33.
47. Ranganathan M., Nirmala B.P., Padankatti B.S. (1991) Problems of the families of the chronic mentally ill: relevance of the social work approach. In: Bharat S. (ed.) *Research on Families with Problems in India*, vol. 1. Tata Institute of Social Sciences, Bombay, pp. 121–127.
48. Raj L., Kulhara P., Avasthi A. (1991) Social burden of positive and negative schizophrenia. *Int. J. Soc. Psychiatry*, **37**, 242–250.
49. Gopinath P.S., Chaturvedi S.K. (1992) Distressing behavior of schizophrenics at home. *Acta Psychiatr. Scand.*, **86**, 185–188.
50. Gautam S., Nijhawan M. (1984) Burden on families of schizophrenic and chronic lung disease patients. *Indian J. Psychiatry*, **26**, 156–159.
51. Chakrabarti S., Kulhara P. (1999) Family burden of caring for people with mental illness. *Br. J. Psychiatry*, **174**, 463.
52. Hatfield A.B. (1994) Family education. Theory and practice in family interventions in mental illness. In: Hatfield A.B. (ed.) *New Directions for Mental Health Services*. Jossey-Bass, San Francisco, CA, pp. 3–11.
53. Lefley P.H. (2002) Helping families cope with mental illness. Future international directions. In: Lefley H.P., Johnson D.L. (eds) *Family Interventions in Mental Illness: International Perspectives*. Praeger, Westport, CT, pp. 222–234.
54. McFarlane W.R., Dunne E., Lukens E.P., Newmark M., McLaughlin-Toran J., Deakins S.M., Horan B. (1993) From research to clinical practice; dissemination

of New York State's family psychoeducation project. *Hosp. Commun. Psychiatry*, **44**, 265–270.

55. Fadden G.B., Birchwood M. (2002) British models for expanding family psychoeducation in routine practice. In: Lefley H.R., Johnson D.L. (eds) *Family Interventions in Mental Illness: International Perspectives*. Praeger, Westport, CT, pp. 25–41.

56. Trivedi J.K. (2002) Need for family interventions in schizophrenia. *Indian J. Psychiatry*, **44**, 199.

57. Kulhara P., Chakrabarthi S., Ramana A.L. (1999) Management of schizophrenia: minimum standards of care—psychosocial treatment. *Indian J. Soc. Psychiatry*, **14**, 1–4.

58. Bhargava S.C., Kataria D.K., Vohra A.K. (2001) The coping strategies in the families of schizophrenic patients. *Indian J. Psychiatry*, **43**(Suppl.), 113.

59. Chakrabarti S., Gill S. (2002) Coping and its correlates among caregivers of patients with bipolar disorder: a preliminary study. *Bipolar Disord.*, **4**, 50–60.

60. Magliano L., Guarneri M., Marasco C., Tosini P., Morosini P., Maj M. (1996) A new questionnaire assessing coping strategies in relatives of patients with schizophrenia. Development and factor analysis. *Acta Psychiatr. Scand.*, **94**, 224–228.

61. Varma V.K. (1982) Present state of psychotherapy in India. *Indian J. Psychiatry*, **174**, 154–158.

62. Birchwood M., Cochrane R. (1990) Families coping with schizophrenia: coping styles. Their origins and correlates. *Psychol. Med.*, **20**, 857–865.

63. Rammohan A., Rao K., Subbakrishna D.K. (2002) Religious coping and psychological well being in carers of relatives with schizophrenia. *Acta Psychiatr. Scand.*, **105**, 356–362.

64. Nagaswami V., Valecha V., Thara R., Rajkumar S., Menon M.S. (1985) Rehabilitation needs of schizophrenic patients: a preliminary report. *Indian J. Psychiatry*, **27**, 213–220.

65. Gopinath P.S., Sharma P.S.V.N., Reddy M.V. (1987) Patients who discontinue day hospitalization—an analysis. *Indian J. Psychiatry*, **29**, 197–201.

66. Shankar R., Kamath S. (1991) Needs based interventions with families of the chronic mentally ill. Presented at the Congress of the World Association of Psychosocial Rehabilitation, Montreal, 14–18 October.

67. Elangovan S., Verghese M., Murali T. (1997) Assessment of needs and disability in chronic schizophrenia and bipolar affective disorder. *NIMHANS J.*, **15**, 199–200.

68. Shrivastava A., Sakel G., Iyer S. (2001) Experience of working with relatives of schizophrenia: evolving caregivers program for advocacy and intervention. *Indian J. Psychiatry*, **43**, 105.

69. Srinivasan N. (2000) Families as partners in care. Perspectives from AMEND. *Indian J. Soc. Work*, **61**, 352–365.

70. Kulhara P., Avasthi A., Sharan P., Sharma P., Malhotra S., Gill S. (2001) Assessment of needs of patients of schizophrenia. *Indian J. Psychiatry*, **43**(Suppl.), 10.

71. Murthy R.S. (1998) Rural psychiatry in developing countries. *Psychiatr. Serv.*, **49**, 967–969.

72. Leff J.N.N., Wig H., Bedi D.K., Menon L., Kuipers A., Korten G., Ernberg R., Day N., Sartorius N., Jablensky A. (1990) Relatives' expressed emotion and the course of schizophrenia in Chandigarh. A two year follow up of a first contact sample. *Br. J. Psychiatry*, **156**, 351–356.

73. Bharat S. (1991) Research on family structure and problems: review, implications and suggestions. In: Bharat S. (ed.) *Research on Families with Problems in India: Issues and Implications*, vol. 1. Tata Institute of Social Sciences, Bombay, pp. 33–67.

74. Sinha D. (1984) Some recent changes in the Indian family and their implications for socialization. *Indian J. Soc. Work*, **45**, 271–286.

75. Indian Council of Medical Research (1990) *Final Report on the Longitudinal Study of Functional Psychosis in an Urban Community*. Indian Council of Medical Research, New Delhi.

76. Padmavathi R., Rajkumar S., Srinivasan T.N. (1998) Schizophrenic patients who were never treated. A study in an Indian urban community. *Psychol. Med.*, **28**, 1113–1117.

77. Bhaskaran K. (1970) The unwanted patient. *Indian J. Psychiatry*, **12**, 1–12.

78. Gupta S.P., Yadav B.S., Bharadwaj R.C., Sharma R.P. (1980) Psychosocial problems of long stay mental patients. *Indian J. Psychiatry*, **22**, 251–255.

79. Thangarajan C.M. (1994) Coping with schizophrenia in the family. PhD dissertation, Tata, Institute of Social Sciences, Bombay.

80. Gore M.S. (1968) *Urbanisation and Family Change in India*. Popular Prakashan, Bombay.

81. Lefley P.H. (1988) Training professionals to work with families of chronic patients. *Commun. Ment. Health J.*, **24**, 338–357.

82. Lopez S.R., Kopelowicz A., Canive J.M. (2002) Strategies in developing culturally congruent interventions for schizophrenia; the case of Hispanics. In: Lefley H.P., Johnson D.L. (eds) *Family Interventions in Mental Illness: International Perspectives*. Praeger, Westport, CT, pp. 62–90.

83. Campion J., Bhugra D. (1997) Experiences of religious healing in psychiatric patients in South India. *Soc. Psychiatry Psychiatr. Epidemiol.*, **32**, 215–221.

84. Tewari D., Panchal B., Patel K., Vankar G.K. (1997) Perception about schizophrenia among key relatives. *Indian J. Psychiatry*, **39**, 49.

85. Raguram R., Venkateswaran A., Ramakrishna J., Weiss M.G. (2002) Traditional community resources for mental health: a report of temple healing from India. *Br. Med. J.*, **325**, 38–40.

86. Prema T.P., Kodandaram P. (1998) Impact of mental health education on the attitudes of the families of mentally ill. *Indian J. Clin. Psychol.*, **25**, 27–31.

87. Shankar R., Menon M.S. (1993) Development of a framework of interventions with families in the management of schizophrenia. *Psychosoc. Rehabil. J.*, **16**, 75–91.

88. Verghese A. (1988) Families' participation in mental health care—The Vellore experiment. *Indian J. Psychiatry*, **30**, 117–121.

89. Verghese M., Chandra P.S., Ananthram Z. (1991) Working with families of people with schizophrenia. Experiences at the Family Psychiatry Center at the National Institute of Mental Health Bangalore. In: *Families and Schizophrenia: Developing Strategies for Interventions*. Schizophrenia Care and Research Foundation, Chennai, pp. 45–48.

90. Sarkar A., Nagpal J., Apte M., Anand R. (1997) Therapeutic process in group intervention with the families of schizophrenic patients. *Indian J. Psychiatry*, **39**, 48.

91. Pai S., Kapur R.I. (1983) Evaluation of home care treatment for schizophrenic patients. *Acta Psychiatr. Scand.*, **67**, 80–83.

92. Pai S., Channabasavanna S.M., Nagarajaiah M., Raghuram R. (1985) Home care for chronic mental illness in Bangalore: an experiment in the prevention of repeated hospitalization. *Br. J. Psychiatry*, **147**, 175–179.

93. Sharma P.S.V.N., Gopinath P.S., Reddy M.V. (1987) Patients attending a psychiatric day hospital: analysis of one year's referrals. *NIMHANS J.*, **5**, 39–45.
94. Rao K., Barnabas I.P., Gopinath P.S. (1988) Family burden in chronic schizophrenia: the role of the day hospital. *Indian J. Psychol. Med.*, **11**, 131–135.
95. Lam D.H. (1991) Psychosocial family intervention in schizophrenia: a review of empirical studies. *Psychol. Med.*, **21**, 423–441.
96. Barbato A., D'Avanzo B. (2000) Family intervention in schizophrenia and related disorders: a critical review. *Acta Psychiatr. Scand.*, **102**, 81–97.
97. Pitschel–Walz G., Leucht S., Bauml J., Kissling W., Engel R.R. (2001) The effect of family interventions on relapse and rehospitalization in schizophrenia—a meta-analysis. *Schizophr. Bull.*, **27**, 73–91.
98. Bebbington P., Kuipers L. (1994) The predictive utility of expressed emotion in schizophrenia: an aggregate analysis. *Psychol. Med.*, **24**, 707–718.
99. Jenkins J.H., Karno M. (1992) The meaning of expressed emotion. Theoretical issues raised by cross-cultural research. *Am. J. Psychiatry*, **149**, 9–21.
100. Barrowclough C., Tarrier N., Lewis S., Sellwood W., Mainwaring J., Quinn J., Hamlin C. (1999) Randomized controlled trial of needs based psychosocial intervention service for carers of people with schizophrenia. *Br. J. Psychiatry*, **174**, 505–511.
101. Xiang M., Ran M., Li S. (1994) A controlled evaluation of psycho educational family intervention in a rural Chinese community. *Br. J. Psychiatry*, **165**, 544–548.
102. Kleinman A. (1982) Clinically applied anthropology on a psychiatric consultation liaison service. In: Chrisman N.J., Martezki T.W. (eds) *Clinically Applied Anthropology*. Reidel, Dordrecht, pp. 83–115.
103. Littlewood R. (1990) From categories to contexts: a decade of the new cross-cultural psychiatry. *Br. J. Psychiatry*, **156**, 308–327.
104. Shankar R., Menon M.S. (1991) Interventions with families of people with schizophrenia: the issues facing a community based rehabilitation in India. *Psychosoc. Rehabil. J.*, **15**, 85–89.
105. Wijngaarden B.V., Schene A.H., Koeter M. (2002) Caregiving consequences in the Netherlands and other European countries. The development and use of the Family Involvement Questionnaire. In: Lefley H.P., Johnson D.L. (eds) *Family Interventions in Mental Illness: International Perspectives*. Praeger, Westport, CT, pp. 145–169.
106. Lefley H.P., Johnson D.L. (2002) Introduction. In: Lefley H.P., Johnson D.L. (eds) *Family Interventions in Mental Illness: International Perspectives*. Praeger, Westport, CT, pp. vii–ix.
107. Johnson D.L. (2002) A brief history of the international family movement of family organizations for persons with mental illness. In: Lefley H.P., Johnson D.L. (eds) *Family Interventions in Mental Illness: International Perspectives*. Praeger, Westport, CT, pp. 209–219.
108. Kapur R.L. (1992) The family and schizophrenia. Priority areas for intervention research in India. *Indian J. Psychiatry*, **34**, 3–7.
109. Lefley H.P. (1992) Discussion on family and social support system in the care of the mentally ill. In: Murthy R.S., Burns B.J. (eds) *Community Mental Health*. NIMHANS, Bangalore, pp. 289–295.

Index

Note: page numbers in *italics* refer to tables

advance directives 31
advocacy
  drug abuse *182–3*
  groups for *see* family organizations
aggressive behaviours, dementia 40
agoraphobia *see* panic disorder with
    agoraphobia
alcohol abuse
  family burden 162–3
  family interventions 248, 250
  see also drug abuse
alcohol-related problems 136
  see also alcohol abuse
Alzheimer's disease 25, 26
  clinical course 26–8
  family caregivers 28–32
    cultural variations 30–1, 37
    effects of caregiving 32–8
    ethnic variations 30–1, 37
    guardianship 31–2
    help for 38–42, 43–4
    interventions 42–5, 228
    living wills 31
    patterns of care 29
    power of attorney 31
  prevalence 26
anorexia nervosa
  confidentiality 123
  effect on families 114, 115, 116, 122
  family burden 117–18, 122
  family coping strategies 118
  family effects on 116–17, 122
  family interventions 119–21, 122–3
  onset 113
anxiety disorders 87–107
  in childhood 148–50

interventions 96–107, 148–50, 247–8,
    250
obsessive–compulsive disorder 87
  in childhood 150
  clinical picture 88–9
  couples' relationships 92, 97, 103
  expressed emotion 96, 98–101, 103
  family constellations 91–3
  family effects on 92, 93–4, 95–6, 106
  family factors in treatment 96–101
  family interventions 101–5, 106–7,
    247
  heritability 92, 93
panic disorder with agoraphobia 87
  clinical picture 87–8
  couples' relationships 90–1, 97, 99,
    100, 102
  expressed emotion 95, 98–100
  family constellations 89–91, 92–3
  family effects on 90, 93–5, 106
  family factors in treatment 96–100
  family interventions 101–2, 106–7
  heritability 90, 93
  panic attacks 87–8
anxiety management training 149
applied behavioural analysis (ABA)
    146–7
applied family management *12*
appraisals
  research issues 221
  transactional model of coping 3–4, 5
attention deficit/hyperactivity disorder
    (ADHD)
  family burden 130–1, 132, 133, 134,
    136–7
  interventions 145–6, 151

Families and Mental Disorders. Edited by Norman Sartorius, Julian Leff, Juan José López-Ibor, Mario Maj and
Ahmed Okasha. © 2005 John Wiley & Sons Ltd. ISBN 0-470-02382-1